Advances in Imaging of Multiple Sclerosis

Editor

ÀLEX ROVIRA

NEUROIMAGING CLINICS
OF NORTH AMERICA

www.neuroimaging.theclinics.com

Consulting Editor
SURESH K. MUKHERJI

May 2017 • Volume 27 • Number 2

ELSEVIER

1600 John F. Kennedy Boulevard • Suite 1800 • Philadelphia, Pennsylvania, 19103-2899

http://www.neuroimaging.theclinics.com

NEUROIMAGING CLINICS OF NORTH AMERICA Volume 27, Number 2
May 2017 ISSN 1052-5149, ISBN 13: 978-0-323-52850-4

Editor: John Vassallo (j.vassallo@elsevier.com)
Developmental Editor: Casey Potter

Neuroimaging Clinics of North America (ISSN 1052-5149) is published quarterly by Elsevier Inc., 360 Park Avenue South, New York, NY 10010-1710. Months of issue are February, May, August, and November. Business and editorial offices: 1600 John F. Kennedy Blvd., Suite 1800, Philadelphia, PA 19103-2899. Business and editorial offices: 6277 Sea Harbor Drive, Orlando, FL 32887-4800. Periodicals postage paid at New York, NY, and additional mailing offices. Subscription prices are USD 365 per year for US individuals, USD 581 per year for US institutions, USD 100 per year for US students and residents, USD 415 per year for Canadian individuals, USD 740 per year for Canadian institutions, USD 525 per year for international individuals, USD 740 per year for international institutions and USD 260 per year for Canadian and foreign students and residents. To receive student/resident rate, orders must be accompanied by name of affiliated institution, date of term, and the *signature* of program/residency coordinator on institution letterhead. Orders will be billed at individual rate until proof of status is received. Foreign air speed delivery is included in all *Clinics* subscription prices. All prices are subject to change without notice. POSTMASTER: Send address changes to *Neuroimaging Clinics of North America*, Elsevier Health Sciences Division, Subscription **Customer Service, 3251 Riverport Lane, Maryland Heights, MO 63043. Telephone: 1-800-654-2452 (U.S. and Canada); 314-447-8871 (outside U.S. and Canada). Fax: 314-447-8029. E-mail: journalscustomer service-usa@elsevier.com (for print support); journalsonlinesupport-usa@elsevier.com (for online support).**

Reprints. For copies of 100 or more of articles in this publication, please contact the Commercial Reprints Department, Elsevier Inc., 360 Park Avenue South, New York, NY 10010-1710. Tel.: 212-633-3874; Fax: 212-633-3820; E-mail: reprints@elsevier.com.

Neuroimaging Clinics of North America is covered by *Excerpta Medical/EMBASE,* the RSNA Index of Imaging Literature, *MEDLINE/PubMed (Index Medicus),* MEDLINE/MEDLARS, SciSearch, Research Alert, and Neuroscience Citation Index.

PROGRAM OBJECTIVE

The goal of *Neuroimaging Clinics of North America* is to keep practicing radiologists and radiology residents up to date with current clinical practice in radiology by providing timely articles reviewing the state of the art in patient care.

TARGET AUDIENCE

Practicing radiologists, radiology residents, and other healthcare professionals who utilize neuroimaging findings to provide patient care.

LEARNING OBJECTIVES

Upon completion of this activity, participants will be able to:
1. Review developing techniques in multiple sclerosis imaging.
2. Discuss the use of MRI in pediatric and adult multiple sclerosis.
3. Recognize the use of neuroimaging in predicting and monitoring treatment response in multiple sclerosis.

ACCREDITATION

The Elsevier Office of Continuing Medical Education (EOCME) is accredited by the Accreditation Council for Continuing Medical Education (ACCME) to provide continuing medical education for physicians.

The EOCME designates this enduring material for a maximum of 15 *AMA PRA Category 1 Credit*(s)™. Physicians should claim only the credit commensurate with the extent of their participation in the activity.

All other health care professionals requesting continuing education credit for this enduring material will be issued a certificate of participation.

DISCLOSURE OF CONFLICTS OF INTEREST

The EOCME assesses conflict of interest with its instructors, faculty, planners, and other individuals who are in a position to control the content of CME activities. All relevant conflicts of interest that are identified are thoroughly vetted by EOCME for fair balance, scientific objectivity, and patient care recommendations. EOCME is committed to providing its learners with CME activities that promote improvements or quality in healthcare and not a specific proprietary business or a commercial interest.

The planning committee, staff, authors and editors listed below have identified no financial relationships or relationships to products or devices they or their spouse/life partner have with commercial interest related to the content of this CME activity:

Tetsuya Akaishi, MD; Cristina Auger, MD; Massimiliano Calabrese, MD; Marco Castellaro, PhD; Iris Dekker, MD; Christian Enzinger, MD; Franz Fazekas, MD; Anjali Fortna; Marcello Moccia, MD; Suresh K. Mukerjhi, MD, MBA, FACR; Deborah Pareto, PhD; Daniel S. Reich, MD, PhD; Stefan Ropele, PhD; Pascal Sati, PhD; Matthew K. Schindler, MD, PhD; Karthik Subramaniam; Toshiyuki Takahashi, MD; Silvia N. Tenembaum, MD; John Vassallo; Katie Widmeier; Amy Williams.

The planning committee, staff, authors and editors listed below have identified financial relationships or relationships to products or devices they or their spouse/life partner have with commercial interest related to the content of this CME activity:

Olga Ciccarelli, PhD, FRCP is a consultant/advisor for Biogen; Novartis AG; Genzyme Corporation; Hoffmann-La Roche Ltd; Teva Pharmaceutical Industries Ltd; and General Electric Company, and has research support from The Engineering and Physical Sciences Research Council; the Multiple Sclerosis Society; and the National Institute for Health Research.

Massimo Filippi, MD, FEAN is on the speakers' bureau for, and is a consultant/advisor for, Teva Pharmaceutical Industries Ltd; Biogen; Novartis AG; and EMD Serono, Inc, and has research support from Biogen; Teva Pharmaceutical Industries Ltd; and Novartis AG.

Kazuo Fujihara, MD is on the speakers' bureau for Biogen; Mitsubishi Tanabe Pharma Corporation; Takeda Pharmaceuticals; Novartis AG; Bayer AG; Asahi Kasei Medical Co.; Ltd; and Nikkei Radio, and is a consultant/advisor for Biogen; Mitsubishi Tanabe Pharma Corporation; Takeda Pharmaceuticals; Novartis AG; Alexion; Chugai Pharmaceutical Co., Ltd; Dai-Nippon; and Zushioh.

Douglas Kazutoshi Sato, MD is on the speakers' bureau for EMD Serono, Inc; Bayer AG; Hoffmann-La Roche Ltd; Teva Pharmaceutical Industries Ltd; and Biogen, and is a consultant/advisor for EMD Serono, Inc; Teva Pharmaceutical Industries Ltd; and Shire.

Xavier Montalban, MD, PhD is a consultant/advisor for Actelion Pharmaceuticals US, Inc; Almirall, S.A.; Bayer AG; Biogen; Celgene Corporation; Genzyme Corporation; Hoffmann-La Roche Ltd; Merck & Co., Inc; Novartis AG; Oryzon Genomics; and Teva Pharmaceutical Industries Ltd.

Ichiro Nakashima, MD is on the speakers' bureau for Mitsubishi Tanabe Pharma Corporation, and has research support from LSI Medience Corporation.

Darin T. Okuda, MD, MS, FAAN, FANA is on the speakers' bureau for Acorda Therapeutics; Gentech, A Member of the Roche Group; Genzyme Corporation; and Teva Pharmaceutical Industries Ltd, and is a consultant/advisor for EMD Serono, Inc; Gentech, A Member of the Roche Group; Genzyme Corporation; and Novartis AG, and has research support from Biogen.

Paolo Preziosa, MD is on the speakers' bureau for EXCEMED.

Jordi Río, MD is on the speakers' bureau for Novartis AG and Teva Pharmaceutical Industries Ltd, and is a consultant/advisor for Biogen; Genzyme Corporation; and EMD Serono, Inc.

Maria A. Rocca, MD is on the speakers' bureau for Biogen; EMD Serono, Inc; Teva Pharmaceutical Industries Ltd; Sanofi-Aventis; Genzyme Corporation; and Novartis AG.

Àlex Rovira, MD is on the speakers' bureau for Biogen; Novartis AG; Genzyme Corporation; Teva Pharmaceutical Industries Ltd; Bracco; and Bayer AG, and is a consultant/advisor for Biogen; Novartis AG; Genzyme Corporation; Bracco; and Olea Medical.

Jaume Sastre-Garriga, MD, PhD is on the speakers' bureau for Genzyme Corporation; Novartis AG; and Merck & Co., Inc, is a consultant/advisor for Genzyme Corporation; Novartis AG; Biogen; Merck & Co., Inc; and Celgene Corporation, and has research support from Genzyme corporation.

Angela Vidal-Jordana, MD, PhD is on the speakers' bureau for Novartis AG; Hoffmann-La Roche Ltd.; Biogen; and Stendhal, and is a consultant/advisor for Hoffmann-La Roche Ltd. and Sanofi-Aventis.

Mike P. Wattjes, MD is a consultant/advisor for Biogen; Genzyme Corporation; Novartis AG; and Hoffmann-La Roche Ltd.

UNAPPROVED/OFF-LABEL USE DISCLOSURE

The EOCME requires CME faculty to disclose to the participants:

1. When products or procedures being discussed are off-label, unlabelled, experimental, and/or investigational (not US Food and Drug Administration [FDA] approved); and
2. Any limitations on the information presented, such as data that are preliminary or that represent ongoing research, interim analyses, and/or unsupported opinions. Faculty may discuss information about pharmaceutical agents that is outside of FDA-approved labelling. This information is intended solely for CME and is not intended to promote off-label use of these medications. If you have any questions, contact the medical affairs department of the manufacturer for the most recent prescribing information.

TO ENROLL

To enroll in the *Neuroimaging Clinics of North America* Continuing Medical Education program, call customer service at 1-800-654-2452 or sign up online at http://www.theclinics.com/home/cme. The CME program is available to subscribers for an additional annual fee of USD $235.

METHOD OF PARTICIPATION

In order to claim credit, participants must complete the following:

1. Complete enrolment as indicated above.
2. Read the activity.
3. Complete the CME Test and Evaluation. Participants must achieve a score of 70% on the test. All CME Tests and Evaluations must be completed online.

CME INQUIRIES/SPECIAL NEEDS

For all CME inquiries or special needs, please contact elsevierCME@elsevier.com.

NEUROIMAGING CLINICS OF NORTH AMERICA

THE CLINICS ARE AVAILABLE ONLINE!
Access your subscription at:
www.theclinics.com

Contributors

CONSULTING EDITOR

SURESH K. MUKHERJI, MD, MBA, FACR
Professor and Chairman, Walter F. Patenge
Endowed Chair, Department of Radiology,
Michigan State University, Chief Medical
Officer & Director of Health Care Delivery,
Michigan State University Health Team,
Department of Radiology, Michigan State
University, East Lansing, Michigan

EDITOR

ÀLEX ROVIRA, MD
Head of Neuroradiology and Magnetic
Resonance Units, Department of Radiology
(IDI), Professor of Radiology and
Neuroimmunology, Vall d'Hebron University
Hospital, Autonomous University of Barcelona,
Barcelona, Spain

AUTHORS

TETSUYA AKAISHI, MD
Department of Neurology, Tohoku University
Graduate School of Medicine, Aobaku, Sendai,
Japan

CRISTINA AUGER, MD
Neuroradiology and Magnetic Resonance
Units, Department of Radiology (IDI), Hospital
Universitari Vall d'Hebron, Autonomous
University of Barcelona, Barcelona, Spain

MASSIMILIANO CALABRESE, MD
Neurology B, Department of Neurosciences,
Biomedicine and Movement Sciences,
University of Verona, Verona, Italy

MARCO CASTELLARO, PhD
Department of Information Engineering,
University of Padova, Italy

OLGA CICCARELLI, PhD, FRCP
NMR Research Unit, Queen Square MS
Centre, University College London, Institute of
Neurology; NIHR University College London
Hospitals Biomedical Research Centre,
London, United Kingdom

IRIS DEKKER, MD
Department of Radiology and Nuclear
Medicine; Department of Neurology,
Neuroscience Amsterdam, VUmc MS Center
Amsterdam, VU University Medical Center,
Amsterdam, The Netherlands

CHRISTIAN ENZINGER, MD
Department of Neurology, Medical University
of Graz, Graz, Austria

FRANZ FAZEKAS, MD
Department of Neurology, Medical University
of Graz, Graz, Austria

MASSIMO FILIPPI, MD, FEAN
Neuroimaging Research Unit, Institute of
Experimental Neurology, Division of
Neuroscience, San Raffaele Scientific Institute,
Vita-Salute San Raffaele University, Milan, Italy

KAZUO FUJIHARA, MD
Departments of Neurology and Multiple
Sclerosis Therapeutics, Tohoku University
Graduate School of Medicine, Aobaku, Sendai;
Department of Multiple Sclerosis Therapeutics,
Multiple Sclerosis & Neuromyelitis Optica
Center, Southern TOHOKU Research Institute
for Neuroscience, Fukushima Medical
University School of Medicine, Yatsuyamada,
Koriyama, Japan

MARCELLO MOCCIA, MD
NMR Research Unit, Queen Square MS
Centre, University College London, Institute of
Neurology, London, United Kingdom; MS
Clinical Care and Research Centre,
Department of Neuroscience, Federico II
University, Naples, Italy

XAVIER MONTALBAN, MD, PhD
Professor, Department of Neurology-
Neuroimmunology, Multiple Sclerosis Centre
of Catalonia, Edifici Cemcat, Hospital
Universitari Vall d'Hebron, Universitat
Autònoma de Barcelona, Barcelona, Spain

ICHIRO NAKASHIMA, MD
Department of Neurology, Tohoku University
Graduate School of Medicine, Aobaku, Sendai,
Japan

DARIN T. OKUDA, MD, MS, FAAN, FANA
Director, Neuroinnovation Program; Director,
Multiple Sclerosis and Neuroimmunology
Imaging Program, Associate Professor of
Neurology, Department of Neurology and
Neurotherapeutics, Deputy Director, Clinical
Center for Multiple Sclerosis, University of
Texas Southwestern Medical Center, Dallas,
Texas

DEBORAH PARETO, PhD
Neuroradiology and Magnetic Resonance
Units, Department of Radiology (IDI), Hospital
Universitari Vall d'Hebron, Autonomous
University of Barcelona, Barcelona, Spain

PAOLO PREZIOSA, MD
Neuroimaging Research Unit, Institute of
Experimental Neurology, Division of
Neuroscience, San Raffaele Scientific
Institute, Vita-Salute San Raffaele University,
Milan, Italy

JORDI RÍO, MD
Department of Neurology/Neuroimmunology,
Centre d'Esclerosi Múltiple de Catalunya
(Cemcat), Hospital Universitari Vall d'Hebron,
Autonomous University of Barcelona,
Barcelona, Spain

DANIEL S. REICH, MD, PhD
Translational Neuroradiology Section, National
Institute of Neurological Disorders and Stroke,
National Institutes of Health, Bethesda,
Maryland

MARIA A. ROCCA, MD
Neuroimaging Research Unit, Institute of
Experimental Neurology, Division of
Neuroscience, San Raffaele Scientific
Institute, Vita-Salute San Raffaele University,
Milan, Italy

STEFAN ROPELE, PhD
Department of Neurology, Medical University
of Graz, Graz, Austria

ÀLEX ROVIRA, MD
Head of Neuroradiology and Magnetic
Resonance Units, Department of Radiology
(IDI), Professor of Radiology and
Neuroimmunology, Vall d'Hebron University
Hospital, Autonomous University of Barcelona,
Barcelona, Spain

JAUME SASTRE-GARRIGA, MD, PhD
Department of Neurology/Neuroimmunology,
Centre d'Esclerosi Múltiple de Catalunya
(Cemcat), Hospital Universitari Vall d'Hebron,
Autonomous University of Barcelona,
Barcelona, Spain

PASCAL SATI, PhD
Translational Neuroradiology Section, National
Institute of Neurological Disorders and Stroke,
National Institutes of Health, Bethesda,
Maryland

DOUGLAS KAZUTOSHI SATO, MD
Departments of Neurology and Multiple
Sclerosis Therapeutics, Tohoku University
Graduate School of Medicine, Aobaku, Sendai,
Japan; Brain Institute, The Pontifical Catholic
University of Rio Grande do Sul, Porto Alegre,
Rio Grande do Sul, Brazil

MATTHEW K. SCHINDLER, MD, PhD
Translational Neuroradiology Section,
National Institute of Neurological Disorders
and Stroke, National Institutes of Health,
Bethesda, Maryland

TOSHIYUKI TAKAHASHI, MD
Department of Neurology, Tohoku University
Graduate School of Medicine, Aobaku, Sendai;
Department of Neurology, Yonezawa National
Hospital, Yonezawa, Japan

SILVIA N. TENEMBAUM, MD
Member of Executive Board, International
Child Neurology Association; Pediatric
Neurologist, Head of Clinic and Director of
Referral Center for Pediatric MS and Related
Disorders, Department of Neurology, National
Pediatric Hospital Dr. Juan P. Garrahan,
Ciudad Autónoma de Buenos Aires, Argentina;
Member of Steering Committee, International
Pediatric MS Study Group, Foundation for
Neurologic Disease, Newburyport,
Massachusetts

ANGELA VIDAL-JORDANA, MD, PhD
Department of Neurology-Neuroimmunology,
Multiple Sclerosis Centre of Catalonia, Edifici
Cemcat, Hospital Universitari Vall d'Hebron,
Universitat Autònoma de Barcelona,
Barcelona, Spain

MIKE P. WATTJES, MD
Department of Radiology and Nuclear
Medicine, Neuroscience Amsterdam,
VUmc MS Center Amsterdam,
VU University Medical Center, Amsterdam,
The Netherlands

Contents

> Multiple sclerosis (MS) is a chronic autoimmune and degenerative disease of the central nervous system that affects young people. MS develops in genetically susceptible individuals exposed to different unknown triggering factors. Different phenotypes are described. About 15% of patients present with a primary progressive course and 85% with a relapsing-remitting course. An increasing number of disease-modifying treatments has emerged. Although encouraging, the number of drugs challenges the neurologist because each treatment has its own risk–benefit profile. Patients should be involved in the decision-making process to ensure good treatment and safety monitoring adherence.

> Multiple sclerosis (MS) is a disabling disease, with the first symptoms mostly appearing early in life. In addition to the clinical and laboratory findings, imaging has become increasingly important for diagnosis, prognosis, and monitoring. Because of its importance for these purposes, a high level of knowledge of imaging MS pathology and a standardization of the imaging acquisition, interpretation, and reporting is necessary. Here we will describe the MR imaging characteristics of MS pathology, the current imaging protocols, diagnostic criteria, and the differential diagnosis of MS.

> This article presents an overview of evolving diagnostic criteria of pediatric multiple sclerosis and related disorders, emphasizing distinguishing clinical and neuroimaging features that should be considered for differential diagnosis in childhood and adolescence. New data on the integrity of brain tissue in children with MS provided by advanced MR imaging techniques are addressed as well.

> Neuromyelitis optica (NMO) is clinically characterized by severe optic neuritis and transverse myelitis, but recent studies with anti-aquaporin-4-antibody specific to NMO have revealed that the clinical spectrum is wider than previously thought.

International consensus diagnostic criteria propose NMO spectrum disorders (NMOSD) as the term to define the entire spectrum including typical NMO, optic neuritis, acute myelitis, brain syndrome, and their combinations. NMOSD is now divided into anti-aquaporin-4-antibody-seropositive NMOSD and -seronegative NMOSD (or unknown serostatus). MR imaging and optical coherence tomography are indispensable in the diagnosis and evaluation of NMOSD. This article reviews the clinical and MR imaging findings of anti-aquaporin-4-antibody-seropositive and anti-myelin oligodendrocyte glycoprotein-antibody-seropositive NMOSD.

Remarkable advances in the understanding of the biology of multiple sclerosis have been achieved through the use of conventional and novel MR imaging techniques of the central nervous system. With improvements in access by patients and utilization of MR imaging technology in health care, an increasing number of unanticipated structural anomalies are being appreciated. In certain instances, white matter abnormalities within the brain and spinal cord are discovered in subjects with no prior history of neurologic symptoms supportive of inflammatory demyelinating events.

MR imaging is the most sensitive tool for identifying lesions in patients with multiple sclerosis (MS). MR imaging has also acquired an essential role in the detection of complications arising from these treatments and in the assessment and prediction of efficacy. In the future, other radiological measures that have shown prognostic value may be incorporated within the models for predicting treatment response. This article examines the role of MR imaging as a prognostic tool in patients with MS and the recommendations that have been proposed in recent years to monitor patients who are treated with disease-modifying drugs.

There is evidence of a neurodegenerative process running in parallel with or as a consequence of the inflammatory phenomenon in multiple sclerosis (MS). MR imaging has been central in the generation of such knowledge and has played a pivotal role in investigating the neurodegenerative process. However, there is insufficient evidence supporting MR imaging–measured brain atrophy as a biomarker of the neurodegenerative component of MS in the daily care of patients with MS. This article discusses the prognostic value of brain volume measurements and their potential role in monitoring treatment response in patients with MS.

Several neuropathologic and imaging studies have consistently confirmed that multiple sclerosis affects both white (WM) and gray matter (GM) and that GM damage plays a key role in disability progression. However, differently from WM damage, the less inflammatory cell infiltration, the absence of significant blood-brain barrier damage, the low myelin density in upper cortical layers, as well as technical constraints, make the GM damage almost undetectable by means of conventional MR imaging.

Foreword
Imaging in Multiple Sclerosis: Diagnosis and Management

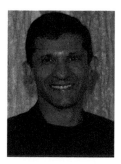

Suresh K. Mukherji, MD, MBA, FACR
Consulting Editor

I would like to thank Dr Àlex Rovira for guest editing this issue of *Neuroimaging Clinics*. This state-of-the-art issue provides new information on both conventional and different advanced and quantitative MR techniques in the diagnosis of multiple sclerosis in both the adult and pediatric populations. There are specific articles devoted to epidemiology, monitoring and treatment response, and various new techniques. There is also an article devoted to pediatric multiple sclerosis.

I would like to express my personal gratitude to all of the authors. The articles are beautifully written and are both concise and yet comprehensive. Multiple sclerosis is, unfortunately, a common disease that can have devastating effects. This issue sheds new insights into this disorder that will help us gain new insights into the pathogenesis, diagnosis, and treatment, which will help us improve patient outcome. Thank you again to Dr Àlex Rovira and all of the authors for their outstanding contributions.

Suresh K. Mukherji, MD, MBA, FACR
Department of Radiology
Michigan State University
Michigan State University Health Team
846 Service Road
East Lansing, MI 48824, USA

E-mail address:
mukherji@rad.msu.edu

Neuroimag Clin N Am 27 (2017) xv
http://dx.doi.org/10.1016/j.nic.2017.02.002
1052-5149/17/© 2017 Published by Elsevier Inc.

Preface

Advances in the Diagnosis, Characterization, and Monitoring of Multiple Sclerosis

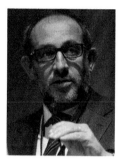

Àlex Rovira, MD

Editor

The high sensitivity of conventional MR imaging techniques in the depiction of brain white matter and spinal cord demyelinating lesions has made this technique the most important paraclinical tool for the diagnosis of multiple sclerosis (MS), for ruling out alternative diagnosis in patients presenting with clinical symptoms suggestive of this disease, and in distinguishing MS from neuromyelitis optica, as this last entity may be aggravated when treated with disease-modifying drugs frequently used for MS.

However, the role of MR imaging goes far beyond the diagnostic workup of these patients. MR imaging can also be used to measure focal lesion burden, inflammatory activity, and brain volume loss, providing useful information for the prediction of disease evolution, and for guiding early treatment decisions on these patients. Moreover, with the availability of a broader range of disease-modifying treatments, conventional MR imaging is commonly used in clinical practice for monitoring treatment efficacy, and for early detection of treatment nonresponders, providing clinicians relevant information for optimizing individualized treatment.

However, conventional MR imaging techniques, such as T2-weighted and gadolinium-enhanced T1-weighted sequences, cannot detect the full extent of the pathophysiological processes associated with MS, including the type and degree of tissue damage within focal white matter lesions, the presence of cortical gray matter lesions, and the extension and severity of diffuse damage in the normal-appearing gray and white matter. This shortcoming is apparent in the poor correlation of conventional MR imaging measures with clinical findings, at least at the individual level, and in their lack of specificity in comparison with histopathological examinations.

Huge efforts are being made to overcome these limitations with the development and implementation of several advanced and quantitative MR techniques, which increase the sensitivity for detecting cortical gray matter lesions, and elucidate the microstructural, metabolic, and functional changes in MS patients.

The combined use of these advanced and quantitative MR techniques could lead to a better understanding of different aspects of the disease process and in the management of MS patients, with the main purpose of providing patients with the most adequate immunomodulatory and/or neuroprotective treatments. However, the implementation in clinical studies of these techniques is still challenging, due to different technical limitations, and is mainly used in the research scenario.

This issue of *Neuroimaging Clinics* provides an up-to-date overview of the value of conventional and different advanced and quantitative MR techniques in the diagnosis of MS in both the adult and

Neuroimag Clin N Am 27 (2017) xvii–xviii
http://dx.doi.org/10.1016/j.nic.2017.02.001
1052-5149/17/© 2017 Published by Elsevier Inc.

pediatric populations, in the surveillance of patients for monitoring and predicting treatment response, in the assessment of the microstructural, metabolic, and functional changes in MS patients, and in the value of ultrahigh field magnets for superior detection of MS abnormality in the white matter and gray matter.

The different articles are preceded by a review of relevant epidemiologic, clinical, and therapeutic aspects of MS that provides the necessary background to understand the important role of MR imaging in the diagnostic process and in the management of these patients in clinical practice.

I would like to express my gratitude to the authors of this issue, all of them well-known experts in the field of MS and other idiopathic inflammatory demyelinating diseases, for immediately accepting their participation in this project, and for their great contribution, which made my task as guest editor very simple. I also would like to thank Suresh K. Mukherji, consulting editor, for inviting me as guest editor of this issue, and to John Vassallo, Associate Publisher, and Casey Potter, Developmental Editor, for the support and patience they demonstrated to me during the entire publication process.

I hope that the readers will enjoy and learn from the different articles that covered some of the cutting-edge aspects of MR imaging in MS.

Àlex Rovira, MD
Section of Neuroradiology
Hospital Universitari Vall d'Hebron
Autonomous University of Barcelona
Pg. Vall d'Hebron 119-129
Barcelona 08035, Spain

E-mail address:
alex.rovira@idi.gencat.cat

Multiple Sclerosis

Epidemiologic, Clinical, and Therapeutic Aspects

 CrossMark

Angela Vidal-Jordana, MD, PhD*, Xavier Montalban, MD, PhD

KEYWORDS

• Multiple sclerosis • Symptoms • Treatment

KEY POINTS

• Multiple sclerosis is a chronic autoimmune and degenerative disease of the central nervous system that affects young people, with a prevalence of 33 per 100,000.
• Multiple sclerosis will develop in genetically susceptible individuals exposed to different triggering environmental factors.
• Based on symptoms onset and their evolution, different phenotypes are described. About 15% of patients will present with a primary progressive course and 85% with a relapsing–remitting course.
• An increasing number of disease-modifying treatments has emerged. Although encouraging, the broad number challenges the clinical neurologist because each treatment has its own risk–benefit profile.
• Patients should be involved in the decision-making process to ensure a good treatment and safety-monitoring adherence.

INTRODUCTION AND EPIDEMIOLOGY

Multiple sclerosis (MS) is a chronic autoimmune disease of the central nervous system (CNS) in which inflammation, demyelination, and axonal loss occurs from the very early stages of the disease. It mainly affects young people, between 20 and 40 years of age, with a female predominance.[1,2]

The global median prevalence of MS is 33 per 100,000 people, with a great variance between different countries. North America and Europe have the highest prevalence (with 140 and 108 per 100,000 people, respectively), and Asia and sub-Saharan Africa countries have the lowest prevalence (2.2 and 2.1 per 100,000 people, respectively).[3]

The ultimate cause of MS is unknown and a multifactorial etiology is accepted. Thus, MS will develop in genetically susceptible individuals exposed to different triggering environmental factors (such as Epstein–Barr virus, tobacco use, and vitamin D).[1–4]

CLINICAL MANIFESTATION AND NATURAL COURSE

MS symptoms vary depending on the area of the CNS affected. Based on symptoms onset and their evolution, 4 MS phenotypes were initially described: relapsing–remitting MS (RRMS), secondary-progressive MS, primary-progressive MS, and relapsing-progressive MS.[5] This classification has been recently reviewed: this last phenotype (relapsing-progressive MS) has been eliminated and the clinically isolated syndrome (CIS) has been added into the classification[6] (Fig. 1). Moreover, additional descriptions of clinical and radiologic disease activity was defined to add information into a static classification based

Department of Neurology-Neuroimmunology, Multiple Sclerosis Centre of Catalonia, Edifici Cemcat, Hospital Universitari Vall d'Hebron, Universitat Autònoma de Barcelona, Ps Vall d'Hebron 119-129, Barcelona 08035, Spain
* Corresponding author.
E-mail address: avidal@cem-cat.org

Neuroimag Clin N Am 27 (2017) 195–204
http://dx.doi.org/10.1016/j.nic.2016.12.001
1052-5149/17/

neuroimaging.theclinics.com

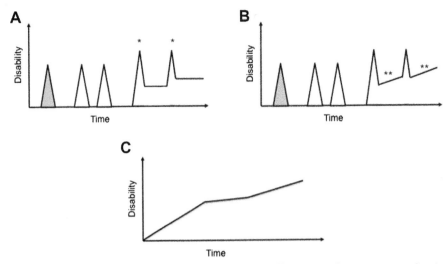

Fig. 1. Multiple sclerosis (MS) phenotypes. The figure shows the different MS phenotypes. In relapsing-remitting MS (*A*), after the first event or clinically isolated syndrome (*light gray*) new relapses will occur. The recovery of these relapses may be complete or partial (*asterisk*). After this initial period, some patients enter a progressive phase of the disease (*double asterisks*), with or without superimposed relapses, that constitutes the secondary progressive MS (*B*). In primary progressive MS (*C*), patients present a sustained and progressive neurologic impairment since onset. (*Adapted from* Lublin FD, Reingold SC. Defining the clinical course of multiple sclerosis results of an international survey. Neurology 1996;46(4):907–11; with permission.)

on symptoms evolution. Thus, patients may be also classified as presenting with or without disease activity based on the presence (or absence) of relapses, progression, new or enlarging T2 lesions, and gadolinium (Gd)-enhancing lesions.[6]

About 15% of patients with MS present with a primary-progressive MS. This phenotype is characterized by a slow progressive neurologic disability from the beginning of the disease (see **Fig. 1**). Most of these patients (80%) present with a gait disorder owing to an spastic paraparesis, which may be accompanied with sensory symptoms and sphincter dysfunction.[7]

In the majority of patients with MS (85%), the disease starts with the RRMS phenotype[8] and they develop relapses (defined as a subacute onset of new neurologic symptoms that last for at least 24 hours in the absence of fever or infection) followed by symptom recovery (see **Fig. 1**). CIS is a term that refers to the first clinical manifestation of the disease that by definition is isolated in time or not preceded by any neurologic event. It usually affects the optic nerves (20%), the brainstem (10%–20%), or the spinal cord (40%) causing an optic neuritis, a brainstem syndrome, or an incomplete transverse myelitis, respectively[8,9] (**Table 1**). These symptoms may also occur in subsequent relapses. Relapse recovery may be complete or lead to neurologic sequelae; in this last scenario, other neurologic signs and symptoms may appear owing to irreversible CNS damage[2] (see **Table 1**). The accumulation of disability is

Table 1
Neurologic symptoms of multiple sclerosis

Relapse neurologic symptoms	
Optic nerve	Mononuclear painful vision loss
Spinal cord	Hemiparesis, mono/paraparesis Hypoesthesia, dysesthesia, parasthesia Urinary and/or fecal sphincter dysfunction
Brainstem and cerebellum	Diplopia, oscillopsy Vertigo Gait ataxia, dismetria Intentional/Postural tremor Facial paresis and/or hypoesthesia
Cerebral hemisphere	Facio–brachial–crural hemiparesis Facio–brachial–crural hemihypoesthesia
Other clinical manifestations	Paroxistic symptoms Painful spasms/spasticity Dysarthria/dysphagia Neuropathic pain Sexual dysfunction Spastic gait Ataxic gait Fatigue Cognitive impairment Depression Seizures

quantified in clinical practice with the Expanded Disability Status Scale (EDSS).[10] The EDSS is an ordinal scale ranging from 0 (normal neurologic examination) to 10 (death owing to MS). EDSS mostly relies in motor function and important milestones are requiring unilateral assistance for walking 100 m (EDSS score of 6.0), requiring bilateral assistance for walking 20 m (EDSS score of 6.5), or requiring a wheelchair most parts of the day (EDSS score of 8.0).

After the occurrence of a CIS, the risk of developing MS depends on the presence of white matter lesions in MR imaging.[2,8] Thus, up to 80% of the patients presenting with typical MS lesions in brain MR imaging develop MS during the follow-up, although only 10% to 20% will do so if baseline brain MR image is normal.[8,11–13] Other clinicodemographic and biological factors, such as a younger age at CIS onset, non-Caucasian patients, the presence of oligoclonal bands in the cerebrospinal fluid, and a greater number of functional systems affected at CIS, have also been related with the risk of developing MS.[8] However, when a multivariate analysis is performed, only a younger age at CIS onset, the presence of oligoclonal bands in the cerebrospinal fluid, and a greater number of white matter lesions in baseline brain MR imaging seems to increase the risk of developing MS.[13]

Natural history studies have demonstrated that after 20 years, about 80% of the patients transition to a progressive phase, which is known as secondary-progressive MS.[8,14–16] Secondary-progressive MS behaves similarly to primary-progressive MS, and patients present with neurologic symptoms that progress over time, mainly gait impairment, with or without superimposed relapses (see **Fig. 1**). Risk factors associated with the development of neurologic disability include being male,[13,15] an older age at CIS onset,[13,15] a higher annualized relapse rate (ARR),[14,15] a short time to the second relapse,[14] presence of oligoclonal bands in the cerebrospinal fluid,[13] and a greater number of white matter lesions in the baseline brain MR image.[13]

DIAGNOSIS AND DIFFERENTIAL DIAGNOSIS

Owing to the absence of a specific test, the diagnosis of MS is established with the fulfilment of a diagnostic criteria. The diagnostic criteria have evolved over time, but all of them are based on demonstrating the involvement of 2 or more areas of the CNS (dissemination in space) in different timepoints (dissemination in time). Classically, the neurologist had to wait for a second relapse to occur. Fortunately, the most recent criteria incorporate the MR imaging to establish the presence of dissemination in space and in time, which allows an earlier diagnosis. In fact, presently, after the occurrence of a CIS, the diagnosis of MS can be established with a single MR image demonstrating dissemination in space and time[17,18] (**Fig. 2**).

It is important to remark that the diagnostic criteria should be only applied when patients present with typical CIS symptoms (see **Table 1**), because these criteria have been developed based on radiologic findings found in prospective

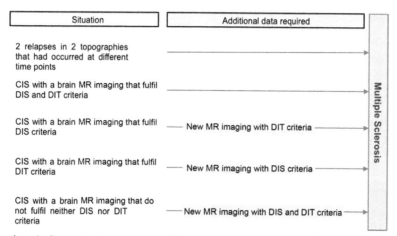

Fig. 2. Multiple sclerosis diagnosis. Figure shows different situations, and the additional data required (if any) to establish the diagnosis of relapsing–remitting multiple sclerosis. CIS, clinically isolated syndrome; DIS, dissemination in space; DIT, dissemination in time. (*Adapted from* Montalban X, Tintore M, Swanton J, et al. MR imaging criteria for MS in patients with clinically isolated syndromes. Neurology 2010;74(5):427–34; and Polman CH, Reingold SC, Banwell B, et al. Diagnostic criteria for multiple sclerosis: 2010 revisions to the McDonald criteria. Ann Neurol 2011;69(2):292–302.)

CIS cohorts.[17] Furthermore, we must be aware that the diagnosis of MS is still considered a diagnosis of exclusion and, therefore, other pathologies should be reasonably ruled out (**Box 1**).

TREATMENT

Over the last years an increasing number of disease-modifying treatments have emerged for treating relapsing MS (**Table 2**). All of these therapies have demonstrated to be effective in reducing clinical and radiologic disease activity and, therefore, modifying the natural history of MS. Although encouraging, the broad number of new drugs challenges the clinical neurologist because each treatment has its own risk–benefit profile. In this review,

we discuss the main results and adverse events of the 10 disease-modifying treatments that both the European Medicines Agency and US Food and Drug Administration have approved for treating relapsing MS as of March 2016.

Injectable Therapies

Interferon beta

Interferon beta (IFN-β), a drug with antiviral, antiproliferative, and immunomodulatory effects,[19] was the first treatment to demonstrate a reduction in the number of relapses and in the development of new T2 lesions in brain MR imaging.[20–24] There are 4 approved formulations of IFN-β (see **Table 2**): subcutaneous IFN-β 1a, subcutaneous IFN-β 1b, intramuscular IFN-β 1a, subcutaneous pegylated IFN-β 1a (sc IFN-β-1a, sc IFN-β-1b, im IFN-β-1a, and sc pegIFN-β-1a, respectively).

Efficacy Compared with placebo, the 3 classical formulations (sc IFN-β-1a, sc IFN-β-1b, and im IFN-β-1a) reduced the ARR by 27% to 33%, reduced the risk of 3-month sustained disability progression (except for the sc IFN-β-1b), and reduced the number of new T2 lesions.[20–23] These older preparations of IFN-β also were demonstrated to be effective in preventing relapses and delaying the diagnosis of definite MS after the occurrence of a CIS.[25–28] More recently, the newest pegylated formulation showed similar results in a 1-year duration phase III clinical trial including patients with RRMS: a 27% reduction in ARR, a 38% reduction in the risk of 3-month sustained disability progression, and a 67% reduction in the new active lesions (a combination of new T2 lesions and Gd-enhancing lesions).[24]

Safety Common adverse events related to IFN-β treatment are injection site reactions (redness, pain, and swelling among others),[29] flulike symptoms (myalgia, arthralgia, and fever), and headache.[30] IFN-β can also produce liver[31] and hematologic abnormalities; a periodic blood test (every 6 months) is recommended.

Glatiramer acetate

Glatiramer acetate (GA) a synthetic polymer composed of 4 amino acids with a complex mechanism of action,[32] demonstrated its efficacy in treating RRMS in a phase III clinical trial.[33]

Efficacy Compared with placebo, daily injections of GA reduced the ARR by 29% and, although patients treated with GA showed a lower disability progression, these differences were not significant.[33] GA treatment also proved to be effective in reducing radiologic disease activity (33% reduction in the number of new T2 lesions, and 29%

Box 1
Differential diagnosis of multiple sclerosis

Inflammatory pathologies of the CNS

Acute disseminated encephalomyelitis

Neuromyelitis optica

Idiopathic transverse myelitis

Susac syndrome

Primary cerebral vasculitis

Systemic inflammatory pathologies with CNS involvement

Small and median vasculitis

Sarcoidosis

Behçets disease

Sjögren syndrome

Erythematous systemic lupus

Noninflammatory pathologies of the CNS

Vascular brain pathology (ischemia, CADASIL, etc)

Metabolic diseases (leukodystrophy, vitamin deficits)

Infectious diseases (HIV, HTLV, syphilis, etc.)

Genetic syndromes[a] (Leber optic neuropathy, hereditary ataxias, leukodystrophy, CADASIL, etc)

Abbreviations: CADASIL, cerebral autosomal dominant arteriopathy with subcortical infarcts and leukoencephalopathy; CNS, central nervous system; HIV, human immunodeficiency virus; HTLV, human T-cell lymphotropicvirus virus.
    [a]Genetic syndromes must be taken into account specially in patients with progressive symptoms from onset.
    Adapted from Compston A, Coles A. Multiple sclerosis. Lancet 2008;372(9648):1502–17.

Table 2
Approved drugs for the treatment of relapsing-remitting multiple sclerosis

Drug	Brand Name	Posology	FDA/EMA Approval
Interferon beta	Betaferon	Subcutaneous / 48 h	1993 / 1995
	Avonex	Intramuscular / week	1996 / 1997
	Rebif	Subcutaneous / 3 per week	2002 / 1998
	Extavia	Subcutaneous / 48 h	2009 / 2008
Pegylated interferon beta	Plegridy	Subcutaneous / 2 wk	2014 / 2014
Glatiramer acetate	Copaxone	Subcutaneous / 24 h / 3 per week	1996 / 2001
			2014 / 2014
Natalizumab	Tysabri	Intravenous / 4 wk	2006 / 2006
Fingolimod	Gilenya	Oral / 24 h	2010 / 2011
Teriflunomida	Aubagio	Oral / 24 h	2012 / 2013
Alemtuzumab	Lemtrada	Intravenous / year	2014 / 2013
Dimethyl fumarate	Tecfidera	Oral / 12 h	2013 / 2014

Abbreviations: EMA, European Medicines Agency; FDA, US Food and Drug Administration.

reduction in the number of Gd-enhancing lesions).[34] In CIS patients, GA treatment delayed conversion to definite MS.[35] Recently, a new formulation with a lower treatment frequency has been approved. This treatment regimen demonstrated similar efficacy results that the daily GA dose.[36]

Safety Injection site reactions (erythema, pruritus, swelling) are the most common adverse event in GA-treated patients, and about 15% to 45% develop lipoatrophy.[29] A transient self-limited systemic reaction, consisting of facial flushing, palpitations, dyspnea, and anxiety may occur in up to 15% of patients.[33]

Monoclonal Antibodies

Natalizumab
Natalizumab is a humanized monoclonal antibody against the alfa4 subunit of the adhesion molecule VLA-4 expressed on the leukocytes surface. This molecule is necessary for the leukocyte migration into the CNS through the blood–brain barrier.[37]

Efficacy Two phase III clinical trials evaluated natalizumab's efficacy as monotherapy (AFFIRM [Natalizumab Safety and Efficacy in Relapsing-Remitting Multiple Sclerosis][38]) or as add-on therapy to im IFN-β-1a (SENTINEL [Safety and Efficacy of Natalizumab in Combination with Interferon Beta-1a in Patients with Relapsing Remitting Multiple Sclerosis][39]). Owing to the associated adverse events natalizumab treatment was finally approved as monotherapy for patients with an active disease. In the AFFIRM trial, compared with placebo, after 1 year of treatment natalizumab reduced by 68% the ARR. At the end of the follow-up (2 years), the

risk of 3-month sustained disability progression was reduced in 42% in natalizumab-treated patients. Regarding MR imaging parameters, natalizumab treatment reduced by 83% and 92% the mean number of new T2 lesions and Gd-enhancing lesions, respectively.[38] Similar results, although with a lower magnitude, were reported for the SENTINEL trial.[39]

Safety Natalizumab treatment is associated with a higher risk of developing progressive multifocal leukoencephalopathy (PML), a rare but severe CNS opportunistic infection caused by the JC virus. The overall incidence of PML in natalizumab-treated patients is estimated in 2.1 in 1000. Risk factors for PML include evidence of prior exposure to the JC virus, number of natalizumab infusions, and prior use of immunosuppressant treatment.[40,41] Thus, a patient with the 3 risk factors will have a PML risk as high as 11.1 in 1000. This risk stratification strategy may help to counsel patients about starting or discontinuing treatment, and to establish different monitoring strategies to include a more frequent brain MR images schedule to detect presymptomatic PML, which has been associated with better outcomes.[42]

Alemtuzumab
Alemtuzumab is a humanized monoclonal antibody against the CD52 antigen present in the B and T lymphocytes, natural killer cells, monocytes, macrophages, and most of the granulocytes except for neutrophils. The binding of alemtuzumab with the CD52 antigen will produce a profound and prolonged depletion of these cells.[43]

Efficacy Alemtuzumab demonstrated it efficacy as first-line and second-line treatments in 2 clinical trials: CARE-MS-I (Comparison of Alemtuzumab and Rebif Efficacy in Multiple Sclerosis, Study One; enrolling treatment naïve patients)[44] and CARE-MS-II (enrolling patient who had failed to a previous disease-modifying treatments; Comparison of Alemtuzumab and Rebif® Efficacy in Multiple Sclerosis, Study Two).[45] Compared with sc IFN-β-1a treatment, alemtuzumab reduced in about 50% the ARR (54.9% reduction in CARE-MS-I and 49.4% reduction in CARE-MS-II). In the CARE-MS-II trial, but not in the CARE-MS-I, alemtuzumab reduced by 42% the risk of 6-month sustained disability progression. As for MR imaging parameters, 17% and 32% fewer patients presented new T2 lesions, and 63% and 61% fewer patients presented Gd-enhancing lesions in the CARE-MS-I and CARE-MS-II trials, respectively.[44,45]

Safety Owing to the cytokine release, up to 90% of patients present an infusion reaction that may cause fever, headache, and skin reactions; pre-medication is recommended to minimize this reaction. Infectious diseases were reported generally with a greater frequency in alemtuzumab-treated patients; herpes simplex reactivation is seen in up to 20% of patients and it may be prevented with acyclovir treatment. The most serious adverse events were thyroid, renal, and platelet autoimmune events that may affect up to 30% of patients.[44,45] These autoimmunity events may occur long after the last alemtuzumab dose, and therefore a close and prolonged laboratory test monitoring is mandatory.

Oral Therapies

Fingolimod
Fingolimod was the first oral treatment approved for treating RRMS. As an sphingosine 1-phosphate analogue, it blocks the lymphocyte egression from the lymph nodes and ultimately prevents autoreactive lymphocytes to enter into the CNS.[46]

Efficacy Fingolimod's efficacy has been demonstrated in 3 clinical trials, 2 of them compared with placebo,[47,48] and 1 of them compared with im IFN-β-1a.[49] In both situations, the dose of 0.5 mg (the dose that has been finally approved) reduced in about 50% the ARR 54% and 48% reduction compared with placebo in FREEDOMS (Efficacy and Safety of Fingolimod in Patients With Relapsing-remitting Multiple Sclerosis) and FREEDOMS II (Efficacy and Safety of Fingolimod (FTY720) in Patients With Relapsing-remitting Multiple Sclerosis)[47,48]; and a 51% reduction compared with im IFN-β-1a in TRANSFORMS (Efficacy and Safety of Fingolimod in Patients With Relapsing-remitting Multiple Sclerosis With

Optional Extension Phase)[49] clinical trial. As for disability, in the FREEDOMS trial but not in the other trials, fingolimod reduced by 30% the risk of 3-month sustained disability progression.[47] Compared with placebo, and after 2 years of treatment, fingolimod reduced the presence of new T2 lesions in 32% and 37% in the FREEDOMS II and FREEDOMS trials, respectively, and reduced the presence of patients presenting with Gd-enhancing lesions in 62% and 70% in the FREEDOMS II and FREEDOMS trials, respectively.[47,48] In the TRANSFORMS trial, after 1 year of treatment and compared with im IFN-β-1a, the radiologic disease activity reduction was also in favor of fingolimod.[49]

Safety Owing to the ubiquity of the sphingosine 1-phosphate receptor, a number of adverse events have been reported with fingolimod treatment. The most important adverse event is the occurrence of bradycardia the first hours after treatment onset that is usually asymptomatic. Other adverse events reported with higher frequency in the fingolimod-treated arms were macular edema, liver function abnormalities, skin cancer, hypertension, and herpes virus infections.[47–49] Therefore, before starting fingolimod treatment, the physician should rule out cardiac contraindications and test for varicella zoster virus serology. Patients should receive the first dose of fingolimod under cardiac monitoring. Last, during the postmarketing monitoring, a few cases of PML in patients treated with fingolimod have been reported.

Dimethyl fumarate
Dimethyl fumarate (DMF) is a fumaric acid derivative that demonstrated its efficacy in 2 phase III clinical trials.[50,51] Its mechanism of action is not well-elucidated, but it seems to have both an immunomodulatory effect through cytokine modulation, and a neuroprotective effect by reducing the oxidative cellular stress.[52,53]

Efficacy In both trials, a dose of 240 mg administered twice daily (the dose that has been finally approved) reduced in about 50% the ARR (44% and 53% reduction in the CONFIRM [Comparator and an Oral Fumarate in RRMS] and DEFINE [Efficacy and Safety of Oral BG00012 in Relapsing-Remitting Multiple Sclerosis] trials, respectively).[50,51] In the DEFINE, but not in the CONFIRM trial, DMF also reduced the risk of 3-month sustained disability by 38%.[50] DMF proved to be effective in reducing radiologic disease activity too, with reductions of 71% and 85% in the number of new T2 lesions, and a reduction of 74% and 90% in the number of

Gd-enhancing lesions (in the CONFIRM and DEFINE trials, respectively).[50,51]

Safety Gastrointestinal events and flushing occurred more frequently in DMF-treated patients. These events usually occurred shortly after treatment onset and resolved few weeks later.[54] About one-third of patients present with lymphopenia, and it may be severe in up to 5% of DMF-treated patients.[50,51] Recently, a few cases of PML have been reported in patients with MS treated with DMF.

Teriflunomide
Teriflunomide exerts its action by inhibiting the mitochondrial enzyme dihydroorotate-dehydrogenase. This enzyme is involved in the synthesis of pyrimidines in proliferating cells such as T and B lymphocytes.[55] Thus, teriflunomide action in MS is mediated by reducing the proliferation of T and B lymphocytes.

Efficacy Compared with placebo, the 2 doses of teriflunomide (7 and 14 mg) reduced the ARR in about 30% (31% reduction for both doses in the TEMSO [Study of Teriflunomide in Reducing the Frequency of Relapses and Accumulation of Disability in Patients With Multiple Sclerosis] trial,[56] and 22% and 36% for the 7-mg and 14-mg doses in the TOWER [An Efficacy Study of Teriflunomide in Participants With Relapsing Multiple Sclerosis] trial[57]). The higher dose, but not the 7-mg dose, reduced by 30% the risk of 3-month sustained disability progression.[56,57] Only the TEMSO trial evaluated teriflunomide MR imaging effects proving to be effective in reducing the number of new T2 lesions (by 39% and 67% for the 7-mg and 14-mg doses, respectively) and it also reduced the number of Gd-enhancing lesions (by 57% and 80% for the 7-mg and 14-mg doses, respectively).[56] In the TENERE clinical trial (A Study Comparing the Effectiveness and Safety of Teriflunomide and Interferon Beta-1a in Patients With Relapsing Multiple Sclerosis), sc IFN-β-1a was included as an active comparator.[58] In this trial, no differences were detected for the primary outcome, namely, time to treatment failure

(defined as either presenting a relapse or treatment withdrawal owing to any cause).[58]

Safety The adverse events that were more frequently reported in teriflunomide-treated patients were liver function abnormalities, hair thinning, hypertension, and gastrointestinal events.[56–58] Owing to the higher frequency of liver abnormalities, a close liver function monitoring is recommended.

SUMMARY

The diagnosis and treatment of MS has changed broadly in the last years. The incorporation of conventional MR imaging into the diagnostic criteria has allowed for an earlier diagnosis. Consequently, patients are also treated earlier, when treatments are more effective.[59] Treatment options have been expanding over the last years (see **Table 2**). All treatment options have demonstrated to be effective in reducing clinical and radiologic disease activity, and with the newer therapies a new concept of no evidence of disease activity has emerged. Natalizumab was the first drug to report a great number of patients meeting no evidence of disease activity criteria,[60] defined as the absence of relapses, absence of disability progression, and absence of radiologic disease activity (absence of new or enlarged T2 lesions and/or Gd-enhancing lesions). This concept is used extensively currently, and all the newest therapies have reported it[61] (**Table 3**).

Thanks to the development of newer and more effective treatments, we are starting to move toward a more personalized medicine, where the therapeutic strategy may be different for each patient. In this regard, an induction therapy or a step-down strategy may be used in patients with highly active disease or with poor prognostic factors at disease onset. In contrast, the standard escalation or step-up strategy may be a good option for patients with a less aggressive disease, or patients not willing to accept greater treatment risks.[62,63] Nevertheless, the assessment of treatment options should be reevaluated longitudinally,

Table 3 NEDA outcomes for each drug					
	Natalizumab	Fingolimod	Teriflunomide	Dimethyl Fumarate	Alemtuzumab
Proportion of patients presenting NEDA at 2 y	37%	33%	23%	23%	32%

Abbreviation: NEDA, no evidence of disease activity.

because treatment and disease risks, as well as treatment benefits, may change over time.

This new treatment scenario, with a large number of treatment options and specific risk-benefit profiles, makes treatment decision more complex. Moreover, the risk–benefit balance may be perceived differently between individual patients owing to different personal expectations and disease perception. Therefore, patient should be involved in the decision making process to ensure a good treatment and safety monitoring adherence.[64,65]

REFERENCES

1. Noseworthy JH, Lucchinetti C, Rodriguez M, et al. Medical progress: multiple sclerosis. N Engl J Med 2000;343:938–52.

2. Compston A, Coles A. Multiple sclerosis. Lancet 2008;372(9648):1502–17.

3. Belbasis L, Bellou V, Evangelou E, et al. Environmental risk factors and multiple sclerosis: an umbrella review of systematic reviews and meta-analyses. Lancet Neurol 2015;14(3):263–73.

4. Handel AE, Giovannoni G, Ebers GC, et al. Environmental factors and their timing in adult-onset multiple sclerosis. Nat Rev Neurol 2010;6(3):156–66.

5. Lublin FD, Reingold SC. Defining the clinical course of multiple sclerosis results of an international survey. Neurology 1996;46(4):907–11.

6. Lublin FD, Reingold SC, Cohen JA, et al. Defining the clinical course of multiple sclerosis: the 2013 revisions. Neurology 2014;83(3):278–86.

7. Miller DH, Leary SM. Primary-progressive multiple sclerosis. Lancet Neurol 2007;6(10):903–12.

8. Miller DH, Chard DT, Ciccarelli O. Clinically isolated syndromes. Lancet Neurol 2012;11(2):157–69.

9. Miller D, Barkhof F, Montalban X, et al. Clinically isolated syndromes suggestive of multiple sclerosis, part I: natural history, pathogenesis, diagnosis, and prognosis. Lancet Neurol 2005;4(5):281–8.

10. Kurtzke JF. Geography in multiple sclerosis. J Neurol 1977;215(1):1–26.

11. Fisniku LK, Brex PA, Altmann DR, et al. Disability and T2 MRI lesions: a 20-year follow-up of patients with relapse onset of multiple sclerosis. Brain 2008;131(3):808–17.

12. Tintoré M, Rovira A, Rio J, et al. Baseline MRI predicts future attacks and disability in clinically isolated syndromes. Neurology 2006;67(6):968–72.

13. Tintore M, Rovira À, Río J, et al. Defining high, medium and low impact prognostic factors for developing multiple sclerosis. Brain 2015;138(7):1863–74.

14. Degenhardt A, Ramagopalan SV, Scalfari A, et al. Clinical prognostic factors in multiple sclerosis: a natural history review. Nat Rev Neurol 2009;5(12):672–82.

15. Scalfari A, Neuhaus A, Daumer M, et al. Onset of secondary progressive phase and long-term evolution of multiple sclerosis. J Neurol Neurosurg Psychiatry 2014;85(1):67–75.

16. Rovaris M, Confavreux C, Furlan R, et al. Secondary progressive multiple sclerosis: current knowledge and future challenges. Lancet Neurol 2006;5(4):343–54.

17. Montalban X, Tintore M, Swanton J, et al. MRI criteria for MS in patients with clinically isolated syndromes. Neurology 2010;74(5):427–34.

18. Polman CH, Reingold SC, Banwell B, et al. Diagnostic criteria for multiple sclerosis: 2010 revisions to the McDonald criteria. Ann Neurol 2011;69(2):292–302.

19. Dhib-Jalbut S, Marks S. Interferon-β mechanisms of action in multiple sclerosis. Neurology 2010;74(1 Supplement 1):S17–24.

20. Interferon beta-1b is effective in relapsing-remitting multiple sclerosis. I. Clinical results of a multicenter, randomized, double-blind, placebo-controlled trial. The IFNB Multiple Sclerosis Study Group. Neurology 1993;43(4):655–61.

21. Interferon beta-1b in the treatment of multiple sclerosis: final outcome of the randomized controlled trial. The IFNB Multiple Sclerosis Study Group and The University of British Columbia MS/MRI Analysis Group. Neurology 1995;45(7):1277–85.

22. Jacobs LD, Cookfair DL, Rudick RA, et al. Intramuscular interferon beta-1a for disease progression in relapsing multiple sclerosis. The Multiple Sclerosis Collaborative Research Group (MSCRG). Ann Neurol 1996;39(3):285–94.

23. Ebers GC. Randomised double-blind placebo-controlled study of interferon β-1a in relapsing/remitting multiple sclerosis. Lancet 1998;352(9139):1498–504.

24. Calabresi PA, Kieseier BC, Arnold DL, et al. Pegylated interferon β-1a for relapsing-remitting multiple sclerosis (ADVANCE): a randomised, phase 3, double-blind study. Lancet Neurol 2014;13(7):657–65.

25. Jacobs LD, Beck RW, Simon JH, et al. Intramuscular interferon beta-1a therapy initiated during a first demyelinating event in multiple sclerosis. N Engl J Med 2000;343(13):898–904.

26. Comi G, Filippi M, Barkhof F, et al. Effect of early interferon treatment on conversion to definite multiple sclerosis: a randomised study. Lancet 2001;357(9268):1576–82.

27. Kappos L, Polman CH, Freedman MS, et al. Treatment with interferon beta-1b delays conversion to clinically definite and McDonald MS in patients with clinically isolated syndromes. Neurology 2006;67(7):1242–9.

28. Comi G, De Stefano N, Freedman MS, et al. Comparison of two dosing frequencies of subcutaneous interferon beta-1a in patients with a first clinical demyelinating event suggestive of multiple sclerosis

(REFLEX): a phase 3 randomised controlled trial. Lancet Neurol 2012;11(1):33–41.

29. Balak DM, Hengstman GJ, Çakmak A, et al. Cutaneous adverse events associated with disease-modifying treatment in multiple sclerosis: a systematic review. Mult Scler 2012;18(12):1705–17.

30. Calabresi PA. Considerations in the treatment of relapsing-remitting multiple sclerosis. Neurology 2002;58(8 Suppl 4):S10–22.

31. Chan S, Kingwell E, Oger J, et al. High-dose frequency beta-interferons increase the risk of liver test abnormalities in multiple sclerosis: a longitudinal study. Mult Scler 2011;17(3):361–7.

32. Racke MK, Lovett-Racke AE, Karandikar NJ. The mechanism of action of glatiramer acetate treatment in multiple sclerosis. Neurology 2010;74(1 Supplement 1): S25–30.

33. Johnson KP, Brooks BR, Cohen JA, et al. Copolymer 1 reduces relapse rate and improves disability in relapsing-remitting multiple sclerosis: results of a phase III multicenter, double-blind placebo-controlled trial. The Copolymer 1 Multiple Sclerosis Study Group. Neurology 1995;45(7):1268–76.

34. Comi G, Filippi M, Wolinsky JS. European/Canadian multicenter, double-blind, randomized, placebo-controlled study of the effects of glatiramer acetate on magnetic resonance imaging–measured disease activity and burden in patients with relapsing multiple sclerosis. European/Canadian Glatiramer Acetate Study Group. Ann Neurol 2001;49(3):290–7.

35. Comi G, Martinelli V, Rodegher M, et al. Effect of glatiramer acetate on conversion to clinically definite multiple sclerosis in patients with clinically isolated syndrome (PreCISe study): a randomised, double-blind, placebo-controlled trial. Lancet 2009; 374(9700):1503–11.

36. Khan O, Rieckmann P, Boyko A, et al. Three times weekly glatiramer acetate in relapsing-remitting multiple sclerosis. Ann Neurol 2013;73(6):705–13.

37. Ransohoff RM. Natalizumab for multiple sclerosis. N Engl J Med 2007;356(25):2622–9.

38. Polman CH, O'Connor PW, Havrdova E, et al. A randomized, placebo-controlled trial of natalizumab for relapsing multiple sclerosis. N Engl J Med 2006;354(9):899–910.

39. Rudick RA, Stuart WH, Calabresi PA, et al. Natalizumab plus interferon beta-1a for relapsing multiple sclerosis. N Engl J Med 2006;354(9):911–23.

40. Bloomgren G, Richman S, Hotermans C, et al. Risk of natalizumab-associated progressive multifocal leukoencephalopathy. N Engl J Med 2012;366(20): 1870–80.

41. Plavina T, Subramanyam M, Bloomgren G, et al. Anti-JC virus antibody levels in serum or plasma further define risk of natalizumab-associated progressive multifocal leukoencephalopathy: anti-JCV antibody and PML risk. Ann Neurol 2014;76(6):802–12.

42. McGuigan C, Craner M, Guadagno J, et al. Stratification and monitoring of natalizumab-associated progressive multifocal leukoencephalopathy risk: recommendations from an expert group. J Neurol Neurosurg Psychiatry 2016;87(2):117–25.

43. Coles AJ. Alemtuzumab therapy for multiple sclerosis. Neurotherapeutics 2013;10(1):29–33.

44. Cohen JA, Coles AJ, Arnold DL, et al. Alemtuzumab versus interferon beta 1a as first-line treatment for patients with relapsing-remitting multiple sclerosis: a randomised controlled phase 3 trial. Lancet 2012;380(9856):1819–28.

45. Coles AJ, Twyman CL, Arnold DL, et al. Alemtuzumab for patients with relapsing multiple sclerosis after disease-modifying therapy: a randomised controlled phase 3 trial. Lancet 2012;380(9856):1829–39.

46. Pelletier D, Hafler DA. Fingolimod for multiple sclerosis. N Engl J Med 2012;366(4):339–47.

47. Kappos L, Radue EW, O'Connor P, et al. A placebo-controlled trial of oral fingolimod in relapsing multiple sclerosis. N Engl J Med 2010;362(5):387–401.

48. Calabresi PA, Radue EW, Goodin D, et al. Safety and efficacy of fingolimod in patients with relapsing-remitting multiple sclerosis (FREEDOMS II): a double-blind, randomised, placebo-controlled, phase 3 trial. Lancet Neurol 2014;13(6):545–56.

49. Cohen JA, Barkhof F, Comi G, et al. Oral fingolimod or intramuscular interferon for relapsing multiple sclerosis. N Engl J Med 2010;362(5):402–15.

50. Gold R, Kappos L, Arnold DL, et al. Placebo-controlled phase 3 study of oral BG-12 for Relapsing multiple sclerosis. N Engl J Med 2012;367(12):1098–107.

51. Fox RJ, Miller DH, Phillips JT, et al. Placebo-Controlled Phase 3 Study of Oral BG-12 or Glatiramer in Multiple Sclerosis. N Engl J Med 2012; 367(12):1087–97.

52. Linker RA, Lee DH, Ryan S, et al. Fumaric acid esters exert neuroprotective effects in neuroinflammation via activation of the Nrf2 antioxidant pathway. Brain 2011;134(Pt 3):678–92.

53. Gold R, Linker RA, Stangel M. Fumaric acid and its esters: an emerging treatment for multiple sclerosis with antioxidative mechanism of action. Clin Immunol 2012;142(1):44–8.

54. Kappos L, Giovannoni G, Gold R, et al. Time course of clinical and neuroradiological effects of delayed-release dimethyl fumarate in multiple sclerosis. Eur J Neurol 2015;22(4):664–71.

55. Claussen MC, Korn T. Immune mechanisms of new therapeutic strategies in MS — Teriflunomide. Clin Immunol 2012;142(1):49–56.

56. O'Connor P, Wolinsky JS, Confavreux C, et al. Randomized trial of oral teriflunomide for relapsing multiple sclerosis. N Engl J Med 2011;365(14): 1293–303.

57. Confavreux C, O'Connor P, Comi G, et al. Oral teriflunomide for patients with relapsing multiple sclerosis

(TOWER): a randomised, double-blind, placebo-controlled, phase 3 trial. Lancet Neurol 2014;13(3):247–56.

58. Vermersch P, Czlonkowska A, Grimaldi LM, et al. Teriflunomide versus subcutaneous interferon beta-1a in patients with relapsing multiple sclerosis: a randomised, controlled phase 3 trial. Mult Scler 2014;20(6):705–16.

59. Gold R, Wolinsky JS, Amato MP, et al. Evolving expectations around early management of multiple sclerosis. Ther Adv Neurol Disord 2010;3(6):351–67.

60. Havrdova E, Galetta S, Hutchinson M, et al. Effect of natalizumab on clinical and radiological disease activity in multiple sclerosis: a retrospective analysis of the Natalizumab Safety and Efficacy in Relapsing-Remitting Multiple Sclerosis (AFFIRM) study. Lancet Neurol 2009;8(3):254–60.

61. Milo R. Effectiveness of multiple sclerosis treatment with current immunomodulatory drugs. Expert Opin Pharmacother 2015;16(5):659–73.

62. Giovannoni G. Multiple sclerosis should be treated using a step-down strategy rather than a step-up strategy–YES. Mult Scler 2016;22(11):1397–400.

63. Naismith RT. Multiple sclerosis should be treated using a step-down strategy rather than a step-up strategy–NO. Mult Scler 2016;22(11):1400–2.

64. Johnson FR, Van Houtven G, Ozdemir S, et al. Multiple sclerosis patients—benefit-risk preferences: serious adverse event risks versus treatment efficacy. J Neurol 2009;256(4):554–62.

65. Heesen C, Solari A, Giordano A, et al. Decisions on multiple sclerosis immunotherapy: New treatment complexities urge patient engagement. J Neurol Sci 2011;306(1–2):192–7.

Brain and Spinal Cord MR Imaging Features in Multiple Sclerosis and Variants

Iris Dekker, MD[a,b], Mike P. Wattjes, MD[a],*

KEYWORDS

- Multiple sclerosis • MR imaging • Protocol • Diagnostic criteria • Differential diagnosis

KEY POINTS

- Multiple sclerosis pathology has certain imaging characteristics that have been incorporated into diagnostic criteria.
- Focal multiple sclerosis lesions are ovoid shaped, perivascularly located, have specific locations throughout the central nervous system, and are not restricted to the white matter.
- MR imaging plays a crucial role in diagnosing multiple sclerosis, in predicting the prognosis, and monitoring of the disease course (treatment efficacy and safety).
- Standardized imaging acquisition, reading, and reporting according to recent expert panel guidelines is highly recommended.
- Diagnostic criteria are crucial for the correct diagnosis of multiple sclerosis.

INTRODUCTION

Multiple sclerosis (MS) is the most frequent chronic, inflammatory, demyelinating disease of the central nervous system in young adults leading to long-term disability.[1] In addition to the clinical presentation, including the neurologic examination and cerebrospinal fluid (CSF) markers (eg, the demonstration of oligoclonal bands), MR imaging of the brain and spinal cord plays a crucial role for diagnostic and disease-monitoring purposes.[2] In 2001, for the first time, brain and spinal cord MR imaging have been incorporated into the MS diagnostic criteria (McDonald criteria) for the demonstration of both dissemination in space (DIS) and in time (DIT).[3] The 2005 and the 2010 revisions of the McDonald criteria have further reinforced the crucial role of MR imaging in the diagnosis of MS, allowing the diagnosis of MS in patients with clinically isolated syndrome (CIS) with only 1 MR imaging scan.[4,5] Although MS pathology has some characteristic imaging characteristics and follows a certain distribution pattern, other pathologies (eg, vascular, inflammatory) can mimic MS pathology clinically as well as radiologically, leading to a broad spectrum of differential diagnoses. MR imaging, in particular spinal cord imaging, can aid in making the correct diagnosis, and exclude relevant differential diagnoses.[6,7] Unfortunately, MR imaging pathology does not correlate well with the clinical presentation and disease progression with respect to clinical outcome measures such as physical disability and cognitive performance, which has

Disclosures: M.P. Wattjes has received consultancy fees from Biogen, Novartis and Roche.
a Department of Radiology and Nuclear Medicine, Neuroscience Amsterdam, VUmc MS Center Amsterdam, VU University Medical Center, De Boelelaan 1117, Amsterdam 1081 HV, The Netherlands; b Department of Neurology, Neuroscience Amsterdam, VUmc MS Center Amsterdam, VU University Medical Center, De Boelelaan 1117, Amsterdam 1081 HV, The Netherlands
* Corresponding author. Department of Radiology, VU University Medical Center, De Boelelaan 1117, Amsterdam 1081 HV, The Netherlands.
E-mail address: m.wattjes@vumc.nl

coined the term "clinico-radiological paradox" in MS.[8,9] This is probably because MS pathology on MR imaging is heterogeneous with respect to pathology distribution involving gray and white matter structures of the brain and spinal cord to different degrees. In addition to focal pathology, diffuse white and gray matter changes (diffusively abnormal white matter [DAWM] and gray matter [DAGM]), as well as pathology that is not visible on conventional MR imaging (normal-appearing gray and white matter), contribute substantially to the clinical presentation and the functional outcome.[10–14]

In addition to the MS diagnosis and differential diagnosis, there is increasing and conclusive evidence that MR imaging is also useful for prognostic classification and for monitoring the disease progression, treatment efficacy, and safety.[15]

The aim of this review was to give a comprehensive overview of brain and spinal cord imaging in MS with special regard to different MR imaging approaches for diagnosing MS and distinguishing MS variants.

IMAGING OF MULTIPLE SCLEROSIS, MR IMAGING PROTOCOLS OF BRAIN, SPINAL CORD, AND TREATMENT MONITORING

Because imaging has become increasingly important for the diagnosis and monitoring of MS, there is an unmet medical need for the standardization of the MR imaging acquisition, timing of MR imaging scanning, and image interpretation/reporting.[5] The need for standardization goes beyond the diagnostic process and is of special clinical relevance for those patients with an established diagnosis of MS and being treated with MS therapeutics. In 2015, evidence-based guidelines were published by the Magnetic Resonance Imaging in MS (MAGNIMS) study group (www.magnims.eu) and the Consortium of MS Centers (CMSC), creating a framework for clinical MR imaging sequences necessary for the diagnostic and monitoring processes.[15,16]

MR Imaging Protocol of the Brain

Table 1 shows the recommended MR imaging acquisition protocol, including mandatory and optional brain MR imaging sequences for baseline assessment and follow-up examination as proposed by the MAGNIMS and the CMSC panel. Due to the higher detection of white and gray matter MS lesions in the brain, the use of an MR imaging system operating at 3 T is recommended, applying standard spatial resolution parameters (slice thickness of 3 mm, in-plane resolution of 1 × 1 mm) for diagnostic and monitoring purposes.[17–20]

Mandatory sequences in the MR imaging protocols for diagnosing, disease monitoring, and treatment include T2-weighted imaging, T2-fluid-attenuated inversion recovery (T2-FLAIR), and T1-weighted imaging, including contrast

Table 1
Protocols for brain MR imaging acquisition for diagnostic purposes

MR Imaging sequences	Baseline MR Imaging MAGNIMS	Baseline MR Imaging CMSC	Follow-up MR Imaging MAGNIMS
Axial PD and/or T2-FLAIR/T2-weighted	Yes	Yes, 3D	Highly recommended
Sagittal 2D or 3D T2-FLAIR	Yes	Yes[b]	Optional
2D or 3D contrast-enhanced T1-weighted[a]	Yes	Yes,[b] precontrast and postcontrast	Yes
Unenhanced 2D or high-resolution isotropic 3D T1-weighted	Optional	Yes[b]	Optional
2D and/or 3D DIR	Optional	No	Optional
Axial diffusion-weighted imaging	Optional	Yes	No

Abbreviations: CMSC, Consortium of MS Centers; DIR, double inversion recovery; FLAIR, fluid-attenuated inversion recovery; MAGNIMS, Magnetic Resonance Imaging in MS; PD, proton density; 2D, 2 dimensional; 3D, 3 dimensional.
  [a] Standard contrast administration: single dose, 0.1 mmol/kg body weight.
  [b] Three-dimensional acquisition precontrast and postcontrast.
  Adapted from Traboulsee A, Simon JH, Stone L, et al. Revised recommendations of the Consortium of MS Centers task force for a standardized MRI protocol and clinical guidelines for the diagnosis and follow-up of multiple sclerosis. AJNR Am J Neuroradiol 2016;37(3):394–401; and Rovira A, Wattjes MP, Tintore M, et al. Evidence-based guidelines: MAGNIMS consensus guidelines on the use of MRI in multiple sclerosis-clinical implementation in the diagnostic process. Nat Rev Neurol 2015;11(8):471–82.

administering. The choice of the recommended sequences is based on the pulse sequences with higher detection rates in certain anatomic areas. For instance, T2-FLAIR shows a higher lesion load in the periventricular white matter because of CSF attenuation, whereas T2-weighted (turbo/fast) spin echo sequences show higher detection rates in the posterior fossa.[21]

New/active lesions may show enhancement after gadolinium administration, and detection of an enhancing lesion could complete the dissemination in time with a single MR imaging scan when at the same moment also nonenhancing lesions are present.[5]

It has been suggested that diffusion-weighted imaging (DWI) may be useful in MS imaging with respect to the detection of acute inflammation and for the differentiation between demyelinating lesions and (sub)acute vascular white matter lesions (eg, lacunar infarcts).[22] However, DWI is not recommended for clinical routine setting for MS diagnosis. In particular, it should not replace the contrast-enhanced T1-weighted sequences for detecting active lesions.[15,23]

In addition to white matter lesions, cortical gray matter lesions are of clinical relevance for diagnostic purposes and in predicting cognitive decline and future disability.[13] Recently, it has been suggested to incorporate cortical gray matter lesions into future diagnostic criteria with respect to the demonstration of DIS.[24] However, their location close to the CSF and white matter impedes the detection of cortical gray matter lesions and leads to a high interrater variability.[25]

Brain atrophy is a better representation of physical disability and cognitive decline than can be measured by focal lesion load. Measurements of atrophy are a promising tool for treatment trials as well.[2,26] In addition, ultra–high-field imaging is a promising method for lesion differentiation purposes, to better understand the in vivo MS pathology and to further increase the sensitivity of MS lesion detection (in particular gray matter lesions).[25–27] However, although the number of ultra–high-field (≥7T) whole-body MR imaging systems increases, these systems are not yet available in most clinics, and ultra–high-field MR acquisition protocols are not standardized.

MR Imaging Protocol of the Spinal Cord

The clinical relevance of spinal cord imaging in the (differential) diagnosis of MS has conclusively been demonstrated, and should be performed routinely in the diagnostic workup of patients with suspected demyelination.[28] Presence of spinal cord lesions further increases the sensitivity of the diagnosis in all types of disease courses and is predictive for the conversion to clinically definite MS in radiologically isolated syndrome (RIS) as well as in patients with CIS.[6,29,30] Furthermore, spinal cord lesions have a strong impact in fulfilling the diagnostic criteria for DIS and in ruling out other diseases. The clinical relevance of spinal cord imaging in MS is further reinforced by a broad spectrum of indications for spinal cord imaging as listed in **Table 2**.

However, compared with brain imaging, spinal cord imaging is technically more difficult and quite challenging with respect to image interpretation, caused by its long, thin, and flexible anatomy and the higher propensity to show artifacts caused by breathing and pulsation and/or flow of CSF and blood vessels.[31] **Table 3** summarizes the MR imaging acquisition for spinal cord imaging according to both expert panel guidelines. Sagittal T2-weighted imaging covering the whole spinal cord is necessary for diagnostic purposes and

Table 2
Indications for spinal cord imaging

Clinical Presentation	Added Value of Spinal Cord Imaging
CIS	Predictive for conversion to CDMS
• Spinal cord symptoms	Excluding other diseases (eg, malignancy)
• No spinal cord symptoms but inconclusive brain MR imaging	Detection of asymptomatic lesions: • Could attribute to fulfill DIS/DIT
Normal brain MR imaging but clinically suspected for MS	No spinal cord lesions: diagnosis MS unlikely
Nonspecific brain MR imaging findings	Presence of spinal cord lesions, support diagnosis of MS
RIS	Presence of spinal cord lesions predict conversion to CDMS
PPMS	Excluding other diseases

Abbreviations: CDMS, clinically definite multiple sclerosis; CIS, clinically isolated syndrome; DIS, dissemination in space; DIT, dissemination in time; MS, multiple sclerosis; PPMS, primary progressive multiple sclerosis; RIS, radiologically isolated syndrome.

Modified from Rovira A, Wattjes MP, Tintore M, et al. Evidence-based guidelines: MAGNIMS consensus guidelines on the use of MRI in multiple sclerosis-clinical implementation in the diagnostic process. Nat Rev Neurol 2015;11(8):471–82.

Table 3
Protocols for spinal cord MR imaging acquisition

MR Imaging sequences	Baseline MR Imaging MAGNIMS	Baseline MR Imaging CMSC
Single-echo T2	Sagittal (if combined with STIR) (axial optional)	Sagittal, axial through lesions
Dual-echo PD/T2	Sagittal	Alternative for T2
STIR	Alternative for PD	Sagittal
2D or 3D contrast-enhanced T1	Sagittal	Sagittal, optional
PSIR	Sagittal, optional	(PST1-IR)

Abbreviations: CMSC, Consortium of MS Centers; MAGNIMS, Magnetic Resonance Imaging in MS; PD, proton density; PSIR, phase sensitive inversion recovery; PST1-IR, Phase Sensitive T1 inversion recovery; STIR, short-tau inversion recovery; 2D, 2 dimensional; 3D, 3 dimensional.
Modified from Traboulsee A, Simon JH, Stone L, et al. Revised recommendations of the Consortium of MS Centers task force for a standardized MRI protocol and clinical guidelines for the diagnosis and follow-up of multiple sclerosis. AJNR Am J Neuroradiol 2016;37(3):394–401; and Rovira A, Wattjes MP, Tintore M, et al. Evidence-based guidelines: MAGNIMS consensus guidelines on the use of MRI in multiple sclerosis-clinical implementation in the diagnostic process. Nat Rev Neurol 2015;11(8):471–82

should be performed as a double echo (proton density [PD]/T2).[23] Short-tau inversion recovery (STIR) could be used as an alternative if PD-weighted sequences are not reliable.[32,33]

Because sagittal images could fail in detecting spinal cord lesions, axial imaging should be performed as well.[34] Contrast administering is advised to be performed right after the brain MR imaging, this reduces time and patient discomfort.[7,23] Enhancing lesions are less frequently seen in the spinal cord compared with the brain, and are mostly symptomatic when visible.[31]

T2-FLAIR imaging is not sensitive for spinal cord lesions and therefore not performed.[23,35]

In contrast to brain MR imaging, it has not been proven that a higher field strength of 3T MR imaging is superior to 1.5 T in terms of MS lesion detection.[36]

MR Imaging Protocol of the Optic Nerve

For the imaging of the optic nerve, a standardized MR imaging protocol has been composed as well. However, optic nerve imaging is not recommended on a regular basis in the clinical routine setting because it is restricted to certain clinical conditions and for research purposes.[37]

MR Imaging Protocol for Treatment Monitoring

The most frequent indications for serial imaging in the setting of MS disease or treatment monitoring

Table 4
MR imaging for treatment monitoring

MR Imaging sequences	Treatment Efficacy and Monitoring. Yearly	Screening PML in Case of High Risk of PML. Every 3–4 months
Axial PD and/or T2-FLAIR/ T2-weighted	Yes	Yes
Sagittal 2D or 3D T2-FLAIR	Optional	Yes
2D or 3D contrast-enhanced T1-weighted	Yes	No
Axial diffusion-weighted imaging	No	Yes

Abbreviations: FLAIR, fluid attenuation inversion recovery; PD, proton density; PML, progressive multifocal leukoencephalitis; 2D, 2 dimensional; 3D, 3 dimensional.
Data from Refs.[2,15,16]

includes the assessment of treatment efficacy, the prediction of treatment response, and drug safety monitoring (eg, the detection of comorbidities, unexpected severe disease progression, and screening for opportunistic infections such as progressive multifocal leukoencephalopathy [PML]).[2,15] The MR imaging acquisition protocol is strongly dependent on the specific indication, and different protocols used for MS treatment monitoring purposes are summarized in **Table 4**. It has been recommended to monitor disease-modifying therapy (DMT) efficacy just after the initiation of therapy and on a yearly basis.[15] The disease monitoring is often dependent on clinical status, but imaging is showing clinical silent changes (new/enlarged T2 lesions, contrast-enhancing lesions) and is more sensitive for disease activity than the neurologic examination.[2] A special indication for brain MR imaging follow-up are patients with a higher risk of developing PML (patients treated with natalizumab with a positive John Cunningham virus serostatus and a treatment duration of ≥18 months). Current guidelines and the recommendations from the regulatory authorities state that these high-risk patients should be screened every 3 to 4 months[15] or 3 to 6 months[16] (depending on the specific guidelines protocol followed), with an abbreviated scan protocol including T2-FLAIR, T2, and DWI sequences.[15,38] This follow-up is also recommended for patients switching from natalizumab to another therapy.[15,39,40] Both spinal cord imaging and quantitative MR imaging have no additive value for monitoring in clinical routine setting and are therefore not recommended.[15]

MULTIPLE SCLEROSIS PATHOLOGY IN THE BRAIN AND SPINAL CORD
Imaging Brain Pathology

White matter pathology: focal lesions
The pathophysiology and histopathology of MS is characterized by an inflammation crossing the blood-brain barrier via venous vessels leading to inflammation, demyelination, and neurodegeneration[41] (**Fig. 1**). In this context, it is worth stressing that MS is not based on a chronic venous obstruction, as recently suggested.[42]

Focal MS lesions appear on different locations throughout the brain and spinal cord, showing a characteristic but not specific distribution pattern. Characteristically, MS focal lesions are ovoid shaped and have sharp borders[41] (**Fig. 2**). One histopathological hallmark of focal MS lesions is the perivascular (perivenous) inflammation pattern in the white matter leading to this characteristic location of focal MS lesions along a vein.[43] This lesion

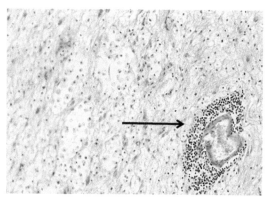

Fig. 1. Vein surrounded by infiltration and macrophages destroying myelin (*arrow*). (*Courtesy of* Prof Dr Paul van der Valk, MD, PhD, Amsterdam, Netherlands.)

distribution pattern is most impressive for periventricular lesions leading to a fingerlike shape on axial images, first described by Dawson in 1916,[44] the so called "Dawson fingers" (Dawson 1916). The demonstration of this perivascular location of MS lesions is increasingly being used for diagnostic/lesion differentiation purposes. By combining T2-FLAIR with susceptibility weighted imaging (SWI), 3T,[45] and in particular 7T, MR imaging are well suited to demonstrate the central veins in white matter lesions.[27,46] **Fig. 3** demonstrates a central vein on a 7T MR image. These central veins are most frequently seen in periventricular lesions and less in peripheral lesions.[47] However, it is important to note that this central vein sign is not 100% specific for MS pathology. In larger vascular lesions in the deep white matter and/or in the periventricular white matter, vessels may be visible on MR imaging as well.[27] In other words, the demonstration of the central vein in these white matter lesions is rather specific for MS pathology because this is not present in other disease entities mimicking MS pathology (eg, neuromyelitis optica, Susac syndrome, and rather not in vascular diseases).[27,48,49]

Infratentorial lesions can be located in the brainstem and cerebellum, and the importance lies in their contribution to predict future disability accumulation and progression.[50] Infratentorial lesions were studied in a CIS cohort, which showed that both cerebellar and brainstem lesions predicted conversion to clinically definite MS (CDMS), and brainstem lesions predicted disability progression as well.[51] Besides the characteristic MS lesion location, white matter lesions in the corpus callosum and temporal stem are frequently present in MS and this could help in differentiating from white matter lesions of other origin[41] (see **Tables 6** and **7**).

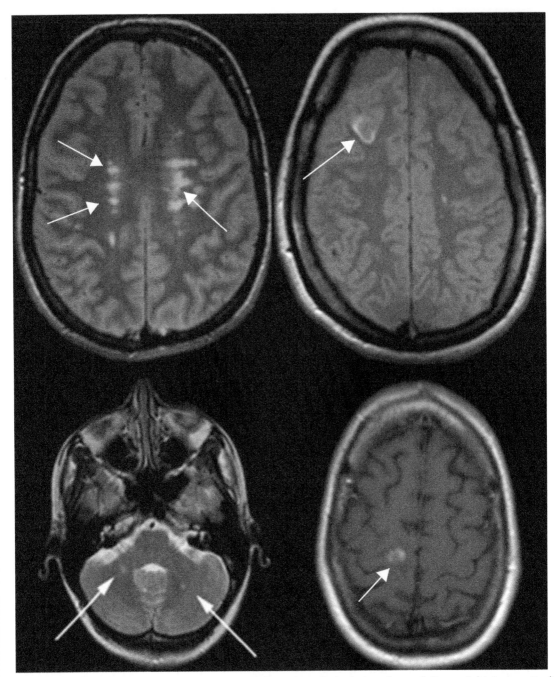

Fig. 2. MS lesions at characteristic locations. Upper left: periventricular lesions (*arrows*). Upper right: juxtacortical lesion (*arrow*). Bottom left: infratentorial lesions (*arrows*). Bottom right: contrast enhancing, juxtacortical lesion (*arrow*).

Gadolinium-enhancing lesions represent recently developed lesions, and is seen only in the first 3 weeks (sometimes up to 3 months) after the development of focal inflammation. Due to the breakdown of the blood-brain barrier in new lesions, gadolinium enters the area of inflammation and shows enhancement on a T1-weighted image.[52] Usually, the enhancement is nodular or homogeneous, but also may appear like a ring. The presence of enhancing and nonenhancing lesions is commonly seen.[53] In case enhancement lasts longer than 3 months, other diagnoses should be taken into consideration (see also MS variants and differential diagnosis).

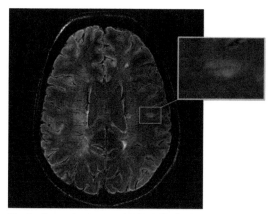

Fig. 3. Central vein on 7T. Magnified a focal lesion with a central vein. (*Courtesy of* Iris D. Kilsdonk, MD, PhD, Amsterdam, Netherlands.)

White matter pathology: diffuse abnormalities

MS pathology goes far beyond focal demyelinating lesions. DAWM reflects demyelination, axonal loss, and chronic gliosis, and is often present in chronic MS, and it is most prominently visible in the deep and periventricular white matter adjacent to focal MS pathology[12] (**Fig. 4**). Conventional MR imaging sequences are able to detect DAWM, but because quantification of DAWM is difficult, incorporation in the diagnostic criteria has not been accomplished so far.[12] DAWM may be more extensive in secondary progressive MS (SPMS) compared with primary progressive MS (PPMS).[54] Histopathological studies showed that white matter damage is more extensively affected than is visible on conventional MR imaging. White matter appearing normal on conventional MR imaging, but also being affected has been described as "normal-appearing white matter (NAWM)." However, by applying quantitative MR imaging

sequences, such as diffusion tensor imaging, magnetization transfer ratio (MTR), and proton magnetic resonance spectroscopy (^{1}H-MRS), these diffuse changes can be detected and quantified in vivo. Even in very early disease stages, such as in CIS, ^{1}H-MRS and MTR are able to show the subtle changes in areas of NAWM suggestive of axonal loss and glial cell activity.[55–57]

Gray matter pathology: cortical lesions

MS has been considered as a white matter disease for a long time; however, it has been conclusively shown by histopathology that MS pathology occurs abundantly in the gray matter, in particular in the cortical gray matter.[8] Although cortical pathology is much more prominent in later disease stages, frequently cortical gray matter lesions are already visible at very early disease stages, even in RIS.[41] Although quite challenging, the detection of cortical lesions is very interesting and clinically relevant, because they correlate with certain clinical outcome measures such as cognition.[13] Different cortical gray matter lesion types have been defined: type 1: a mixed gray matter, white matter lesion (juxtacortical lesion) (**Fig. 5**); type 2: a pure intracortical and full gray matter lesion, which does not touch the borders of the gray matter; type 3: a subpial cortical gray matter lesion; and type 4: a gray matter lesion reaching out of the full cortex but not involving white matter.[58] Unfortunately, only a small portion of the gray matter lesions can be detected on conventional MR imaging sequences (T2-weighted/PD-weighted, T2-FLAIR).[12] Approximately one-third of the cortical lesions can be detected with PD/T2 and T2-FLAIR, of which type 1 cortical lesions are best detectable, followed by type 4 cortical lesions. The reason for this is that the gray matter contains less myelin than white matter,[59] it shows

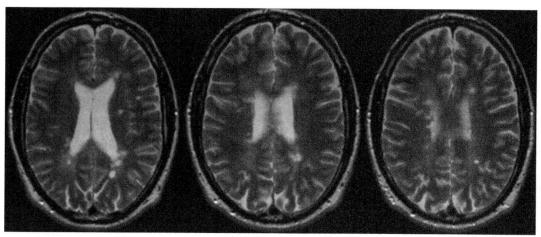

Fig. 4. DAWM.

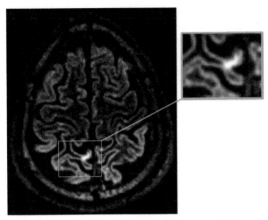

Fig. 5. Magnified a mixed gray/white matter lesion on DIR.

minor glial reaction,[60] there is no lymphocyte infiltration,[61] blood-brain barrier is intact,[62] and no complement deposition is present.[63] Even though the histopathology differences with white matter lesions make the detection of gray matter lesions difficult, the lesion size rather than the underlying histopathology determines if a cortical lesion is detectible on conventional MR imaging. Cortical lesion volume is reflected by the number, location, and size of cortical lesions.[64]

Dedicated pulse sequences, such as double inversion recovery (DIR) and phase sensitive inversion recovery (PSIR), can further increase the sensitivity in the detection of cortical gray matter lesions[65–67] (examples in **Fig. 6**). In addition, the combination, of (ultra)high-field MR imaging and these pulse sequences can further increase the detection of cortical lesions in vivo and in the postmortem setting.[20,68–71] However, still only a small number of the total cortical lesions are visible with these MR imaging techniques. Besides the cortical gray matter, also the subcortical gray

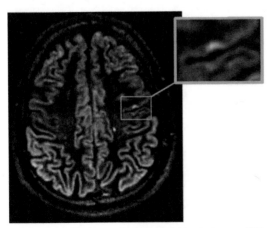

Fig. 6. Magnified a cortical gray matter lesion on DIR.

matter structures show extensive demyelination and loss of axons and neurons.[72]

Gray matter pathology: brain atrophy
Starting slowly early in the disease, when the demyelination seems to dominate, brain atrophy later overrules the demyelination[72] and goes faster than age-related brain atrophy.[73] Brain atrophy is an irreversible neurologic change that predicts both cognitive decline and physical disability but lacks a standardized protocol, thus is not yet useful for clinical use.[2,26,74]

Imaging Spinal Cord Pathology

Focal lesions
Spinal cord lesions are frequently seen in MS, and MR imaging of the spinal cord is important for (differential) diagnosis and prognosis of the disease. Presence of asymptomatic spinal cord lesions at baseline was predictive for conversion from CIS to clinically definite MS.[6,75] Spinal cord lesions can differentiate between MS and other diseases, because it is uncommon, for example, for vascular diseases, to have spinal cord abnormalities.[28]

As is shown in **Fig. 7**, the upper cervical cord and in lesser degree also the lower thoracic cord are most frequently affected, but lesions are seen on any level. Gadolinium-enhanced lesions are rare but mostly seen in the cervical spine.[7,76] Due to the anatomy of the spinal cord, lesions are wedge shaped and mostly located in the lateral and posterior columns of the spinal cord (**Fig. 8**), although they are not restricted to the white matter, so gray matter is involved as well.[77] Physical disability was shown to be related to gray matter lesion load, independently from cord atrophy.[78] Although many nonconventional sequences have been tried to identify the gray matter lesions, like PSIR, DIR, and STIR, no standard has yet been found.[77]

Diffuse abnormalities
Besides focal lesions, diffuse white matter abnormalities are frequently seen in MS, and seem to be independent of T2-hyperintensities.[79] Borders of these abnormalities are not well defined but show a hyperintense signal compared with the surrounding structures.[7] Diffuse abnormalities are not easily seen on T2-weighted images because the CSF is disturbing the signal. PD-weighted imaging can be helpful to image these diffuse spinal cord abnormalities.[76,80] Generally, diffuse abnormalities are an indication of a progressive disease course.[81,82]

Atrophy
Atrophy of the spinal cord has been described mostly in the cervical spinal cord and differs

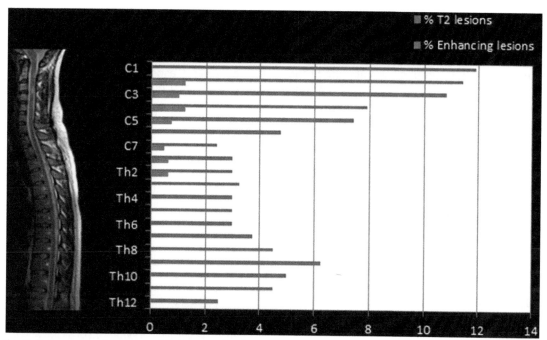

Fig. 7. Percentage of spinal cord lesions per level. (*Modified from* Bot JC, Barkhof F, Polman CH, et al. Spinal cord abnormalities in recently diagnosed MS patients: added value of spinal MRI examination. Neurology 2004;62(2):226–33.)

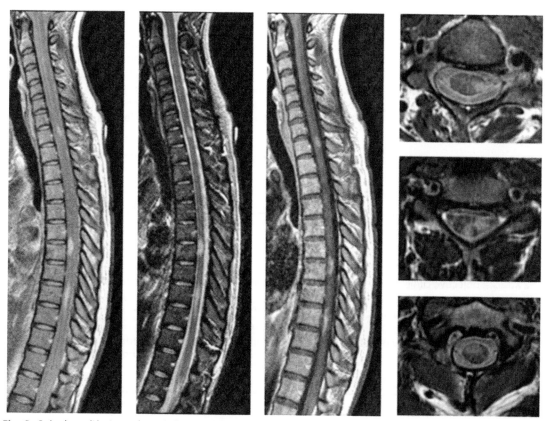

Fig. 8. Spinal cord lesions, from left to right: T2-weighted image, PD T2-weighted image, T1-weighted image post-gadolinium, and 3 axial images at the level of lesions.

between the different MS subtypes.[31] The annual change of cross-sectional area of the upper cervical cord has shown to be higher in patients showing disease progression over that period. Spinal cord atrophy, in particular atrophy of the cervical spine, is evident and is related to clinical disability,[83–85] which makes it interesting for clinical trials to be used as an outcome measure.

DIAGNOSTIC CRITERIA
Radiologically Isolated Syndrome

It has been repeatedly demonstrated that healthy individuals may show asymptomatic lesions in the brain and/or in the spinal cord suggestive of inflammatory demyelination, known as an RIS.[86] Special criteria have been proposed to define RIS in patients.[86] These criteria describe lesion characteristics that should be met (ovoid shaped, well circumscribed, and no vascular pattern of lesions), and fulfilling at least 3 of 4 MR imaging criteria for DIS.[87] Further demyelinating lesions should not be the result of other diseases or drugs.[86] One-third of patients with RIS have a first clinical event in the first 5 years after detection of demyelination on MR imaging. Patients with RIS with (asymptomatic) spinal cord lesions[29] or gadolinium-enhancing lesions have a higher risk of having a clinical event, and also an age younger than 37 and male sex were recognized as independent predictors.[88]

Clinically Isolated Syndrome and Relapsing-Remitting Multiple Sclerosis

Over the past decades, the diagnostic criteria for MS have been changing and MR imaging has gained an important role in diagnosing and differentiating between diseases.[89] Different subtypes of MS are distinguished according to the clinical manifestation of the disease in combination with the radiological aspect. The current diagnostic criteria are based on demonstration of DIT and DIS (Table 5), which, after presentation of the first clinical sign suspect for demyelination, can be achieved by a second clinical attack at a different location as well as by imaging criteria.[5] Since the revision of the McDonald criteria in 2010 (Box 1), DIT can be achieved by a single MR image showing asymptomatic enhancing T1 lesions and nonenhancing T2 lesions or by a new T2 lesion or gadolinium-enhancing lesion on a follow-up scan. DIS (Box 2) requires at least one T2 lesion at 2 specific locations: juxtacortical, periventricular, infratentorial, and spinal cord. For DIS, symptomatic enhancing spinal cord or brainstem lesions are not included in the count. Presenting with a single neurologic symptom and not fulfilling DIS and DIT is defined as a CIS.[5] An optic neuritis is often the initial clinical symptom of a CIS, and for this reason, new proposed criteria incorporate the optic nerve as an MS-specific location. Further, these proposed criteria by the MAGNIMS group expect that at least 3 periventricular lesions are needed instead of 1 periventricular lesion, because only a single periventricular lesion is also often seen in patients not suspected for demyelinating events. Cortical lesions are added to the area of juxtacortical lesions because distinction between these lesion types is often difficult. Furthermore, no differences are made for symptomatic or asymptomatic lesions, which simplifies

Table 5
McDonald criteria 2010

Clinical Presentation	Additional Data Needed for Diagnosis
≥2 attacks; objective clinical evidence of ≥2 lesions or objective clinical evidence of 1 lesion with reasonable historical evidence of a prior attack	None
≥2 attacks; objective clinical evidence of 1 lesion	DIS: see MR imaging criteria; or await a second clinical attack implicating a different CNS site
1 attack; objective clinical evidence of ≥2 lesions	DIT: see MR imaging criteria; or await a second clinical attack
1 attack; objective clinical evidence of 1 lesion (CIS)	DIS: see MR imaging criteria; or await a second clinical attack implicating a different CNS site DIT: see MR imaging criteria; or await a second clinical attack

Abbreviations: CIS, clinically isolated syndrome; CNS, central nervous system; DIS, dissemination in space; DIT, dissemination in time.

Data from Polman CH, Reingold SC, Banwell B, et al. Diagnostic criteria for multiple sclerosis: 2010 revisions to the McDonald criteria. Ann Neurol 2011;69(2):292–302.

Box 1

Criteria for dissemination in time (DIT)

DIT demonstrated by the following:

1. A new T2 and/or gadolinium-enhancing lesion(s) on follow-up MR imaging, with reference to baseline scan, irrespective of the timing of the baseline MR imaging

2. Simultaneous presence of asymptomatic gadolinium-enhancing and nonenhancing lesions at any time

Data from Polman CH, Reingold SC, Banwell B, et al. Diagnostic criteria for multiple sclerosis: 2010 revisions to the McDonald criteria. Ann Neurol 2011;69(2):292–302; and *Adapted from* Swanton JK, Rovira A, Tintore M, et al. MRI criteria for multiple sclerosis in patients presenting with clinically isolated syndromes: a multicentre retrospective study. Lancet Neurol 2007;6(8):677–86.

diagnosing for both the radiologist and neurologist, as it is sometimes difficult to decide whether a lesion is symptomatic or not.[24]

In patients with a single clinical attack not fulfilling the DIS or DIT, or in case of spinal cord symptoms, spinal cord MR imaging should always be performed (see also the paragraph in the above section "IMAGING OF MULTIPLE SCLEROSIS, MR IMAGING PROTOCOLS OF BRAIN, SPINAL CORD, AND TREATMENT MONITORING" about imaging guidelines).

Progressive Disease Courses

Progressive course of the disease follows after a relapsing onset or starts from the onset. The first being defined as SPMS, in which relapses diminish

Box 2

Criteria for dissemination in space (DIS)

DIS demonstrated by $\geq$1 T2 lesion in at least 2 of the following central nervous system areas:

- Periventricular
- Juxtacortical
- Infratentorial
- Spinal cord

Data from Polman CH, Reingold SC, Banwell B, et al. Diagnostic criteria for multiple sclerosis: 2010 revisions to the McDonald criteria. Ann Neurol 2011;69(2):292–302; and *Adapted from* Swanton JK, Rovira A, Tintore M, et al. MRI criteria for multiple sclerosis in patients presenting with clinically isolated syndromes: a multicentre retrospective study. Lancet Neurol 2007;6(8):677–86.

but neurologic deterioration is continuing. The start of this phase is sometimes difficult to determine in the disease course, and often retrospectively recognized.[90] PPMS is diagnosed in patients having 1 year of disease progression and separated from patients with a relapsing onset of the disease. Two of 3 of the following criteria have to be met: (1) fulfilling the DIS criteria, at least 1 T2 brain lesion periventricular, juxtacortical, or infratentorial; (2) DIS in the spinal cord by confirmation of at least 2 T2 lesions in the spinal cord; (3) CSF positive for oligoclonal bands and or an elevated IgG index.[5]

MULTIPLE SCLEROSIS VARIANTS AND DIFFERENTIAL DIAGNOSIS

Clinically and radiologically, the differential diagnosis of MS consists of a broad spectrum of diseases, including variants of idiopathic inflammatory demyelinating pathology, other inflammatory disease entities, vascular disease, and neoplasms (**Tables 6** and **7**).[99] The detailed description of these diseases goes far beyond this review article. Many of these differential diagnoses may mimic MS on MR imaging; therefore, distinguishing these diseases is crucial for treatment and prognosis. MR imaging can be a tool, alone or together with clinical and laboratory findings, in distinguishing MS variants and other diseases from MS. No specific test is available to prove MS as the diagnosis, which makes it important to consider different diagnoses. Imaging the spinal cord is important in the differential diagnosis, because spinal cord involvement is frequently seen in MS, but rarely present in other diseases, or has a different configuration.[28] Also, cortical gray matter lesions are thought to be quite MS specific, but the previously described difficulties in visualizing these lesions is impeding the use of these lesions in differentiating from other diseases.[68] MS lesions can be present at all sites of the brain, are bilaterally present, but not symmetrically distributed. Characteristic for MS are lesions in the corpus callosum (Dawson fingers), and lesions involving the U-fibers in juxtacortical lesions. Lesions in the brainstem are not located in the center, as is seen in other diseases, but more at the periphery. The basal ganglia are rarely involved in MS.[91]

Multiple Sclerosis Variants

MS variants include acute disseminated encephalomyelitis (ADEM) and tumefactive MS and its variants; these are summarized in **Table 6**. Here we discuss the different MS variants followed by some of the major differential diagnoses that should be considered.

Table 6
Most important MR imaging differences for MS variants versus MS

MS variants	Clinical Characteristics of the Disease	Differences on MR Imaging Compared with MS	Other Differences Between Disease and MS
RRMS[5,28,41,43,68,91]	• Symptoms progressively starting in hours/days. Decline of symptoms	MS characteristic: • Fulfilling criteria for DIS and DIT • Ovoid shaped, sharp borders • Bilateral, but not symmetrically distributed lesions • Periventricular, juxtacortical, infratentorial, and spinal cord lesions • Dawson fingers (periventricular lesions following a perivascular distribution pattern) • U-fibers are involved in juxtacortical lesions • Brainstem lesions, located peripheral • Cortical and deep gray matter lesions • Basal ganglia are rarely involved	• OCBs in CSF • Elevated IgG index
ADEM[89,91–97]	• Multifocal neurologic symptoms, including encephalopathy • Typically first clinical episode • Fever, confusion, headache, seizures	• Bilateral, symmetric distributed lesions • Usually large and confluent lesions • Bilateral deep gray matter involvement • Subcortical WM lesions • No DIT, no new lesions at FU • Gadolinium enhancement of all lesions at the same moment, enhancement not always present • Poorly circumscribed lesions • Periventricular regions are spared	• No OCBs in CSF • CSF mainly with lymphocytes in younger patients, mainly neutrophils in older patients • Often seen in children • Following vaccination or viral infection

Tumefactive MS and variants[89,91,98,99]	• Clinical presentation is dependent of lesion size and location • Symptoms including headache, confusion, seizures • Variants are clinically more severe	• Large lesions (≥2 cm) • Edema and mass effect • Open ring enhancement
Marburg variant	Acute, severe, progressive neurologic decline	• Imaging is suggestive for MS, but presence of ≥1 large (tumefactive) lesion
Balo concentric sclerosis	Cognitive/behavioral alterations, seizures	• Rings of demyelination and spared myelin (hyper and iso T2 signal intensity rings)

Abbreviations: ADEM, acute disseminated encephalomyelitis; CSF, cerebrospinal fluid; DIS, dissemination in space; DIT, dissemination in time; FU, follow-up; MS, multiple sclerosis; OCBs, Oligoclonal bands; RRMS, relapsing-remitting multiple sclerosis; WM, white matter.

Table 7
Most important MR imaging difference for differential diagnosis versus MS

Disease entitity	Clinical Characteristics	Differences on MR Imaging Compared with MS	Other differences between disease and MS
Vascular diseases (small-vessel disease)[27,91,100]	• Acute symptoms	• Lacunar infarcts • Nonspecific WM lesions, U-fibers are not affected • Nonlobar microbleeds (seen on SWI or gradient echo) • No involvement of temporal lobes, corpus callosum, and spinal cord • Brainstem lesions are centrally located • No contrast enhancement • No perivascular orientation of WM lesions	• Cardiovascular risk factors • Older age
CADASIL[91,96,100–103]	• Recurrent transient ischemic attacks • Features including: depression, dementia, strokes, migraine	• Multiple bilateral lacunar infarcts • Microbleeds • Early involvement of • Subcortical U-fibers • Anterior temporal, inferior frontal lobes, external capsule, insular regions involved Relatively spared: • Cortex, corpus callosum, cerebellum	• Positive family history • No OCBs in CSF • NOTCH3 mutation

			Presence of serum:
NMOSD[49,104–106]	Core clinical characteristics indicating the following regions: • Optic neuritis (bilateral, involving the optic chiasm, severe visual loss) • Acute myelitis (complete) • Area postrema syndrome of dorsal medulla (hiccups or nausea and vomiting) • Brainstem • Diencephalon • Cerebrum	Spinal cord imaging Acute myelitis • LETM, increased signal on sagittal T2, extending over ≥3 segments. • Central cord predominance • Rostral extension to the brainstem • Cord swelling • Decreased T1 signal at site of T2 lesion • Bright spotty lesions (Yonezu et al.[105] 2014) Chronic • Spinal cord atrophy Brain imaging • Possibility of no brain lesions • Lesions in dorsal medulla • Large subcortical or deep white matter lesions • Periependymal lesions around third and fourth ventricle • Long corticospinal tract lesion Rarely seen in NMOSD but seen in MS: • Dawson fingers, periventricular lesions in temporal lobe, cortical lesions, central vein[49]	• AQ4 antibodies • MOG antibodies
Sarcoidosis[90,91,96,100,107]	• Almost always respiratory involvement • Chronic basilar leptomeningitis	• T2/FLAIR high signal in parenchyma and GM/WM junction • Enhancement >3 mo • Simultaneous enhancement of multiple lesions • Meningeal and punctiform parenchymal enhancement • Hydrocephalus	• Abnormal chest radiograph • Multisystem granulomatous disease

(continued on next page)

Table 7
(continued)

Disease entitity	Clinical Characteristics	Differences on MR Imaging Compared with MS	Other differences between disease and MS

Susac syndrome[48,96,108,109]	• Clinical triad
	  • Encephalopathy
	  • Hearing loss
	  • Visual deficits (branch retinal artery occlusion)
		• Small multifocal microinfarcts
		• "Snowball-like" lesions in corpus callosum
		• Parenchymal and meningeal enhancement
		• No central vein in WM lesions
		• Discrete lesions in basal ganglia and thalamus	

Behçet[91,100,103,110,111]	• Mucosal ulcers • Uveitis anterior	• Diffuse WM involvement • Cerebral venous sinus thrombosis • Large, infiltrating brainstem and basal ganglia lesions, accompanied by swelling and enhancement; can reduce at FU • Punctiform parenchymal enhancement	
PML[91,100,112–120]	• Immunocompromised patients, for example, after DMT use (natalizumab, dimethyl fumarate, fingolimod) • Asymptomatic, or later symptomatic and fulminant compared with MS	• New lesion in clinically stable patients on natalizumab • Frequently located frontal and parietal-occipital lobes • Cortical GM and juxtacortical and deep WM lesions, progressively expanding • Punctate lesions in the vicinity of the main PML lesions • Enhancement in up to 30% of natalizumab-associated PML • Large, multifocal (occasionally) and asymmetrical lesions without mass effect • Spinal cord and optic nerve not involved	• JCV seropositive

Abbreviations: AQ4, Aquaporin-4 antibodies; CADASIL, cerebral autosomal dominant arteriopathy subcortical infarcts and leukoencephalopathy; CSF, cerebrospinal fluid; DMT, disease-modifying treatment; FLAIR, fluid attenuation inversion recovery; FU, follow-up; GM, gray matter; JCV, John Cunningham virus; LETM, long extensive transverse myelitis; MOG, myelin oligodendrocyte glucoprotein antibodies; MS, multiple sclerosis; NMOSD, neuromyelitis optica spectrum disorders; OCB, oligoclonal bands; PML, progressive multifocal leukoencephalitis; SWI, susceptibility weighted imaging; WM, white matter.

Even though ADEM is mostly seen in children,[92] it occurs in adults as well. Usually ADEM is monophasic with multiple neurologic symptoms at the same moment, often including an encephalopathic syndrome. ADEM is a not well defined disease, which makes the differentiation with MS difficult. No radiological features are completely characteristic for ADEM, but MR imaging could help in distinguishing ADEM from MS.[93] Usually ADEM is a clinically monophasic disease; even when a new relapse occurs, the MR imaging shows enlargement of the previous lesion(s) but no evidence for DIT. Therefore, follow-up MR imaging is highly recommended to exclude DIT, that could lead to diagnosis of MS, and besides this, ADEM lesions sometimes diminish, which distinguishes them from MS lesions.[89,94–96] Other radiological findings are subcortical white matter lesions and early involvement of the deep gray matter.[97] Enhancement is not always seen, but all lesions can be enhancing at the same moment. Further lesions are poorly circumscribed and periventricular areas and the corpus callosum are rarely affected, and lesions are commonly distributed symmetrically.

Tumefactive multiple sclerosis, acute multiple sclerosis (Marburg disease), and Balo concentric sclerosis

Tumefactive MS, acute MS (Marburg disease [MD]), and Balo concentric sclerosis (BCS) are clinically different from typical MS, and commonly present with headache, confusion, and seizures, which are uncommon symptoms for MS.

MD (also termed malignant MS) is a rare, acute MS variant that occurs predominantly in young adults. Because MD is often preceded by a febrile illness, this disease also may be considered a fulminant form of ADEM. In MD, MR imaging typically shows multiple focal T2 lesions of varying size, which may coalesce to form large white matter plaques disseminated throughout the hemispheric white matter and brainstem.

BCS is also a rare subtype of MS, with characteristic radiological and pathologic features. The pathologic hallmarks of the disease are large demyelinated lesions showing a peculiar pattern of alternating layers of preserved and destroyed myelin, which can be identified with T2-weighted sequences that typically show thick concentric hyperintense bands corresponding to areas of demyelination and gliosis, alternating with thin isointense bands corresponding to normal myelinated white matter. Contrast enhancement and decreased diffusivity are frequent in the outer rings (inflammatory edge) of the lesion.[89,99]

Tumefactive multiple sclerosis

Tumefactive MS can be defined as demyelinating lesions larger than 2 cm, normally with a ring-enhancing or open ring–enhancing pattern, but without the layering that defines BCS. Clues that can help to differentiate these lesions from a brain tumor include a relatively minor mass effect or vasogenic edema, and incomplete ring enhancement on T1-weighted gadolinium-enhanced images with the open border facing the cortical/subcortical gray matter, sometimes associated with a rim of peripheral hypointensity on T2-weighted sequences.[89,91,98]

Differential Diagnosis

Besides these MS variants, other diagnoses also should be considered; these are summarized in **Table 7**. Due to a high prevalence, small-vessel disease is the most challenging differential diagnosis, especially in older patients.[91,100] Vascular events are typically characterized by acute symptoms, and patients are mainly older at onset of symptoms and have cardiovascular risk factors. Lacunar infarcts, nonspecific white matter lesions, micro bleeds (seen on SWI and gradient-echo T2* sequences), and sparing of the U-fibers, are suspicious for vascular origin of the lesions. The corpus callosum, temporal lobes, and spinal cord are usually not involved. Brainstem lesions are centrally located compared with the peripheral location of MS brainstem lesions. Enhancement is rarely seen after contrast administration.[91,100] MR imaging does not show perivascular orientation in most white matter lesions.[27]

Another vasculopathy that could mimic MS is cerebral autosomal dominant arteriopathy subcortical infarcts and leukoencephalopathy (CADASIL). This is distinguished from MS mostly by location of the white matter lesions in the anterior temporal and inferior frontal lobes, external capsule, and early involvement of the subcortical U-fibers is seen. The periventricular and juxtacortical regions, the cortex, corpus callosum, and cerebellum are relatively spared in CADASIL.[101] Bilateral lacunar infarcts could be seen and micro bleeds can occur.[91] Clinically, CADASIL is characterized by recurrent transient ischemic attacks or features including depression, dementia, migraine, and strokes and the presence of NOTCH 3 mutation.[102] Furthermore, a family history of CADASIL and CSF without oligoclonal bands is helpful in the diagnosis.[103]

In patients showing extensive spinal cord lesions, more than 3 segments long, located centrally in the spinal cord, neuromyelitis optica spectrum disorders (NMOSD) should be considered.

NMOSD is clinically distinct from MS in that bilateral and extensive optic neuritis occurs, or complete rather than incomplete myelitis.

Radiologically, brain lesions can be present or not. Most brain lesions are located in the periependymal white matter, around the ventricles, area postrema of the dorsal medulla (producing hiccups or nausea and vomiting) or are extensive lesions in the corticospinal tract, or subcortical or deep white matter. Although the corpus callosum can be involved, Dawson fingers are not present, and further cortical lesions and periventricular lesions in the temporal lobe are rarely seen in NMOSD.[104,105] High-field MR imaging shows no central vein in patients with NMOSD,[49] which is suggestive for another pathologic origin of the disease. Spinal cord lesions are present, but are distinguished from MS lesions because they extend over 3 or more segments, have a central cord predominance, sometimes extend to the brainstem, and cord swelling can be seen. In the long term, spinal cord atrophy can be present.[105] Furthermore, on axial T2-weighted imaging, the spinal cord lesions can appear as "bright spotty lesions," which, together with longitudinally extensive transverse myelitis differentiates NMOSD from MS lesions.[106]

In case of (clinical) respiratory involvement, the possibility of sarcoidosis should be kept in mind. Although the most common radiologic findings in neurosarcoidosis are meningeal involvement and granulomatous lesions (commonly found in the hypothalamus or pituitary gland), asymptomatic periventricular and subcortical nonenhancing multifocal hyperintense lesions on T2-weighted images, mimicking those seen in MS, have also been commonly described on T2/T2-FLAIR images.[90,107]

Multifocal hyperintense lesions on T2-weighted images, mimicking those seen in MS, can also be identified in Susac syndrome, but the clinical triad (encephalopathy, branch retinal artery occlusions, and hearing loss) and other MR imaging features can help in diagnosing Susac syndrome. Small and multifocal infarcts and discrete lesions in the thalamus and basal ganglia can be present. T2 and T2-FLAIR sequences show larger lesions in the center of the corpus callosum in the acute stage ("snowball-like"), and differ from MS lesions that are typically located in its inferior margin around the veins.[96,108,109] This is also seen on high-field MR imaging, where a central vein and a T2 hypointense rim is seldom seen in Susac syndrome.[48]

Patients with comprehensive basal ganglia and brainstem lesions, accompanied by swelling and enhancement, should be suspected for Behçet disease. These extensive lesions can reduce in size or disappear over time.[110] Some additional imaging characteristics, like the presence of venous sinus thrombosis, diffuse white matter involvement, and punctiform parenchymal enhancement, should suggest the diagnosis of Behçet disease and make MS less probable.[91,103,111] Clinically, mucosal ulcers and/or uveitis anterior could be suspicious for Behçet disease.[103]

Since natalizumab therapy in MS, PML is also seen in patients with MS due to immunosuppression,[112] and recently also cases have been described in dimethyl fumarate[113,114] and other immunosuppressive therapies of MS.[115] Because the clinical presentation is similar to that of MS, MR imaging plays an important role in detection of PML. Furthermore, lesions can be detected on MR imaging before PML becomes clinically symptomatic.[91] Because asymptomatic PML has a better prognosis than symptomatic PML, early recognition of PML lesions is very important.[116] Symptomatic PML lesions are located in the subcortical white matter affecting the U-fibers and the cortical gray matter. They frequently show small punctuate lesions in the vicinity of the main lesion. Depending on the underlying immunosuppression, PML lesions may show enhancement but no mass effect.[117,118] The spinal cord and optic nerve are not involved.[119] However, in particular, the differentiation between small asymptomatic PML lesions and MS lesions is very challenging.[120]

SUMMARY

MR imaging has become increasingly important in the diagnosis and management of MS. Conventional MR imaging is used to prove DIS and DIT and set the diagnosis, and for monitoring of disease progression and treatment efficacy. Despite the rising number of imaging possibilities, MR imaging is not completely covering the MS pathology and cannot fully explain patient's clinical disability and cognitive decline. High-field MR imaging and other advanced MR imaging techniques are able to get closer to the pathology, but they have technical limitations and are difficult to implement in clinical practice.

Furthermore, for therapeutic and prognostic aims, it is very important to distinguish MS from its variants and differential diagnoses. Together with the clinical presentation and some disease-specific laboratory findings, MR imaging can be helpful in the differentiation.

The future will bring new MR imaging techniques, which will probably facilitate linking the clinical presentation to the underlying pathology seen on MR imaging.

REFERENCES

1. Compston A, Coles A. Multiple sclerosis. Lancet 2008;372(9648):1502–17.
2. Wattjes MP, Steenwijk MD, Stangel M. MRI in the diagnosis and monitoring of multiple sclerosis: an update. Clin Neuroradiol 2015;25(Suppl 2):157–65.
3. McDonald WI, Compston A, Edan G, et al. Recommended diagnostic criteria for multiple sclerosis: guidelines from the International Panel on the Diagnosis of Multiple Sclerosis. Ann Neurol 2001;50(1):121–7.
4. Polman CH, Reingold SC, Edan G, et al. Diagnostic criteria for multiple sclerosis: 2005 revisions to the "McDonald criteria." Ann Neurol 2005;58(6):840–6.
5. Polman CH, Reingold SC, Banwell B, et al. Diagnostic criteria for multiple sclerosis: 2010 revisions to the McDonald criteria. Ann Neurol 2011;69(2):292–302.
6. Sombekke MH, Wattjes MP, Balk LJ, et al. Spinal cord lesions in patients with clinically isolated syndrome: a powerful tool in diagnosis and prognosis. Neurology 2013;80(1):69–75.
7. Bot JC, Barkhof F. Spinal-cord MRI in multiple sclerosis: conventional and nonconventional MR techniques. Neuroimaging Clin N Am 2009;19(1):81–99.
8. Barkhof F. The clinico-radiological paradox in multiple sclerosis revisited. Curr Opin Neurol 2002;15(3):239–45.
9. Hackmack K, Weygandt M, Wuerfel J, et al. Can we overcome the 'clinico-radiological paradox' in multiple sclerosis? J Neurol 2012;259(10):2151–60.
10. Wattjes MP, Harzheim M, Lutterbey GG, et al. Axonal damage but no increased glial cell activity in the normal-appearing white matter of patients with clinically isolated syndromes suggestive of multiple sclerosis using high-field magnetic resonance spectroscopy. AJNR Am J Neuroradiol 2007;28(8):1517–22.
11. Wattjes MP, Harzheim M, Lutterbey GG, et al. High field MR imaging and 1H-MR spectroscopy in clinically isolated syndromes suggestive of multiple sclerosis: correlation between metabolic alterations and diagnostic MR imaging criteria. J Neurol 2008;255(1):56–63.
12. Seewann A, Vrenken H, van der Valk P, et al. Diffusely abnormal white matter in chronic multiple sclerosis: imaging and histopathologic analysis. Arch Neurol 2009;66(5):601–9.
13. Geurts JJG, Calabrese M, Fisher E, et al. Measurement and clinical effect of grey matter pathology in multiple sclerosis. Lancet Neurol 2012;11(12):1082–92.
14. Geurts JJ. The neurologist's dilemma: MS is a grey matter disease that standard clinical and MRI measures cannot assess adequately–yes. Mult Scler 2012;18(5):559–60.
15. Wattjes MP, Rovira A, Miller D, et al. Evidence-based guidelines: MAGNIMS consensus guidelines on the use of MRI in multiple sclerosis–establishing disease prognosis and monitoring patients. Nat Rev Neurol 2015;11(10):597–606.
16. Traboulsee A, Simon JH, Stone L, et al. Revised recommendations of the consortium of MS centers task force for a standardized MRI protocol and clinical guidelines for the diagnosis and follow-up of multiple sclerosis. AJNR Am J Neuroradiol 2016;37(3):394–401.
17. Wattjes MP, Harzheim M, Lutterbey GG, et al. Does high field MRI allow an earlier diagnosis of multiple sclerosis? J Neurol 2008;255(8):1159–63.
18. Simon B, Schmidt S, Lukas C, et al. Improved in vivo detection of cortical lesions in multiple sclerosis using double inversion recovery MR imaging at 3 Tesla. Eur Radiol 2010;20(7):1675–83.
19. Wattjes MP, Barkhof F. High field MRI in the diagnosis of multiple sclerosis: high field-high yield? Neuroradiology 2009;51(5):279–92.
20. Kilsdonk ID, de Graaf WL, Barkhof F, et al. Inflammation high-field magnetic resonance imaging. Neuroimaging Clin N Am 2012;22(2):135–57, ix.
21. Wattjes MP, Lutterbey GG, Harzheim M, et al. Imaging of inflammatory lesions at 3.0 Tesla in patients with clinically isolated syndromes suggestive of multiple sclerosis: a comparison of fluid-attenuated inversion recovery with T2 turbo spin-echo. Eur Radiol 2006;16(7):1494–500.
22. Schaefer PW, Grant PE, Gonzalez RG. Diffusion-weighted MR imaging of the brain. Radiology 2000;217(2):331–45.
23. Rovira A, Wattjes MP, Tintore M, et al. Evidence-based guidelines: MAGNIMS consensus guidelines on the use of MRI in multiple sclerosis-clinical implementation in the diagnostic process. Nat Rev Neurol 2015;11(8):471–82.
24. Filippi M, Rocca MA, Ciccarelli O, et al. MRI criteria for the diagnosis of multiple sclerosis: MAGNIMS consensus guidelines. Lancet Neurol 2016;15(3):292–303.
25. Geurts JJ, Roosendaal SD, Calabrese M, et al. Consensus recommendations for MS cortical lesion scoring using double inversion recovery MRI. Neurology 2011;76(5):418–24.
26. De Stefano N, Airas L, Grigoriadis N, et al. Clinical relevance of brain volume measures in multiple sclerosis. CNS Drugs 2014;28(2):147–56.
27. Kilsdonk ID, Wattjes MP, Lopez-Soriano A, et al. Improved differentiation between MS and vascular brain lesions using FLAIR* at 7 Tesla. Eur Radiol 2014;24(4):841–9.
28. Bot JC, Barkhof F, Lycklama à Nijeholt G, et al. Differentiation of multiple sclerosis from other inflammatory disorders and cerebrovascular disease: value of spinal MR imaging. Radiology 2002;223(1):46–56.

29. Okuda DT, Mowry EM, Cree BA, et al. Asymptomatic spinal cord lesions predict disease progression in radiologically isolated syndrome. Neurology 2011; 76(8):686–92.

30. Swanton JK, Fernando KT, Dalton CM, et al. Early MRI in optic neuritis: the risk for clinically definite multiple sclerosis. Mult Scler 2010;16(2):156–65.

31. Gass A, Rocca MA, Agosta F, et al. MRI monitoring of pathological changes in the spinal cord in patients with multiple sclerosis. Lancet Neurol 2015; 14(4):443–54.

32. Bot JC, Barkhof F, Lycklama a Nijeholt GJ, et al. Comparison of a conventional cardiac-triggered dual spin-echo and a fast STIR sequence in detection of spinal cord lesions in multiple sclerosis. Eur Radiol 2000;10(5):753–8.

33. Philpott C, Brotchie P. Comparison of MRI sequences for evaluation of multiple sclerosis of the cervical spinal cord at 3 T. Eur J Radiol 2011; 80(3):780–5.

34. Weier K, Mazraeh J, Naegelin Y, et al. Biplanar MRI for the assessment of the spinal cord in multiple sclerosis. Mult Scler 2012;18(11):1560–9.

35. Lycklama G, Thompson A, Filippi M, et al. Spinal-cord MRI in multiple sclerosis. Lancet Neurol 2003;2(9):555–62.

36. Stankiewicz JM, Neema M, Alsop DC, et al. Spinal cord lesions and clinical status in multiple sclerosis: a 1.5 T and 3 T MRI study. J Neurol Sci 2009;279(1–2):99–105.

37. Petzold A, Wattjes MP, Costello F, et al. The investigation of acute optic neuritis: a review and proposed protocol. Nat Rev Neurol 2014;10(8):447–58.

38. McGuigan C, Craner M, Guadagno J, et al. Stratification and monitoring of natalizumab-associated progressive multifocal leukoencephalopathy risk: recommendations from an expert group. J Neurol Neurosurg Psychiatry 2016;87(2):117–25.

39. Fine AJ, Sorbello A, Kortepeter C, et al. Progressive multifocal leukoencephalopathy after natalizumab discontinuation. Ann Neurol 2014;75(1): 108–15.

40. Killestein J, Vennegoor A, van Golde AE, et al. PML-IRIS during fingolimod diagnosed after natalizumab discontinuation. Case Rep Neurol Med 2014;2014:307872.

41. Matthews PM, Roncaroli F, Waldman A, et al. A practical review of the neuropathology and neuroimaging of multiple sclerosis. Pract Neurol 2016; 16(4):279–87.

42. Valdueza JM, Doepp F, Schreiber SJ, et al. What went wrong? The flawed concept of cerebrospinal venous insufficiency. J Cereb Blood Flow Metab 2013;33(5):657–68.

43. Fog T. The topography of plaques in multiple sclerosis with special reference to cerebral plaques. Acta Neurol Scand Suppl 1965;15:1–161.

44. Dawson JD. The Histology of Disseminated Sclerosis. Transactions of the Royal Society of Edinburgh 1916;50:517–740.

45. Sati P, George IC, Shea CD, et al. FLAIR*: a combined MR contrast technique for visualizing white matter lesions and parenchymal veins. Radiology 2012;265(3):926–32.

46. Kilsdonk ID, Lopez-Soriano A, Kuijer JP, et al. Morphological features of MS lesions on FLAIR* at 7 T and their relation to patient characteristics. J Neurol 2014;261(7):1356–64.

47. Tallantyre EC, Brookes MJ, Dixon JE, et al. Demonstrating the perivascular distribution of MS lesions in vivo with 7-Tesla MRI. Neurology 2008;70(22): 2076–8.

48. Wuerfel J, Sinnecker T, Ringelstein EB, et al. Lesion morphology at 7 Tesla MRI differentiates Susac syndrome from multiple sclerosis. Mult Scler 2012;18(11):1592–9.

49. Sinnecker T, Dorr J, Pfueller CF, et al. Distinct lesion morphology at 7-T MRI differentiates neuromyelitis optica from multiple sclerosis. Neurology 2012; 79(7):708–14.

50. Minneboo A, Barkhof F, Polman CH, et al. Infratentorial lesions predict long-term disability in patients with initial findings suggestive of multiple sclerosis. Arch Neurol 2004;61(2):217–21.

51. Tintore M, Rovira A, Arrambide G, et al. Brainstem lesions in clinically isolated syndromes. Neurology 2010;75(21):1933–8.

52. Cotton F, Weiner HL, Jolesz FA, et al. MRI contrast uptake in new lesions in relapsing-remitting MS followed at weekly intervals. Neurology 2003; 60(4):640–6.

53. Rovaris M, Filippi M. Contrast enhancement and the acute lesion in multiple sclerosis. Neuroimaging Clin N Am 2000;10(4):705–16, viii–ix.

54. Vrenken H, Seewann A, Knol DL, et al. Diffusely abnormal white matter in progressive multiple sclerosis: in vivo quantitative MR imaging characterization and comparison between disease types. AJNR Am J Neuroradiol 2010;31(3): 541–8.

55. West J, Aalto A, Tisell A, et al. Normal appearing and diffusely abnormal white matter in patients with multiple sclerosis assessed with quantitative MR. PLoS One 2014;9(4):e95161.

56. Fernando KT, McLean MA, Chard DT, et al. Elevated white matter myo-inositol in clinically isolated syndromes suggestive of multiple sclerosis. Brain 2004;127(Pt 6):1361–9.

57. Fernando KT, Tozer DJ, Miszkiel KA, et al. Magnetization transfer histograms in clinically isolated syndromes suggestive of multiple sclerosis. Brain 2005;128(Pt 12):2911–25.

58. Bo L, Vedeler CA, Nyland HI, et al. Subpial demyelination in the cerebral cortex of multiple sclerosis

patients. J Neuropathol Exp Neurol 2003;62(7): 723–32.

59. Geurts JJ, Bo L, Pouwels PJ, et al. Cortical lesions in multiple sclerosis: combined postmortem MR imaging and histopathology. AJNR Am J Neuroradiol 2005;26(3):572–7.

60. Wegner C, Esiri MM, Chance SA, et al. Neocortical neuronal, synaptic, and glial loss in multiple sclerosis. Neurology 2006;67(6):960–7.

61. Bo L, Vedeler CA, Nyland H, et al. Intracortical multiple sclerosis lesions are not associated with increased lymphocyte infiltration. Mult Scler 2003; 9(4):323–31.

62. van Horssen J, Brink BP, de Vries HE, et al. The blood-brain barrier in cortical multiple sclerosis lesions. J Neuropathol Exp Neurol 2007;66(4):321–8.

63. Brink BP, Veerhuis R, Breij EC, et al. The pathology of multiple sclerosis is location-dependent: no significant complement activation is detected in purely cortical lesions. J Neuropathol Exp Neurol 2005;64(2):147–55.

64. Seewann A, Vrenken H, Kooi EJ, et al. Imaging the tip of the iceberg: visualization of cortical lesions in multiple sclerosis. Mult Scler 2011;17(10):1202–10.

65. Geurts JJ, Pouwels PJ, Uitdehaag BM, et al. Intracortical lesions in multiple sclerosis: improved detection with 3D double inversion-recovery MR imaging. Radiology 2005;236(1):254–60.

66. Wattjes MP, Lutterbey GG, Gieseke J, et al. Double inversion recovery brain imaging at 3T: diagnostic value in the detection of multiple sclerosis lesions. AJNR Am J Neuroradiol 2007;28(1):54–9.

67. Sethi V, Yousry TA, Muhlert N, et al. Improved detection of cortical MS lesions with phase-sensitive inversion recovery MRI. J Neurol Neurosurg Psychiatry 2012;83(9):877–82.

68. Filippi M, Rocca MA, Calabrese M, et al. Intracortical lesions: relevance for new MRI diagnostic criteria for multiple sclerosis. Neurology 2010; 75(22):1988–94.

69. Kilsdonk ID, Jonkman LE, Klaver R, et al. Increased cortical grey matter lesion detection in multiple sclerosis with 7 T MRI: a post-mortem verification study. Brain 2016;139(Pt 5):1472–81.

70. Nielsen AS, Kinkel RP, Tinelli E, et al. Focal cortical lesion detection in multiple sclerosis: 3 Tesla DIR versus 7 Tesla FLASH-T2. J Magn Reson Imaging 2012;35(3):537–42.

71. Kilsdonk ID, de Graaf WL, Soriano AL, et al. Multicontrast MR imaging at 7T in multiple sclerosis: highest lesion detection in cortical gray matter with 3D-FLAIR. AJNR Am J Neuroradiol 2013; 34(4):791–6.

72. Kutzelnigg A, Lucchinetti CF, Stadelmann C, et al. Cortical demyelination and diffuse white matter injury in multiple sclerosis. Brain 2005;128(Pt 11): 2705–12.

73. Sormani MP, Bruzzi P. MRI lesions as a surrogate for relapses in multiple sclerosis: a meta-analysis of randomised trials. Lancet Neurol 2013;12(7): 669–76.

74. Pareto D, Sastre-Garriga J, Auger C, et al. Juxtacortical lesions and cortical thinning in multiple sclerosis. AJNR Am J Neuroradiol 2015;36(12): 2270–6.

75. Swanton JK, Fernando KT, Dalton CM, et al. Early MRI in optic neuritis: the risk for disability. Neurology 2009;72(6):542–50.

76. Bot JC, Barkhof F, Polman CH, et al. Spinal cord abnormalities in recently diagnosed MS patients: added value of spinal MRI examination. Neurology 2004;62(2):226–33.

77. Kearney H, Miller DH, Ciccarelli O. Spinal cord MRI in multiple sclerosis–diagnostic, prognostic and clinical value. Nat Rev Neurol 2015;11(6):327–38.

78. Gilmore CP, Geurts JJ, Evangelou N, et al. Spinal cord grey matter lesions in multiple sclerosis detected by post-mortem high field MR imaging. Mult Scler 2009;15(2):180–8.

79. Bergers E, Bot JC, De Groot CJ, et al. Axonal damage in the spinal cord of MS patients occurs largely independent of T2 MRI lesions. Neurology 2002; 59(11):1766–71.

80. Nijeholt GJ, van Walderveen MA, Castelijns JA, et al. Brain and spinal cord abnormalities in multiple sclerosis. Correlation between MRI parameters, clinical subtypes and symptoms. Brain 1998; 121(Pt 4):687–97.

81. Bergers E, Bot JC, van der Valk P, et al. Diffuse signal abnormalities in the spinal cord in multiple sclerosis: direct postmortem in situ magnetic resonance imaging correlated with in vitro high-resolution magnetic resonance imaging and histopathology. Ann Neurol 2002;51(5):652–6.

82. Lycklama a Nijeholt G, Barkhof F. Differences between subgroups of MS: MRI findings and correlation with histopathology. J Neurol Sci 2003;206(2): 173–4.

83. Daams M, Weiler F, Steenwijk MD, et al. Mean upper cervical cord area (MUCCA) measurement in long-standing multiple sclerosis: relation to brain findings and clinical disability. Mult Scler 2014; 20(14):1860–5.

84. Lukas C, Knol DL, Sombekke MH, et al. Cervical spinal cord volume loss is related to clinical disability progression in multiple sclerosis. J Neurol Neurosurg Psychiatry 2015;86(4):410–8.

85. Liu Y, Lukas C, Steenwijk MD, et al. Multicenter validation of mean upper cervical cord area measurements from head 3D T1-weighted MR imaging in patients with multiple sclerosis. AJNR Am J Neuroradiol 2016;37(4):749–54.

86. Okuda DT, Mowry EM, Beheshtian A, et al. Incidental MRI anomalies suggestive of multiple

sclerosis: the radiologically isolated syndrome. Neurology 2009;72(9):800–5.

87. Barkhof F, Filippi M, Miller DH, et al. Comparison of MRI criteria at first presentation to predict conversion to clinically definite multiple sclerosis. Brain 1997;120:2059–69.

88. Okuda DT, Siva A, Kantarci O, et al. Radiologically isolated syndrome: 5-year risk for an initial clinical event. PLoS One 2014;9(3):e90509.

89. Karussis D. The diagnosis of multiple sclerosis and the various related demyelinating syndromes: a critical review. J Autoimmun 2014;48-49:134–42.

90. Katz Sand I, Krieger S, Farrell C, et al. Diagnostic uncertainty during the transition to secondary progressive multiple sclerosis. Mult Scler 2014; 20(12):1654–7.

91. Aliaga ES, Barkhof F. MRI mimics of multiple sclerosis. Handb Clin Neurol 2014;122:291–316.

92. Leake JA, Albani S, Kao AS, et al. Acute disseminated encephalomyelitis in childhood: epidemiologic, clinical and laboratory features. Pediatr Infect Dis J 2004;23(8):756–64.

93. Wingerchuk DM, Weinshenker BG. Acute disseminated encephalomyelitis, transverse myelitis, and neuromyelitis optica. Continuum (Minneap Minn) 2013;19(4 Multiple Sclerosis):944–67.

94. Menge T, Kieseier BC, Nessler S, et al. Acute disseminated encephalomyelitis: an acute hit against the brain. Curr Opin Neurol 2007;20(3):247–54.

95. Toledano M, Weinshenker BG, Solomon AJ. A clinical approach to the differential diagnosis of multiple sclerosis. Curr Neurol Neurosci Rep 2015;15(8):57.

96. Bester M, Petracca M, Inglese M. Neuroimaging of multiple sclerosis, acute disseminated encephalomyelitis, and other demyelinating diseases. Semin Roentgenol 2014;49(1):76–85.

97. Rossi A. Imaging of acute disseminated encephalomyelitis. Neuroimaging Clin N Am 2008;18(1): 149–61, ix.

98. Lucchinetti CF, Gavrilova RH, Metz I, et al. Clinical and radiographic spectrum of pathologically confirmed tumefactive multiple sclerosis. Brain 2008;131(Pt 7):1759–75.

99. Zettl UK, Stuve O, Patejdl R. Immune-mediated CNS diseases: a review on nosological classification and clinical features. Autoimmun Rev 2012; 11(3):167–73.

100. Charil A, Yousry TA, Rovaris M, et al. MRI and the diagnosis of multiple sclerosis: expanding the concept of "no better explanation". Lancet Neurol 2006;5(10):841–52.

101. Auer DP, Putz B, Gossl C, et al. Differential lesion patterns in CADASIL and sporadic subcortical arteriosclerotic encephalopathy: MR imaging study with statistical parametric group comparison. Radiology 2001;218(2):443–51.

102. Joutel A, Corpechot C, Ducros A, et al. Notch3 mutations in cerebral autosomal dominant arteriopathy with subcortical infarcts and leukoencephalopathy (CADASIL), a mendelian condition causing stroke and vascular dementia. Ann N Y Acad Sci 1997; 826:213–7.

103. Miller DH, Weinshenker BG, Filippi M, et al. Differential diagnosis of suspected multiple sclerosis: a consensus approach. Mult Scler 2008;14(9): 1157–74.

104. Kim HJ, Paul F, Lana-Peixoto MA, et al. MRI characteristics of neuromyelitis optica spectrum disorder: an international update. Neurology 2015; 84(11):1165–73.

105. Wingerchuk DM, Banwell B, Bennett JL, et al. International consensus diagnostic criteria for neuromyelitis optica spectrum disorders. Neurology 2015;85(2):177–89.

106. Yonezu T, Ito S, Mori M, et al. Bright spotty lesions" on spinal magnetic resonance imaging differentiate neuromyelitis optica from multiple sclerosis. Mult Scler 2014;20(3):331–7.

107. Zajicek JP, Scolding NJ, Foster O, et al. Central nervous system sarcoidosis–diagnosis and management. QJM 1999;92(2):103–17.

108. Susac JO, Murtagh FR, Egan RA, et al. MRI findings in Susac's syndrome. Neurology 2003;61(12):1783–7.

109. Buzzard KA, Reddel SW, Yiannikas C, et al. Distinguishing Susac's syndrome from multiple sclerosis. J Neurol 2015;262(7):1613–21.

110. Lee SH, Yoon PH, Park SJ, et al. MRI findings in neuro-Behcet's disease. Clin Radiol 2001;56(6): 485–94.

111. Akman-Demir G, Mutlu M, Kiyat-Atamer A, et al. Behcet's disease patients with multiple sclerosis-like features: discriminative value of Barkhof criteria. Clin Exp Rheumatol 2015;33(6 Suppl 94):S80–4.

112. Clifford DB, De Luca A, Simpson DM, et al. Natalizumab-associated progressive multifocal leukoencephalopathy in patients with multiple sclerosis: lessons from 28 cases. Lancet Neurol 2010;9(4):438–46.

113. Ermis U, Weis J, Schulz JB. PML in a patient treated with fumaric acid. N Engl J Med 2013; 368(17):1657–8.

114. van Oosten BW, Killestein J, Barkhof F, et al. PML in a patient treated with dimethyl fumarate from a compounding pharmacy. N Engl J Med 2013; 368(17):1658–9.

115. Maas RP, Muller-Hansma AH, Esselink RA, et al. Drug-associated progressive multifocal leukoencephalopathy: a clinical, radiological, and cerebrospinal fluid analysis of 326 cases. J Neurol 2016; 263(10):2004–21.

116. Dong-Si T, Richman S, Wattjes MP, et al. Outcome and survival of asymptomatic PML in natalizumab-treated MS patients. Ann Clin Transl Neurol 2014; 1(10):755–64.

117. Rocha AJ, Littig IA, Nunes RH, et al. Central nervous system infectious diseases mimicking multiple sclerosis: recognizing distinguishable features using MRI. Arq Neuropsiquiatr 2013; 71(9B):738–46.

118. Wattjes MP, Barkhof F. Diagnosis of natalizumab-associated progressive multifocal leukoencephalopathy using MRI. Curr Opin Neurol 2014;27(3): 260–70.

119. Wattjes MP, Richert ND, Killestein J, et al. The chameleon of neuroinflammation: magnetic resonance imaging characteristics of natalizumab-associated progressive multifocal leukoencephalopathy. Mult Scler 2013;19(14):1826–40.

120. Wattjes MP, Vennegoor A, Steenwijk MD, et al. MRI pattern in asymptomatic natalizumab-associated PML. J Neurol Neurosurg Psychiatry 2015;86(7): 793–8.

Pediatric Multiple Sclerosis
Distinguishing Clinical and MR Imaging Features

Silvia N. Tenembaum, MD[a,b,*]

KEYWORDS

- Pediatric multiple sclerosis • Diagnostic criteria • MR imaging
- Acute disseminated encephalomyelitis • Neuromyelitis optica
- Acquired demyelinating syndromes • Children

KEY POINTS

- Overall, 3% to 10% of patients with multiple sclerosis (MS) show their first clinical event during childhood.
- Children with MS have higher relapse rates compared with adult-onset MS.
- As in adult patients, pediatric MS diagnosis requires dissemination in space and time, clinically or by MR Imaging findings.
- Alternative diagnoses such as acute disseminating encephalomyelitis and neuromyelitis optica spectrum disorder must be differentiated from MS.
- Revised MR imaging criteria are a useful tool to discriminate between pediatric MS and mimickers.

INTRODUCTION

Although multiple sclerosis (MS) occurs most commonly in adults, its onset in childhood and adolescence is now increasingly recognized. It has been estimated that pediatric-onset MS accounts for 3% to 10% of all MS patients,[1–4] whereas disease onset before the age of 10 years has been reported in 17% of all pediatric MS patients.[5] Nevertheless, diagnosing MS in a child or adolescent continues to be challenging due to the higher frequency of transient demyelinating events and other disorders with similar symptoms and neuroimaging findings.

In this article, the author gives an overview of the current diagnostic criteria of pediatric MS, key characteristics for differential diagnosis, and distinguishing features of pediatric-onset MS compared with the typical adult-onset disease.

DIAGNOSTIC CRITERIA OF PEDIATRIC MULTIPLE SCLEROSIS

In 2007, the International Pediatric Multiple Sclerosis Study Group (IPMSSG) met to propose consensus definitions for pediatric-onset acquired inflammatory demyelinating disorders of the central nervous system (CNS), including acute

Funding Sources: Dr S.N. Tenembaum: no funding reported.
Conflict of Interest: Dr S.N. Tenembaum served as an advisory board member and speaker for Merck Serono. She serves on the clinical trial advisory board for Genzyme-Sanofi. Professional travel and accommodation expenses have been awarded to Dr S.N. Tenembaum by Merck-Serono.
[a] Department of Neurology, National Pediatric Hospital Dr. Juan P. Garrahan, Combate de los Pozos 1881, Ciudad Autónoma de Buenos Aires C1436AAM, Argentina; [b] International Pediatric MS Study Group, Foundation for Neurologic Disease, 10 State Street, Newburyport, MA 01950, USA
* Corresponding author. Department of Neurology, National Pediatric Hospital Dr. Juan P. Garrahan, Combate de los Pozos 1881, Ciudad Autónoma de Buenos Aires C1436AAM, Argentina.
E-mail address: silviatenembaum@gmail.com

disseminated encephalomyelitis (ADEM), neuro-myelitis optica (NMO), clinically isolated syndromes (CIS), and MS.[6] These definitions were developed to improve consistency in terminology, avoid misclassification, and facilitate epidemiologic studies and clinical research in children.

The diagnosis of MS in childhood, as in adult patients, requires evidence of CNS demyelination with dissemination in space (DIS) and time (DIT). Accordingly, the 2007 criteria for pediatric MS incorporated and expanded the 2005 McDonald criteria for adult-onset MS by including children of all ages and introducing a caveat for an ADEM-like initial event. In this situation, a second non-ADEM event should be accompanied by further evidence of DIT, either with new MR imaging T2 lesions ≥3 months from the second event or with a new clinical relapse.[6]

Several MR imaging criteria specific to pediatric-onset MS were developed to improve the ability to predict a subsequent MS diagnosis in children with acute CNS demyelination, and they are listed in Table 1. The French Kid Sclerose en Plaques Study Group identified 2 MR imaging features on baseline MR imaging that could predict subsequent MS diagnosis. The proposed MS criteria for "Kids with MS" (KIDMUS) were at least one lesion perpendicular to the long axis of the corpus callosum, and the sole presence of well-defined white matter (WM) lesions.[7] Another study that evaluated the KIDMUS criteria and the 2005 McDonald criteria for DIS in a pediatric cohort with acute demyelination demonstrated that both criteria had a high positive predictive value (PPV) and specificity, but low sensitivity, particularly in the youngest patients.[8] Therefore, a study was conducted using a standardized scoring tool, which was applied to MR imaging scans performed in a longitudinal pediatric cohort with CNS demyelination.[9] One set of pediatric criteria was developed to distinguish patients with MS from those with a non-demyelinating disease (migraine and CNS lupus) on baseline MR imaging (see Table 1).[10] Another set of pediatric criteria was developed by the same study group to improve the ability to discriminate between children with monophasic ADEM and those destined for MS (sensitivity 81%, specificity 95%, PPV 95%, negative predictive value 79%)[11] (see Table 1). The performance of these criteria has been replicated in an independent pediatric cohort, particularly focused on children presenting with an ADEM phenotype.[12]

In 2010, the McDonald criteria were further revised by an International Panel in an attempt to simplify neuroimaging requirements necessary in the diagnosis of MS (Table 2). This revision of the McDonald criteria formally addressed the diagnosis of MS in the pediatric population, considering that most pediatric patients with MS

Table 1
Pediatric MR imaging criteria for multiple sclerosis diagnosis

References	Pediatric-Onset MS
Mikaeloff et al,[7] 2004	MR imaging prognostic factors for MS in children with acute demyelination: Two of the following: 1. T2 lesions perpendicular to the long axis of the corpus callosum 2. Sole presence of well-defined T2 lesions
Callen et al,[10] 2009	MR imaging criteria to distinguish pediatric MS from relapsing non-demyelinating disorders Two of the following: 1. >5 T2 lesions 2. >2 T2 periventricular lesions 3. >1 T2 brainstem lesion
Callen et al,[11] 2009	MR imaging criteria to distinguish a first attack of MS from monophasic ADEM Two of the following: 1. Absence of a diffuse bilateral T2 lesion pattern 2. Presence of black holes 3. ≥2 T2 periventricular lesions
Verhey et al,[9] 2011	MR imaging parameters that predict MS in children with acute demyelination Two of the following: 1. ≥1 T2 periventricular lesion 2. ≥1 T1-hypointense lesion

Table 2
2010 revised McDonald MR imaging criteria

Demonstration of DIS	DIS can be demonstrated by ≥1 T2 lesion in at least 2 of 4 areas of the CNS: 1. Periventricular 2. Juxtacortical 3. Infratentorial 4. Spinal cord[a]
Demonstration of DIT	DIT can be demonstrated by: 1. A new T2 and/or gadolinium-enhancing lesion or lesions on follow-up MR imaging, with reference to a baseline scan, irrespective of the timing of the baseline MR imaging 2. Simultaneous presence of asymptomatic gadolinium-enhancing and nonenhancing lesions at any time

[a] Symptomatic lesions are excluded from the criteria in patients with brainstem or spinal cord syndrome, and do not contribute to lesion count.
Data from Polman CH, Reingold S, Banwell B, et al. Diagnostic criteria for multiple sclerosis: 2010 revisions to the McDonald criteria. Ann Neurol 2011;69:292–302.

would meet DIS criteria at the time of their first clinical event, showing at least one lesion in at least 2 of the 4 locations commonly affected in patients with MS.[13] Subsequently, validation studies of the revised 2010 McDonald criteria were performed in pediatric cohorts.[14–18] Taking these studies together showed that the revised 2010 McDonald criteria were sensitive and specific for the diagnosis of pediatric MS, provided that the criteria cannot be applied in the context of an ADEM-like presentation, and with consideration of age at onset. In one of these studies, a prospective cohort of 212 children with an acquired demyelinating syndrome was followed for more than 2 years with serial clinical and MR imagings; the sensitivity of the 2010 criteria assessed at a baseline MR imaging was 100%, with a specificity of 86%, and a PPV for a subsequent diagnosis of MS of 59%.[14] The PPV increased to 76% when the 2010 criteria were applied only to children aged 11 years or older with a non-ADEM presentation.

In another study, DIS and DIT were assessed for both the 2010 McDonald and the 2007 IPMSSG criteria on initial and follow-up MR imagings in children with MS.[15] According to their results, the 2010 McDonald criteria were more sensitive and facilitated the diagnosis of pediatric MS at a first clinical event in at least half of the patients. Additional studies explored the applicability of the 2007 IPMSSG definitions to pediatric cohorts and helped to illustrate their strengths and limitations.[8,19,20]

Accordingly, in 2012, the IPMSSG updated the original consensus definitions, including recent advances to facilitate early diagnosis of MS and decisions concerning the initiation of disease-modifying therapies in children.[21] The 2012

pediatric MS criteria are listed in **Box 1**. In at least 2 studies, the previous 2007 and the revised 2012 IPMSSG criteria were compared in pediatric cohorts.[17,22] According to the reported results, the 2012 IPMSSG criteria applied at the incident event worked better for the subsequent diagnosis of MS, and the inclusion of follow-up MR imaging scans increased both specificity and PPV.

DISTINGUISHING CLINICAL FEATURES

The presenting phenotype of patients with pediatric-onset MS may correspond to the following categories: a clinically monofocal event, with all the symptoms and neurologic findings responding to a single CNS location; a clinically polyfocal event without encephalopathy, when more than one CNS site is required to explain the neurologic findings; or an ADEM-like event, when polyfocal deficits are identified in the context of an acute encephalopathy. These presenting phenotypes are highly variable depending on the age at clinical onset.

In a study of clinical presentation as a function of age at onset, MS patients younger than 11 years were more likely to manifest with multifocal features including encephalopathy, to have clinical attacks affecting the brainstem, and tended to have more severe deficits than older children.[23] In addition, the youngest patients with MS are less likely to have cerebrospinal fluid (CSF) oligoclonal bands.[24] Conversely, adolescents with MS tend to manifest with discrete neurologic symptoms, at presentation and at subsequent relapses, resembling the typical neurologic syndromes of adult-onset MS, such as focal motor or sensory deficits.[25,26] The reported risks of developing MS after an initial clinical event during childhood vary

---

Box 1
2012 International Pediatric Multiple Sclerosis Study Group criteria for pediatric-onset multiple sclerosis

Diagnosis of Pediatric MS can be satisfied by any of the following scenarios

1. Two or more clinical CNS events (without encephalopathy) with presumed inflammatory cause, separated by ≥30 days and affecting more than one area of the CNS.

2. A first, single clinical CNS event (without encephalopathy) consistent with MS with MR imaging findings fulfilling 2010 Revised McDonald criteria for DIS and DIT on baseline MR imaging, in a patient between 12 to 18 years.

3. One clinical CNS event (without encephalopathy) consistent with MS, with MR imaging fulfilling 2010 Revised McDonald criteria for DIS, in which a follow-up MR imaging demonstrates at least one new enhancing or nonenhancing lesion consistent with DIT on a new scan performed >30 days after the initial event.

4. An ADEM-like initial attack followed by a new non-encephalopathic clinical event, three or more months after symptom onset, that is, associated with new MR imaging lesions that fulfill 2010 Revised McDonald criteria for DIS.

Adapted from Krupp LB, Tardieu M, Amato MP, et al. International Pediatric Multiple Sclerosis Study Group criteria for pediatric multiple sclerosis and immune-mediated central nervous system demyelinating disorders: revisions to the 2007 definitions. Mult Scler 2013;19:1261–7.

---

according to the presentation category: 15% to 42% for optic neuritis; 20% for ADEM; 8% for transverse myelitis.[25]

In pediatric MS, different demographic features also show variability according to the age at onset. The reported ratio of girls to boys is 0.8:1 in children less than the age of 6 years and increases to 1.6:1 between 6 and 10 years, reaching ratios of 2:1 to 3:1 in adolescents, similar to adults.[25]

The clinical course in children with MS is relapsing-remitting in 85.7% to 100% of published cases.[3,27] Higher relapse rates in pediatric patients were reported in the first few years after disease onset compared with adults with similar disease duration in a prospective study performed at a large MS center.[28] Another prospective study showed that MS patients with a pediatric onset developed secondary progression on average 10 years later than those with adult onset; however, patients who had had a pediatric-onset MS were 10 years younger when reaching that stage of disability.[27]

DISTINGUISHING MR IMAGING FEATURES
Conventional MR imaging

MR imaging probably represents the single most important diagnostic tool to support the diagnosis of MS in both children and adults. Typical MS lesions appear as well-defined, high-signal ovoid-shaped areas on T2-weighted and T2-fluid-attenuated inversion recovery (FLAIR) images spread throughout the white matter (WM) in different regions, such as the juxtacortical and periventricular areas, corpus callosum, brainstem, and cerebellum (**Figs. 1**A, B and **2**).

Applicability of conventional MR imaging techniques:

- *T2-weighted imaging* is the classic technique to identify MS lesions, with the ability to identify disease activity and lesion formation over time.[29] It allows detection of both supratentorial and infratentorial lesions, but is insensitive to cortical demyelination and to MS-related gray matter (GM) changes.[30] Spinal cord lesions are best identified on T2-weighted images mainly if combined with proton density or STIR (short tau inversion recovery) scans (**Fig. 3**).

- *T2-FLAIR imaging* is a more sensitive sequence for cortical, juxtacortical, and periventricular lesions,[31] but with very poor sensitivity for lesions located in cerebellum, cerebellar peduncles, brainstem, and spinal cord (**Fig. 4**).[30]

- *Proton density-weighted imaging* offers better lesion-tissue contrast, including better identification of periventricular lesions. This sequence is particularly useful in children younger than 2 years of age, who have an incomplete myelinated brain WM.

- *STIR imaging* is frequently used in the detection of subtle spinal cord lesions. STIR sequences provide fat suppression, thus resulting in increased sensitivity for the spinal cord and optic nerve imaging.[30]

- In *contrast-enhanced T1-weighted sequences,* inflammation in acute demyelinating lesions is best identified as a result of increased blood-brain barrier permeability, showing different patterns of contrast

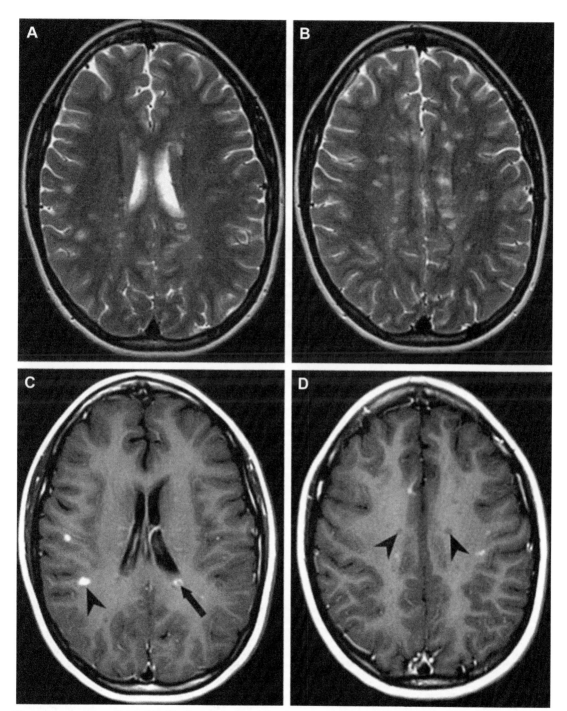

Fig. 1. Images of pediatric MS (*A, B*). Axial T2-weighted images from a 13-year-old girl at the incident clinical event with polyfocal deficits without encephalopathy, showing multiple focal hyperintense lesions with well-defined borders and a bilateral distribution involving the brain WM (*C, D*). Axial post-gadolinium T1-weighted images from the same patient showing focal lesions with different patterns of enhancement; a nodular enhanced lesion is identified by an arrowhead, and a ringlike enhanced lesion is denoted by a arrow in (*C*); the additional simultaneous presence of enhancing and nonenhancing (*arrowheads in D*) hypointense lesions meets MS criteria for DIT at the baseline MR imaging.

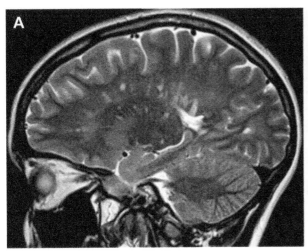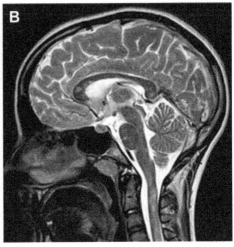

Fig. 2. Images of pediatric MS. (A) Sagittal T2-weighted image showing multiple linear and ovoid T2 hyperintense lesions emanating tangential from the corpus callosum (typical Dawson fingers). Images acquired from the same adolescent as in Fig. 1. (B) Sagittal T2-weighted image depicting hyperintense lesions involving corpus callosum and brainstem. Confluent hyperintense T2 lesions are identified within the cervical spinal cord in a 9-year-old girl with MS by the time of the incident clinical event.

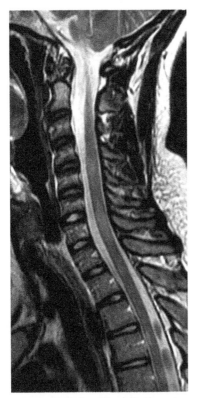

Fig. 3. Images of spinal cord involvement in pediatric MS. Sagittal T2-weighted image depicting multiple spinal cord hyperintense lesions spanning less than 3 vertebral segments within the cervical and thoracic cord. Image acquired from an adolescent with MS at her first clinical event.

enhancement (Fig. 1C). This sequence permits differentiation of active or newly formed lesions from inactive lesions (Fig. 1D). Although lesions typically enhance for approximately 3 weeks, this period may be modified in the context of treatment with methylprednisolone.[32]

Data collected from conventional MR imaging studies performed in pediatric MS cohorts have shown interesting findings:

- Children have a higher lesion burden on their initial brain MR imaging compared with adults, especially in brainstem and cerebellum (Fig. 5).[33]
- Initial brain MR imaging scans in prepubertal children present with atypical MR imaging features compared with adolescents: lesions are frequently larger, confluent, with ill-defined borders, and with deeper GM involvement (Figs. 6 and 7).[34]
- Follow-up brain MR imagings performed in this MS subgroup of prepubertal children show a more than 50% reduction in T2-bright lesions, compared with the more typical ovoid lesions, which persist on serial imaging in adolescents.[34]
- Brain tumefactive lesions (defined as large lesions of >2 cm, with frequent surrounding edema) have been described at initial brain MR imaging in young children with MS (Fig. 8).[35,36]

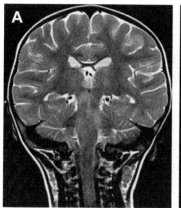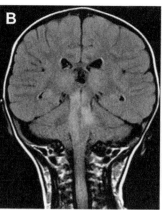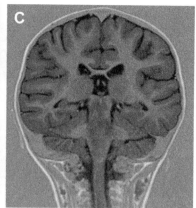

Fig. 4. Images of pediatric acute demyelination. Coronal brain and brainstem image acquired in 3 different sequences: T2-weighted imaging in (A); T2-FLAIR imaging in (B); and T1-weighted inversion-recovery imaging in (C). Multiple lesions involving the entire brainstem, thalami, and the cervical spinal cord can be identified as hyperintense images in (A) and (B), and as hypointense lesions in (C).

Advanced Imaging Techniques

Advanced MR imaging techniques have been developed for a quantitative identification of tissue damage in normal appearing white matter (NAWM) and normal-appearing gray matter (NAGM). These new techniques demonstrated to be more sensitive and specific to evaluate pathologic substrates of clinical disability than conventional MR imaging sequences. Advanced imaging techniques include brain volumetry, magnetization transfer (MT) imaging, cortical imaging techniques, diffusion tensor (DT) imaging, proton MR spectroscopy (^{1}H-MRS), and susceptibility-weighted imaging (SWI).

The application of some of these advanced techniques in pediatric patients with MS has provided novel insights into the structural integrity of brain tissue.

Brain Volumetry

Several cross-sectional studies have been conducted to assess changes in brain volume in

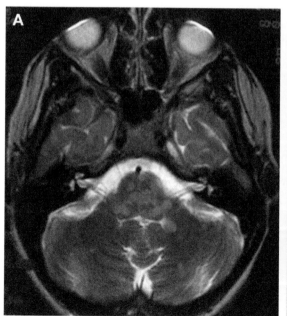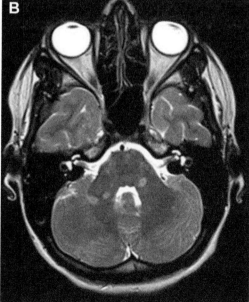

Fig. 5. Images of brainstem involvement in pediatric MS (A, B). Axial T2-weighted images acquired from 2 adolescents with MS presenting with brainstem symptoms at clinical onset. Images show multiple infratentorial T2 lesions involving the pons and the middle cerebellar peduncles.

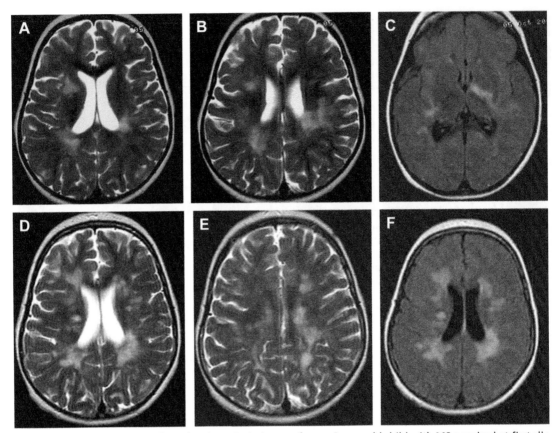

Fig. 6. Images of MS in a prepubertal patient. Brain images from a 3-year-old child with MS acquired at first clinical event (*A–C*) and at 4 years from clinical onset (*D–F*). (*A, B*) Axial T2-weighted images showing multiple, poorly defined lesions with a bilateral distribution within the brain WM. (*C*) Axial T2-FLAIR image showing a diffuse hyperintense signal involving the posterior limb of the left internal capsule. (*D, E*) Axial T2-weighted imaging and (*F*) Axial T2-FLAIR image depicting increase of diffuse hyperintense lesions in addition to new well-defined lesions with an ovoid shape. Evidence of brain volume loss is identified by discrete enlargement of the lateral ventricles and widening of the cortical sulci.

children with MS, comparing those findings with age- and sex-matched healthy controls.

- A recent study demonstrated spatial distribution of brain atrophy in children with MS with a novel approach: regional volumes at each given location in the brain were computed and compared with a database of an age-matched control population.[37]
- Reduced deep GM volume, particularly thalamic atrophy, was detected in children with MS compared with a control group, using voxel-based morphometry to assess the pattern of GM loss. Of note, no differences were detected in normalized brain and cortical GM.[38]
- In a study using a region-of-interest method to evaluate brain volume, a significant reduction in global brain and thalamic volume was detected in children and adolescents with MS

compared with healthy controls, in addition to a reduction in the head size.[39]
- In a longitudinal follow-up study, the authors proposed the following 2 mechanisms to explain the reduced brain volumes in children with MS: failure of age-expected brain growth, and subsequent and progressive reduction of established brain volume.[40]

Magnetization Transfer Imaging

MT imaging is a useful technique to quantify the level of microstructural damage within visible T2 lesions as well as NAWM and NAGM.[41]

- Two preliminary studies using MT imaging evaluated NAWM, NAGM, and cervical spinal cord of children with MS and did not find significant differences when data were compared with age- and sex-matched healthy controls.[42,43]

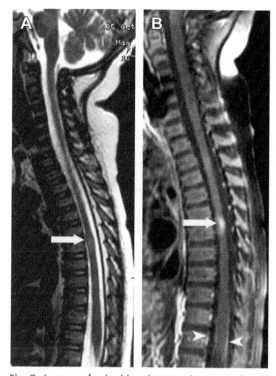

Fig. 7. Images of spinal involvement in a prepubertal patient with MS. (*A*) Sagittal T2-weighted image showing an acute spinal cord lesion at T6-7 level (*arrow*). (*B*) Sagittal postcontrast T1-weighted image depicting a nodular enhancement of the same lesion (*arrow*). An additional linear enhancement surrounding the conus is highlighted by arrowheads.

- In another comparative study using MT imaging, adult patients with pediatric-onset MS showed lower MT ratio values within T2 lesions, NAWM, and NAGM than adult patients with an adult-onset MS.[44] These results suggest a more severe neuroaxonal damage and myelin loss in adult patients with pediatric-onset MS, probably explained by the longer disease duration.

Cortical Imaging Techniques

Several sequences have been shown to improve identification of cortical lesions in adult MS patients when compared with T2-FLAIR or T2-weighted imaging. Double inversion recovery (DIR) sequence, and heavily T1-weighted sequences such as phase-sensitive inversion recovery, 3D spoiled gradient-recalled echo, and 3D magnetization-prepared rapid gradient-echo, are examples of these new techniques.[41]

- In one study, brain cortical lesions could be detected in only 8% of pediatric patients

compared with 66% of adults with MS using DIR techniques.[45] In addition, mean cortical lesion count and median cortical lesion volume were lower in children versus adults.[41,45] These findings suggest that cortical lesion formation is an infrequent initial event in children with MS, considering that the median disease duration was 2 years longer for the adult-onset subgroup.

Diffusion Tensor Imaging

DT imaging is a sensitive technique providing information on the microstructural tissue integrity based on properties of water diffusion. With the diffusion ellipsoid that mathematically represents this information, 4 diffusion parameters are typically calculated and reported in DT imaging studies: mean diffusivity (MD), fractional anisotropy (FA), parallel axial diffusivity (AD), and transverse radial diffusivity (RD). FA is a measure that incorporates both AD and RD and represents the preferential directionality of water diffusion, specifically evaluated in WM tracts. Higher values of AD are considered to indicate axonal loss. RD with higher values is considered to be related to demyelination. Lower FA values are in general an indication of decreased WM microstructural integrity.[41,46]

Several studies using DT imaging have demonstrated widespread abnormalities in children with MS.[42,43,47–53]

- The average MD of normal-appearing brain matter (NABM) was found to be lower in children with MS compared with healthy controls.[42]
- In a follow-up study, it was demonstrated that tissue abnormalities were specific to the NAWM, according to the results showing increased average MD and decreased MD histogram peak height in the NAWM subgroup of children with MS compared with controls.[43]
- Compared with healthy children, the NAWM subgroup also showed lower average FA and higher peak height.[43,53]
- One study used a tract-based approach to evaluate diffusion abnormalities of the callosal, projection, and association pathways in children with MS. In T2-hyperintense lesions, mean apparent diffusion coefficient (ADC) values within corpus callosal, posterior limb of the internal capsule, and long association fiber regions of interest were higher, and FA values were lower in children with MS compared with healthy controls.[47,49] Similar values of ADC and FA were observed in NAWM.[47]

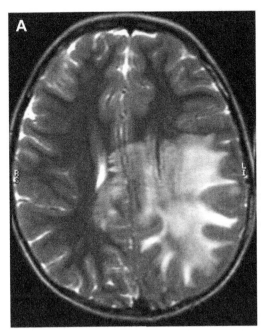
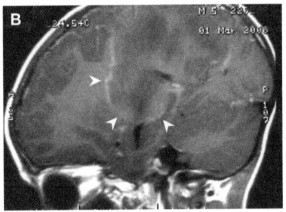

Fig. 8. Images of tumefactive demyelination. (A) Axial T2 imaging reveals a tumefactive lesion involving the parieto-occipital WM of the left brain hemisphere with mass effect, in a young boy presenting with an acute encephalopathy and a focal motor deficit, who was subsequently diagnosed with MS on the basis of numerous further attacks and positive CSF oligoclonal bands. (B) Sagittal postcontrast T1-weighted imaging showing peripheral contrast enhancement from the same patient (arrowheads).

- The functional consequence of damage to the microstructural integrity in children with MS was evaluated using DT imaging and cognitive measures of processing speed in a pediatric MS cohort and age- and sex-matched healthy controls.[54] Lower FA values in the NAWM of the genu and splenium of the corpus callosum, and in the NAWM of the bilateral temporal, parietal, and occipital lobes were found in children with MS compared with controls. Lower FA values in the corpus callosum were clinically relevant given the association with reduced attentional control, slower cognitive processing speed, and poorer math performance.[54,55]
- Recently, a study was conducted to relate DT imaging measures of WM microstructural integrity to resting-state network functional connectivity in children with MS.[46] Compared with healthy controls, children with MS showed lower FA values within the entire WM skeleton. Loss of WM microstructural integrity was associated with increased RS functional connectivity in children with MS, which may reflect a diffuse and potentially compensatory activation process occurring early in the disease.[46]

Proton MR Spectroscopy

^{1}H-MRS acquires information from hydrogen nuclei of molecules or metabolites present in tissues, and this metabolic information has pathologic specificity. MR spectra are identified by their resonance frequency and expressed as a shift in frequency in parts per million (ppm) relative to a reference standard.[41]

Four major metabolite resonances are revealed in the brain at long echo times:

1. The methyl resonance of tetramethylamines, especially the choline-containing phospholipids (Cho) at 3.2 ppm
2. Methyl resonance of creatine (Cr) and phosphocreatine at 3.0 ppm
3. Methyl resonance of N-acetyl (NA)-containing compounds, especially N-acetylaspartate (NAA) at 2.0 ppm
4. Methyl resonance of lactate (Lac) as a doublet at 1.3 ppm (not detected in the normal brain)

Changes in the resonance intensity of Cho can be interpreted as a measure of membrane phospholipids released during active myelin breakdown, whereas Lac increases mainly seem to reflect the metabolism of inflammatory cells or neuronal mitochondrial dysfunction.

NAA is synthesized by neuronal mitochondria and localizes almost exclusively in neurons and neuronal processes. Decreases in NAA peak can result from the following changes: decrease in axonal density secondary to axonal loss of atrophy; mitochondrial dysfunction within neurons and axons; or dilution of NAA secondary to edema or non-NAA-containing cells. In patients with MS, NAA is a specific marker of axonal integrity.[41]

The presence of Cr, which plays a role in energy metabolism and homeostasis, is highest in astrocytes and oligodendrocytes. In the study of patients with MS, the intravoxel NAA/Cr ratio is commonly used as an index of neuronal integrity.[41]

Other metabolites, such as myoinositol (a proposed glial marker likely related to microglial proliferation), glutamate (produced and released by activated leukocytes, macrophages, and microglial cells), and citrulline, which can only be detected at short echo times, play a significant role in the pathophysiology of the inflammatory component and repair mechanisms of MS and have also been proposed as markers of metabolic abnormalities.

The following studies applied ^{1}H-MRS to children with MS:

- The findings reported by the first study applying ^{1}H-MRS to children with MS were similar to the results observed in adult-onset MS: decreased NAA and Cr resonances and increased Cho and myoinositol resonances within lesions.[56]
- Citrullination is a posttranslational modification of myelin basic protein (MBP), by which arginine is converted to citrulline via deamination. Increased citrullination of MBP diminishes its ability to organize lipid bilayers into compact multilayers, thus resulting in myelin instability.[41] A study was conducted in children with MS with ^{1}H-MRS using spectral narrowing to identify the citrulline resonance.[57] A citrulline peak was found in 44% of children with MS compared with only 13% of control patients who were imaged for headache or syncope. In addition, the citrulline peak was observed in both lesional WM and NAWM.[57]
- In an interesting study, children with ADEM were assessed by ^{1}H-MRS in order to identify a signature of monophasic ADEM that could be distinct from the findings reported in MS.[58] The authors reported a reduction in the myoinositol/Cr ratio in children with ADEM, in contrast to observations of increased intralesional myoinositol/Cr ratio reported in patients with MS. Functioning as an osmolyte, decreases in myoinositol could indicate decreases in regulatory volume necessary to reduce cell swelling and normalize edema.

Taken together, these studies suggest that the neurodegenerative aspect of MS pathobiology is occurring in children and adolescents with MS. In addition, these findings demonstrate that the WM integrity disruption is widespread and occurs early in the disease course. Several studies have demonstrated that the early damage to the developing neural networks has functional consequences in children with MS, with impairment in cognition and academic performance.[41,55,59-61]

Susceptibility-Weighted Imaging to Differentiate Acute Disseminated Encephalomyelitis from Multiple Sclerosis

A study was conducted to assess the ability of SWI to discriminate between an initial presentation of pediatric MS and ADEM. Brain MR imagings on a 3-T scanner were performed in 8 children with ADEM and 10 children ultimately diagnosed with MS. Regional brain T2-FLAIR images were coregistered with the corresponding SWI images. Children with MS showed a larger number of T2-FLAIR lesions and SWI abnormalities than children with ADEM. Based on the median percentage of lesions visible on SWI, the authors could establish that 0.2 was the best discriminator to distinguish the 2 groups: children with less than 0.2 were likely to have ADEM and those with greater than 0.2 were likely to have MS.[62,63]

DIFFERENTIAL DIAGNOSIS

After initial presentation with a CNS demyelinating event, children can meet diagnostic criteria for MS if serial changes are documented on MR imaging and other disorders are excluded. However, there is a broad spectrum of pediatric disorders showing WM abnormalities on MR imaging. As an example, in a large prospective cohort of children meeting criteria for acquired demyelinating syndromes, 6% were identified with other causes after performing appropriate diagnostic testing.[64] Because the diagnosis of MS in a child has prognostic and therapeutic implications, including the need for long-term disease-modifying therapy, it is essential to exclude conditions that might resemble MS. The different disorders to be considered in pediatric demyelination have been addressed by several studies.[25,64-67]

Acute Disseminated Encephalomyelitis

ADEM is defined as an acute event of inflammatory demyelination characterized by encephalopathy and polyfocal neurologic findings.[6] Although adults may experience ADEM,[68,69] it occurs more frequently in childhood with a reported incidence

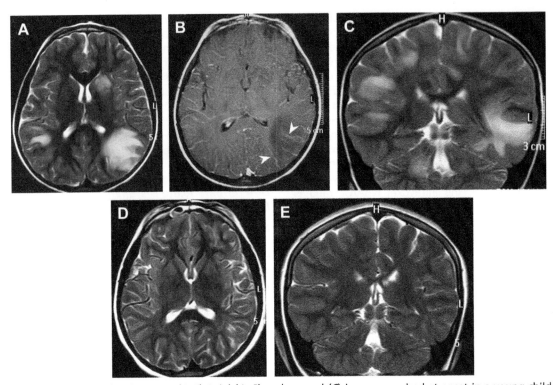

Fig. 9. Images of pediatric ADEM. (*A–C*) Axial (*A, B*) and coronal (*C*) images acquired at onset in a young child with an acute encephalopathy and polyfocal deficits. Multiple large lesions with poorly demarcated borders can be identified in the brain WM and deep GM, and the cerebellum. Postcontrast axial T1-weighted image (*B*) shows a diffuse leptomeningeal enhancement, more prominent around the large left posterior hypointense lesion (*arrowheads*). (*D–E*) Axial and coronal T2-weighted images from the same patient, acquired 12 months after the incident event showing a marked improvement of previous lesions. Based on the absence of further clinical events and no new lesions on follow-up scans, the disorder was diagnosed as monophasic ADEM.

Box 2
2012 International Pediatric Multiple Sclerosis Study Group criteria for pediatric acute disseminated encephalomyelitis

Pediatric ADEM (all are required)

- First event of encephalopathy plus polyfocal deficits
- Presumed inflammatory demyelinating cause
- Encephalopathy cannot be explained by fever
- Brain MR imaging is abnormal during the acute (3-month) phase
- No new clinical and MR imaging findings emerge ≥3 months after initial event
- Typical lesions on brain MR imaging:
  - Diffuse, poorly demarcated, large (>1–2 cm) lesions
  - Involving predominantly cerebral WM
  - T1 hypointense lesions should not be observed
  - Deep gray matter lesions (eg, thalamus or basal ganglia) can be present

Adapted from Krupp LB, Tardieu M, Amato MP, et al. International Pediatric Multiple Sclerosis Study Group criteria for pediatric multiple sclerosis and immune-mediated central nervous system demyelinating disorders: revisions to the 2007 definitions. Mult Scler 2013;19:1261–7.

ranging from 0.1 to 0.6 per 100,000 children per year.[5,70–75]

The key clinical features of ADEM include a diffuse encephalopathy with signs or symptoms of transverse myelitis, optic neuritis, cerebellar involvement, or seizures, particularly in very young children. ADEM may also present a rapid progression of symptoms to coma.[76,77]

Brain MR imaging should be abnormal showing bilateral, large areas of increased signal on T2-weighted and T2-FLAIR images, with ill-defined borders (**Fig. 9**A–C), in contrast to the well-defined focal T2-FLAIR lesions distributed in the periventricular WM, usually associated with MS.[11,77]

ADEM has been used as an umbrella term for any child with noninfectious acute demyelination, regardless of the clinical features. The first set of pediatric diagnostic criteria outlined by the IPMSSG in 2007 was particularly focused on distinguishing ADEM from an ADEM-like initial presentation of MS.[6] **Box 2** summarizes the 2012 revised criteria for pediatric ADEM.

ADEM is typically a monophasic disorder with an active phase lasting no more than 3 months, usually followed by clinical and MR imaging lesion improvement (**Fig. 9**D, E).[76] However, 10% to 29% of children with an initial episode meeting criteria for ADEM may eventually experience a relapsing clinical course.[7,76]

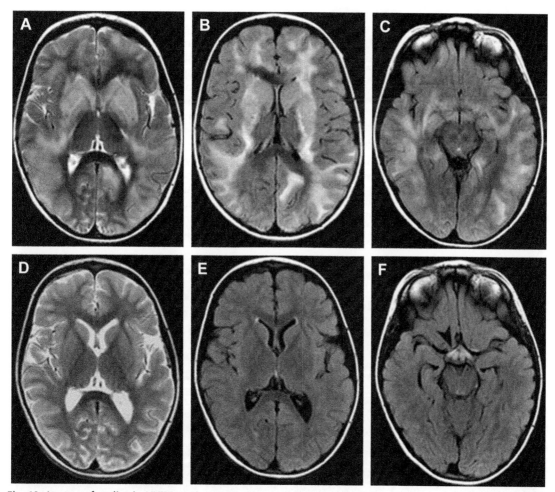

Fig. 10. Images of pediatric ADEM–optic neuritis. Upper row: Axial T2-weighted image in (*A*), and axial T2-FLAIR imaging in (*B*, *C*), acquired at the incident event in a 4-year-old boy, presenting with an acute encephalopathy and polyfocal deficits. Brain images show a bilateral and diffuse involvement of WM and deep GM. Lower row: Axial T2-weighted image in (*D*), and axial T2-FLAIR imaging in (*E*, *F*), acquired from the same young boy 4 months after the initial event, presenting at that time with a bilateral optic neuropathy. Brain images depicted a hyperintense involvement of the optic chiasm (*arrowhead in F*) associated with a marked improvement of previous extensive lesions. Clinical and MR imaging improvement after intravenous corticosteroid treatment, no further relapses, and MOG-IgG seropositivity supported the diagnosis of ADEM–optic neuritis.

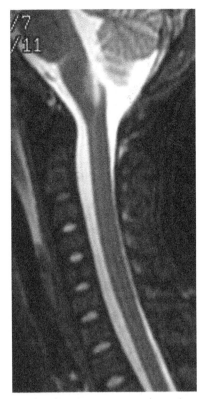

Fig. 11. Image of area postrema syndrome in pediatric NMO spectrum disorder. Sagittal T2-weighted image showing a brainstem lesion involving the area postrema (dorsal medulla), acquired from a 9-year-old girl (AQP4-IgG seropositive) presenting with intractable vomiting.

If the subsequent clinical relapse is a new ADEM event, separated by at least 3 months after symptom onset and not followed by additional events, the condition is classified as multiphasic ADEM.[21]

The diagnostic challenge emerges when an initial event with encephalopathy is followed by clinical episodes without encephalopathy (non-ADEM). The following 3 scenarios should be considered in such cases[78]:

1. According to the revised criteria for pediatric MS, the identification of new MR imaging lesions fulfilling 2010 revised McDonald criteria for DIS[13] with a second non-ADEM event occurring after at least 3 months point to the diagnosis of *pediatric MS* in a patient older than 12 years.[21] In younger patients, the revised criteria require additional clinical or MR imaging evidence for DIT.
2. Recent publications have identified a subset of ADEM patients experiencing single or repeated events of optic neuritis, with complete or almost complete resolution of previous brain T2 lesions on MR imagings, and no new lesions on follow-up studies.[79–81] This new relapsing clinical phenotype is currently known as *ADEM-ON* and has been associated with persistent myelin oligodendrocyte glycoprotein (MOG) antibodies **(Fig. 10)**.[78–82]
3. If the initial ADEM-like event is followed by relapses, including optic neuritis, longitudinally extensive transverse myelitis, or area postrema syndrome **(Fig.11)**, and the MR imaging meets

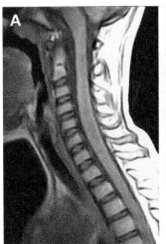
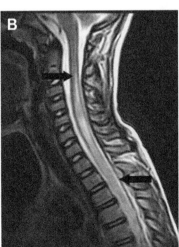
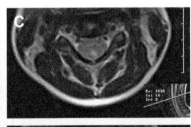
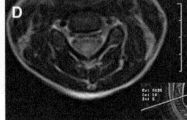

Fig. 12. Images of spinal cord involvement in pediatric NMO spectrum disorder. Spinal MR imaging scans acquired from a 13-year-old boy (AQP4-IgG seropositive) with an acute severe myelopathy. (*A*) Sagittal T1-weighted imaging of the spinal cord showing an edematous and longitudinal extensive cervical cord lesion. (*B*) Sagittal T2-weighted image shows a longitudinally extensive hyperintense cord lesion spanning more than 3 vertebral segments from the same patient (highlighted with *arrows*). (*C, D*) Axial T2-weighted images depicting the central spinal cord involvement at different levels of the longitudinal lesion.

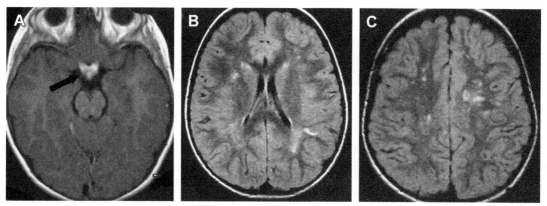

Fig. 13. Images of pediatric NMO spectrum disorder. (*A*) Axial postcontrast T1-weighted image showing optic chiasm enhancement (*arrow*) in a 4-year-old boy presenting with bilateral visual loss. (*B, C*) Axial T2-FLAIR imaging from the same patient showing a bilateral distribution of multiple nonspecific and subclinical hyperintense lesions in the brain WM. AQP4-IgG seropositivity confirmed the diagnosis of NMO spectrum disorder.

Table 3
Revised neuromyelitis optica spectrum disorders diagnostic criteria

A. NMOSD with AQP4-IgG	1. ≥1 Core clinical characteristic 2. Positive AQP4-IgG testing using best available method 3. Exclusion of alternative diagnose

B. NMOSD without AQP4-IgG or with unknown AQP4-IgG status	1. ≥2 core clinical characteristics occurring as a result of ≥1 clinical attacks and meeting all of the following:
	  a. At least 1 clinical characteristic must be optic neuritis, LETM, or area postrema syndrome
	  b. DIS (≥2 different core clinical characteristics)
	  c. Fulfillment of additional MR imaging requirements
	2. Negative tests for AQP4-IgG using best available or testing unavailable
	3. Exclusion of alternative diagnoses

C. Core clinical characteristics	1. Optic neuritis 2. Acute myelitis 3. Area postrema syndrome 4. Acute brainstem syndrome 5. Symptomatic narcolepsy or acute diencephalic syndrome with typical diencephalic MR imaging lesions 6. Symptomatic cerebral syndrome with typical brain lesions
D. Additional MR imaging requirements	
1. Acute optic neuritis	a. Brain MR imaging normal or showing nonspecific white matter lesions, and b. Optic nerve MR imaging with T2-hyperintense or T1-weighted gadolinium-enhancing lesion extending >1/2 optic nerve length or involving optic chiasm
2. Acute myelitis	Requires intramedullary MR imaging lesion extending ≥3 contiguous segments (LETM) or ≥3 contiguous segments of spinal cord atrophy in patients with prior history compatible with acute myelitis
3. Area postrema syndrome	Requires associated dorsal medulla/area postrema lesions
4. Acute brainstem syndrome	Requires associated periependymal brain stem lesions

Abbreviation: LETM, longitudinal extensive transverse myelitis.
 Data from Wingerchuk DM, Banwell B, Bennett JL, et al. International consensus diagnostic criteria for neuromyelitis optica spectrum disorders. Neurology 2015;85:177–89.

the requirements of the revised neuromyelitis optica spectrum disorder (NMOSD) criteria, the diagnosis of pediatric NMOSD may be considered (see **Table 3**).[78,82,83] The identification of a serum-positive aquaporin-4–immunoglobulin G (AQP4-IgG) titer will eventually confirm this diagnosis.[84,85]

Neuromyelitis Optica Spectrum Disorder

NMO and NMOSD are severe autoimmune diseases of the CNS characterized by recurrent inflammatory events primarily involving the optic nerves and spinal cord.[86] A specific biomarker, antibodies (NMO–IgG) targeted against the AQP4 water channel in most adult patients with NMO, identified this disorder as a different autoimmune disease.[87]

NMO is infrequent in children, and current data suggest that pediatric-onset NMO accounts for 3% to 5% of all NMO cases. Of note, children tend to demonstrate a spectrum of clinical attacks involving CNS areas beyond the optic nerves and spinal cord.[86]

Revised IPMSSG consensus criteria for pediatric NMO required the presence of both optic neuritis and transverse myelitis, with at least 2 of the following supportive features[21]:

1. MR imaging evidence of a contiguous spinal cord involvement extending over 3 or more segments (**Fig. 12**)

2. AQP4-IgG seropositive status
3. Brain MR imaging not meeting diagnostic criteria for MS (**Fig. 13**)

According to published data, brain MR imaging lesions appear more frequently in pediatric-onset NMOSD compared with adult-onset patients.[88] These lesions are usually large and tend to localize in areas of high AQP4 expression.[86,88–92] Gadolinium enhancement could be identified in around one-third of children with brain lesions.[88]

NMOSD presents a relapsing course in 53% to 100% of pediatric patients and must be differentiated from MS in order to initiate appropriate immunosuppression to prevent relapses.[84,88] Distinguishing clinical symptoms and MR imaging findings have been highlighted in the recently published revised NMOSD diagnostic criteria (**Table 3**).[83]

MR imaging represents the most important nonserological paraclinical tool to facilitate the diagnosis of NMOSD. The distinct distribution, morphology, and enhancement patterns of brain and spinal cord involvement in patients with NMOSD, with both conventional and advance MR imaging techniques, have been recently addressed by an international panel.[93,94]

Susac Syndrome

Susac syndrome (SuS) consists of the clinical triad of encephalopathy, branch retinal artery occlusions (BRAOs), and hearing loss. Nevertheless,

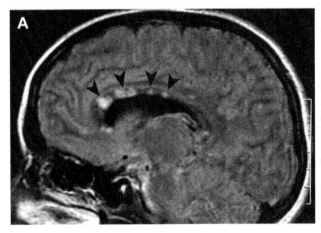
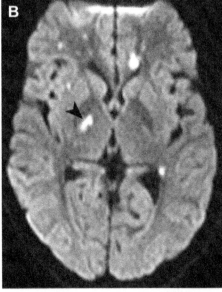

Fig. 14. Images of SuS in children. (*A*) Sagittal T2-FLAIR imaging showing multiple hyperintense lesions within the central portion of the corpus callosum: typical intracallosal "snowballs" (*arrowheads*). Images acquired from a young girl presenting with an acute encephalopathy and polyfocal deficits. (*B*) Axial diffusion-weighted imaging from the same patient depicting a "string of pearls" in the posterior limb of the right internal capsule (*arrowhead*).

Table 4
Clinical red flags to be considered in the differential diagnosis of pediatric demyelination

Atypical Neurologic Findings	Diagnostic Considerations
Hearing loss	SuS, NMOSD
Abnormal extrapyramidal movements	NMDAR encephalitis, organic acid disorders, Wilson disease, amino acid disorders
Hypothalamic symptoms	NMOSD, neurosarcoidosis, histiocytosis
Brainstem syndrome	NMOSD, pontine glioma, vertebrobasilar infarct
Area postrema syndrome	NMOSD
Progressive ataxia	Spinocerebellar ataxia, paraneoplastic syndromes
Cranial neuropathies	Neurosarcoidosis, Lyme disease, mitochondrial diseases
Longitudinally extensive myelopathy	NMOSD, HTLV-1–associated infection, B12 or copper deficiency, juvenile Alexander disease
Recurrent seizures	ADEM, NMDAR encephalitis, SVcPACNS, CNS infection
Recurrent headache	SVcPACNS, SuS, idiopathic intracranial hypertension, tumefactive brain lesion, brain tumor, pachymeningitis
Visual loss (without afferent defect)	LHON, neuroretinitis, psychogenic visual loss
Papilledema without visual loss	Optic disc drusen (pseudopapilledema)
Severe or recurrent optic neuropathy	NMOSD, LHON, CRION
Sudden onset, painless visual loss	Ischemic optic neuropathy
Progressive or relapsing encephalopathy	Leukodystrophies, mitochondrial diseases, gliomatosis cerebri, PML
Peripheral neuropathy	CMTX, CMT2A, Guillain-Barre syndrome

Abbreviations: CMT2A, Charcot-Marie-Tooth type 2A disease; CMTX, X-linked Charcot-Marie-Tooth disease; CRION, chronic relapsing inflammatory optic neuropathy; HTLV-1, human T-cell lymphotropic virus-1; LHON, Leber hereditary optic neuropathy; NMDAR, (N-methyl-D-aspartate-receptor) encephalitis; PML, progressive multifocal leukoencephalopathy; SVcPACNS, small-vessel childhood primary angiitis of the central nervous system.

the condition is often underrecognized because this clinical triad is frequently incomplete. It is considered an autoimmune endotheliopathy affecting the precapillary arterioles of the brain, retina, and inner ear.[95]

Presenting symptoms may include an acute or subacute severe encephalopathy with multifocal neurologic signs, features that may resemble ADEM. Moreover, brain MR imaging findings in the encephalopathic subset of SuS patients reveal multifocal WM lesions, including the corpus callosum, features that can resemble MS. However, the diagnosis of SuS can be made in patients presenting with encephalopathy, even in the

Table 5
MR imaging red flags to be considered in the differential diagnosis of pediatric demyelination

Atypical MR Imaging Findings for MS Diagnosis	Diagnostic Considerations
Leptomeningeal enhancement	CNS infection, neurosarcoidosis, vasculitic process, hemophagocytic lymphohistiocytosis, CNS malignancy
Multiple brain ring–enhancing lesions	CNS tuberculomas, pyogenic abscesses, toxoplasmosis, cysticercosis, fungal infections, CNS lymphoma
Increased size of lesions on serial imaging	Brain tumor, PML, CNS lymphoma, sarcoidosis
Hemorrhage on conventional MR imaging	ANE, CNS stroke, AHLE, SVcPACNS, large-vessel CNS vasculitis

Abbreviations: AHLE, acute hemorrhagic leukoencephalitis; ANE, acute necrotizing encephalopathy.

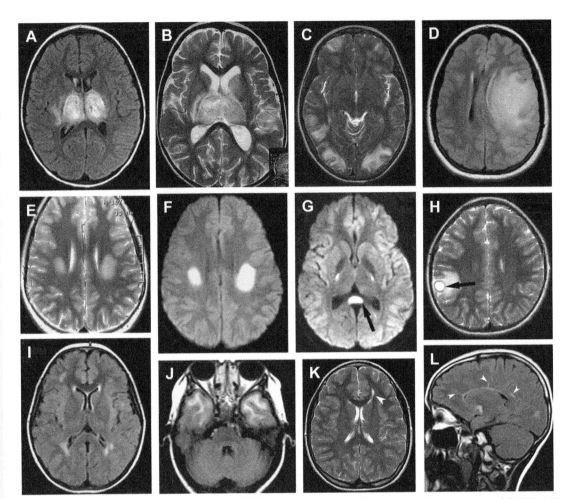

Fig. 15. (A–L) Differential diagnosis of acquired WM and deep GM brain lesions in pediatric patients. (A) T2-FLAIR image depicting a prominent bithalamic involvement in a 2-year-old girl presenting with a febrile acute encephalopathy corresponding to an acute necrotizing encephalopathy. (B) T2-weighted imaging revealed high signal lesions in bilateral thalami, left caudate nucleus, and posterior limb of the right internal capsule in a 3-year-old boy presenting with an acute left hemiparesis. MR venography confirmed the diagnosis of deep cerebral venous thrombosis. (C) A 14-year-old girl was admitted with severe headaches, visual disturbances, and a brief epileptic seizure in the context of a recent-onset kidney disease. T2-weighted brain MR imaging revealed multiple high signal abnormalities in the subcortical WM, predominantly in the parieto-occipital areas, corresponding to the diagnosis of reversible posterior leukoencephalopathy syndrome or posterior reversible encephalopathy syndrome. (D) T2-weighted brain imaging showing a tumefactive lesion with a severe mass effect. Brain biopsy confirmed the diagnosis of multiforme glioblastoma in a 14-year-old girl. (E–G) T2-weighted brain image revealed bilateral high signals involving posterior centrum semiovale (E), with abnormal restricted diffusion with the same distribution (F), including also the splenium of the corpus callosum (arrow in G) on diffusion-weighted imaging in a 10-year-old boy who developed acute-onset weakness in the left lower limb, with signs of a chronic neuropathy with diminished deep tendon reflexes in lower limbs and foot deformities on examination. These MR imaging typical findings led to a diagnosis of X-linked Charcot-Marie-Tooth disease (connexin 32 gene mutation). (H) A 10-year-old boy presented with recent onset headaches and focal motor seizures. Brain T2-weighted image demonstrated a single cortical-subcortical cystic lesion (arrow) with perilesional edema typical of neurocysticercosis, in a young patient coming from an endemic area for cysticercosis. (I, J) A 14-year-old girl presented with 2-year history of walking difficulties, and paraparesis with pyramidal signs on examination. In addition to a spinal cord atrophy (not shown), T2-FLAIR brain imaging depicted multiple hyperintense lesions in the periventricular and subcortical WM (I), more prominent and confluent in temporal lobes (J). Considering the neurologic syndrome (slowly progressive myelopathy) and brain MR imaging findings, CSF and serum immunoreactivity to the human T-cell lymphotropic virus-1 was requested and confirmed by Western blot. (K, L) The diagnosis of MS had been considered in a referred 10-year-old girl showing hyperintense brain WM lesions on T2-weighted images, with a periventricular (arrowhead in K) and Dawson fingerlike (arrowheads in L) distribution. On examination, this girl had reticulated white maculae distributed along Blaschko lines, corresponding to the diagnosis of hypomelanosis of Ito.

absence of BRAO and hearing loss, if the following distinct lesions are identified on brain MR imaging[95]:

- Callosal microinfarcts ("snowballs"), mainly located in the central portion of the corpus callosum, are better identified on sagittal brain T2 and T2-FLAIR-weighted imaging (**Fig. 14**A). These microinfarcts usually evolve into central callosal "holes," better identified on sagittal brain T1-weighted imaging.
- Long-tract involvement by microinfarcts results in a "string-of-pearls" configuration in the internal capsule, lesions that can be easily identified on diffusion-weighted imaging (see **Fig. 14**B). The combination of central callosal "snowballs" and "string of pearls" in the internal capsule is considered diagnostic for SuS.
- Leptomeningeal enhancement may be observed in the cerebellum. This finding is common in SuS and not expected in MS or ADEM.

A recent DT imaging study in SuS revealed damage to the callosal fiber integrity and the prefrontal WM, findings that correlate with the usual clinical severity of the encephalopathy and the long-term neurocognitive decline.[96]

According to the published data, permanent neurologic impairment and hearing loss are more frequent and severe in patients with delayed diagnosis and treatment. Although pediatric-onset SuS is rare, it is important to consider this alternative diagnosis in order to initiate aggressive immunosuppression with agents with fast onset of action such as rituximab.[97]

Some key clinical and imaging features that should raise consideration of other disorders different from MS are listed in **Tables 4** and **5** and are included in **Fig. 15**.

SUMMARY

Pediatric-onset acquired inflammatory demyelinating disorders are increasingly recognized and continue to expand. Nevertheless, MS continues being a challenging diagnosis in children and adolescents. Advances in conventional MR imaging have contributed to improve the identification of distinguishing features of pediatric MS and provided imaging criteria to differentiate between children who will not develop a relapsing disease and children at risk for MS diagnosis. In addition, MR imaging has a key role in the differential diagnosis with a broad spectrum of pediatric disorders, particularly ADEM and NMOSD. Recent research advances in the field of MS and related disorders are providing new insights into the

pathophysiologic mechanisms and immune interactions of this complex disease. Further work is still required to find reliable biomarkers that facilitate a definite diagnosis of pediatric MS at the initial clinical event.

REFERENCES

1. Duquette P, Murray TJ, Pleines J, et al. Multiple sclerosis in childhood: clinical profile in 125 patients. J Pediatr 1987;111:359–63.
2. Ghezzi A, Deplano V, Faroni J, et al. Multiple sclerosis in childhood: clinical features of 149 patients. Mult Scler 1997;3:43–6.
3. Boiko A, Vorobeychik G, Paty D, et al. Early onset multiple sclerosis: a longitudinal study. Neurology 2002;59:1006–10.
4. Simone IL, Carrara D, Tortorella C, et al. Course and prognosis in early-onset MS: comparison with adult-onset forms. Neurology 2002;59:1922–8.
5. Banwell B, Kennedy J, Sadovnick D, et al. Incidence of acquired demyelination of the CNS in Canadian children. Neurology 2009;72:232–9.
6. Krupp LB, Banwell B, Tenembaum S. Consensus definitions proposed for pediatric multiple sclerosis and related disorders. Neurology 2007;68:S7–12.
7. Mikaeloff Y, Adamsbaum C, Husson B, et al. MRI prognostic factors for relapse after acute CNS inflammatory demyelination in children. Brain 2004;127:1942–7.
8. Neuteboom RF, Boon M, Catsman Berrevoets CE, et al. Prognostic factors after a first attack of inflammatory CNS demyelination in children. Neurology 2008;71:967–73.
9. Verhey LH, Branson HM, Shroff MM, et al. MRI parameters for prediction of multiple sclerosis diagnosis in children with acute CNS demyelination: a prospective national cohort study. Lancet Neurol 2011;10:1065–73.
10. Callen DJ, Shroff MM, Branson HM, et al. MRI in the diagnosis of pediatric multiple sclerosis. Neurology 2009;72:961–7.
11. Callen DJ, Shroff MM, Branson HM, et al. Role of MRI in the differentiation of ADEM from MS in children. Neurology 2009;72:968–73.
12. Ketelslegers IA, Neuteboom RF, Boon M, et al. A comparison of MRI criteria for diagnosing pediatric ADEM and MS. Neurology 2010;74:1412–5.
13. Polman CH, Reingold S, Banwell B, et al. Diagnostic criteria for multiple sclerosis: 2010 revisions to the McDonald criteria. Ann Neurol 2011;69:292–302.
14. Sadaka Y, Verhey LH, Shroff MM, et al. 2010 McDonald criteria for diagnosing pediatric multiple sclerosis. Ann Neurol 2012;72:211–23.
15. Sedani S, Lim JM, Hemingway C, et al. Paediatric multiple sclerosis: examining utility of the McDonald 2010 criteria. Mult Scler 2012;18:679–82.

16. Kornek B, Schmitl B, Vass K, et al. Evaluation of the 2010 McDonald multiple sclerosis criteria in children with a clinically isolated syndrome. Mult Scler 2012; 18:1768–74.

17. Hummel HM, Brück W, Dreha-Kulaczewski S, et al. Pediatric onset multiple sclerosis: McDonald criteria 2010 and the contribution of spinal cord MRI. Mult Scler 2013;19:1330–5.

18. Bigi S, Marrie RA, Verhey L, et al. 2010 McDonald criteria in a pediatric cohort: is positivity at onset associated with a more aggressive multiple sclerosis course? Mult Scler 2013;19:1359–62.

19. Dale RC, Pillai SC. Early relapse risk after a first CNS inflammatory demyelination episode: examining international consensus definitions. Dev Med Child Neurol 2007;49:887–93.

20. Peche SS, Alshekhlee A, Kelly J, et al. A long-term follow-up study using IPMSSG criteria in children with CNS demyelination. Pediatr Neurol 2013;49: 329–34.

21. Krupp LB, Tardieu M, Amato MP, et al. International Pediatric Multiple Sclerosis Study Group criteria for pediatric multiple sclerosis and immune-mediated central nervous system demyelinating disorders: revisions to the 2007 definitions. Mult Scler 2013;19: 1261–7.

22. van Pelt ED, Neuteboom RF, Ketelslegers IA, et al, on behalf of the Dutch Study Group for Paediatric MS. Application of the 2012 revised diagnostic definitions for paediatric multiple sclerosis and immune-mediated central nervous system demyelination disorders. J Neurol Neurosurg Psychiatr 2014;85:790–4.

23. Huppke B, Ellenberger D, Rosewich H, et al. Clinical presentation of pediatric multiple sclerosis before puberty. Eur J Neurol 2014;21:441–6.

24. Pohl D. Diagnosing paediatric multiple sclerosis versus acute disseminated encephalomyelitis. Dev Med Child Neurol 2007;49:884.

25. Banwell B, Ghezzi A, Bar-Or A, et al. Multiple sclerosis in children: clinical diagnosis, therapeutic strategies, and future directions. Lancet Neurol 2007;6:887–902.

26. Yeh EA, Chitnis T, Krupp L, et al. Pediatric multiple sclerosis. Nat Rev Neurol 2009;5:621–31.

27. Renoux C, Vukusic S, Mikaeloff Y, et al. Natural history of multiple sclerosis with childhood onset. N Engl J Med 2007;356:2603–13.

28. Gorman MP, Healy BC, Polgar-Turcsanyi M, et al. Increased relapse rate in pediatric-onset compared with adult-onset multiple sclerosis. Arch Neurol 2009;66:54–9.

29. Paty DW, Li DK. Interferon beta-1b is effective in relapsing-remitting multiple sclerosis. II. MRI analysis results of a multicenter, randomized, double-blind, placebo-controlled trial. UBC MS/MRI Study Group, IFNB Multiple Sclerosis Study Group. Neurology 1993;43:662–7.

30. Pirko I. Neuroimaging of demyelinating diseases. Continuum Lifelong Learn Neurol 2008;14:118–43.

31. Filippi M, Yousry T, Baratti C, et al. Quantitative assessment of MRI lesion load in multiple sclerosis. A comparison of conventional spin-echo with fast fluid-attenuated inversion recovery. Brain 1996;119:1349–55.

32. Verhey LH, Narayanan S, Banwell B. Standardized magnetic resonance imaging acquisition and reporting in pediatric multiple sclerosis. Neuroimag Clin N Am 2013;23:217–26.

33. Waubant E, Chabas D. Pediatric multiple sclerosis. Curr Treat Options Neurol 2009;11:203–10.

34. Chabas D, Castillo-Trivino T, Mowry EM, et al. Vanishing MS T2-bright lesions before puberty. A distinct MRI phenotype? Neurology 2008;71:1090–3.

35. Balassy C, Bernert G, Wober-Bingol C, et al. Long-term MRI observations of childhood-onset relapsing-remitting multiple sclerosis. Neuropediatrics 2001;32:28–37.

36. McAdam L, Blaser S, Banwell B. Pediatric tumefactive demyelination: case series and review of the literature. Pediatr Neurol 2002;26:18–25.

37. Aubert-Broche B, Fonov V, Ghassemi R, et al. Regional brain atrophy in children with multiple sclerosis. Neuroimage 2011;58:409–15.

38. Mesaros S, Rocca MA, Absinta M, et al. Evidence of thalamic gray matter loss in pediatric multiple sclerosis. Neurology 2008;70:1107–12.

39. Kerbrat A, Aubert-Broche B, Fonov V, et al. Reduced head and brain size for age and disproportionately smaller thalami in child-onset MS. Neurology 2012; 78:194–201.

40. Aubert-Broche B, Fonov V, Narayanan S, et al. Onset of multiple sclerosis before adulthood leads to failure of age-expected brain growth. Neurology 2014;83: 2140–6.

41. Verhey LH, Sled JG. Advanced magnetic resonance imaging in pediatric multiple sclerosis. Neuroimag Clin N Am 2013;23:337–54.

42. Mezzapesa DM, Rocca MA, Falini A, et al. A preliminary diffusion tensor and magnetization transfer magnetic resonance imaging study of early-onset multiple. Arch Neurol 2004;61:366–8.

43. Tortorella P, Rocca MA, Mezzapesa DM, et al. MRI quantification of gray and white matter damage in patients with early-onset multiple sclerosis. J Neurol 2006;253:903–7.

44. Yeh EA, Weinstock-Guttman B, Ramanathan M, et al. Magnetic resonance imaging characteristics of children and adults with paediatric-onset multiple sclerosis. Brain 2009;132:3392–400.

45. Absinta M, Rocca MA, Moiola L, et al. Cortical lesions in children with multiple sclerosis. Neurology 2011;76:910–3.

46. Akbar N, Giorgio A, Till C, et al. Alterations in functional and structural connectivity in pediatric-onset multiple sclerosis. PLoS One 2016;11:1–14.

47. Vishwas MS, Chitnis T, Pienaar R, et al. Tract-based analysis of callosal, projection, and association pathways in pediatric patients with multiple sclerosis: a preliminary study. AJNR Am J Neuroradiol 2010;31:121–8.

48. Tillema JM, Leach J, Pirko I. Non-lesional white matter changes in pediatric multiple sclerosis and monophasic demyelinating disorders. Mult Scler 2012;18:1754–9.

49. Vishwas MS, Healy BC, Pienaar R, et al. Diffusion tensor analysis of pediatric multiple sclerosis and clinically isolated syndromes. AJNR Am J Neuroradiol 2013;34:417–23.

50. Blaschek A, Keeser D, Muller S, et al. Early white matter changes in childhood multiple sclerosis: a diffusion tensor imaging study. AJNR Am J Neuroradiol 2013;34:2015–20.

51. Rocca MA, Absinta M, Amato MP, et al. Posterior brain damage and cognitive impairment in pediatric multiple sclerosis. Neurology 2014;82:1314–21.

52. Rocca MA, Valsasina P, Absinta M, et al. Intranetwork and internetwork functional connectivity abnormalities in pediatric multiple sclerosis. Hum Brain Mapp 2014;35:4180–92.

53. Absinta M, Rocca MA, Moiola L, et al. Brain macro- and microscopic damage in patients with paediatric MS. J Neurol Neurosurg Psychiatr 2010;81:1357–62.

54. Bethune A, Tipu V, Sled JG, et al. Diffusion tensor imaging and cognitive speed in children with multiple sclerosis. J Neurol Sci 2011;309:68–74.

55. Till C, Deotto A, Tipu V, et al. White matter integrity and math performance in pediatric multiple sclerosis: a diffusion tensor imaging study. Neuroreport 2011;22:1005–9.

56. Bruhn H, Frahm J, Merboldt KD, et al. Multiple sclerosis in children: cerebral metabolic alterations monitored by localized proton magnetic resonance spectroscopy in vivo. Ann Neurol 1992;32:140–50.

57. Oguz KK, Kurne A, Aksu AO, et al. Assessment of citrullinated myelin by 1H-MR spectroscopy in early-onset multiple sclerosis. AJNR Am J Neuroradiol 2009;30:716–21.

58. Ben SL, Miller E, Artzi M, et al. 1H-MRS for the diagnosis of acute disseminated encephalomyelitis: insight into the acute-disease stage. Pediatr Radiol 2010;40:106–13.

59. Amato MP, Goretti B, Ghezzi A, et al, Multiple Sclerosis Study Group of the Italian Neurological Society. Cognitive and psychosocial features of childhood and juvenile MS. Neurology 2008;70:1891–7.

60. Amato MP, Goretti B, Ghezzi A, et al, Multiple Sclerosis Study Group of the Italian Neurological Society. Cognitive and psychosocial features in childhood and juvenile MS: two-year follow-up. Neurology 2010;75:1134–40.

61. Julian L, Serafin D, Charvet L, et al, Network of Pediatric MS Centers of Excellence. Cognitive impairment occurs in children and adolescents with multiple sclerosis: results from a United States network. J Child Neurol 2013;28:102–7.

62. Kelly JE, Mar S, D'Angelo G, et al. Susceptibility-weighted imaging helps to discriminate pediatric multiple sclerosis from acute disseminated encephalomyelitis. Pediatr Neurol 2015;52:36–41.

63. Rubin JP. MRI to discriminate pediatric MS from ADEM. Pediatr Neurol Briefs 2015;29:13.

64. O'Mahony J, Bar-Or A, Arnold DL, et al. Masquerades of acquired demyelination in children: experiences of a national demyelinating disease program. J Child Neurol 2013;28:184–97.

65. Hahn JS, Pohl D, Rensel M, et al, International Pediatric MS Study Group. Differential diagnosis and evaluation in pediatric multiple sclerosis. Neurology 2007;68(Suppl 2):S13–22.

66. Venkateswaran S, Banwell B. Pediatric multiple sclerosis. Neurologist 2010;16:92–105.

67. O'Mahony J, Shroff M, Banwell B. Mimics and rare presentations of pediatric demyelination. Neuroimaging Clin N Am 2013;23:321–36.

68. Schwarz S, Mohr A, Knauth M, et al. Acute disseminated encephalomyelitis: a follow-up study of 40 adult patients. Neurology 2001;56:1313–8.

69. Brinar VV, Poser CM. Disseminated encephalomyelitis in adults. Clin Neurol Neurosurg 2008;110:913–8.

70. Leake JA, Albani S, Kao AS, et al. Acute disseminated encephalomyelitis in childhood: epidemiologic, clinical and laboratory features. Pediatr Infect Dis J 2004;23:756–64.

71. Pohl D, Hennemuth I, von Kries R, et al. Paediatric multiple sclerosis and acute disseminated encephalomyelitis in Germany: results of a nationwide survey. Eur J Pediatr 2007;166:405–12.

72. Torisu H, Kira R, Ishizaki Y, et al. Clinical study of childhood acute disseminated encephalomyelitis, multiple sclerosis, and acute transverse myelitis in Fukuoka Prefecture, Japan. Brain Dev 2010;32:454–62.

73. Van Landingham M, Hanigan W, Vedanarayanan V, et al. An uncommon illness with a rare presentation: neurosurgical management of ADEM with tumefactive demyelination in children. Childs Nerv Syst 2010;26:655–61.

74. Langer-Gould A, Zhang JL, Chung J, et al. Incidence of acquired CNS demyelinating syndromes in a multiethnic cohort of children. Neurology 2011;77(12):1143–8.

75. Absoud M, Lim MJ, Chong WK, et al. Paediatric acquired demyelinating syndromes: incidence, clinical and magnetic resonance imaging features. Mult Scler 2013;19:76–86.

76. Tenembaum S, Chamoles N, Fejerman N. Acute disseminated encephalomyelitis: a long-term follow-up study of 84 pediatric patients. Neurology 2002;59:1224–31.

77. Tenembaum S, Chitnis T, Ness J, et al. Acute disseminated encephalomyelitis. Neurology 2007; 68(16 Suppl 2):S23–36.

78. Pohl D, Alper G, Van Haren K, et al. Acute disseminated encephalomyelitis. Updates on an inflammatory CNS syndrome. Neurology 2016;87(Suppl 2): S38–45.

79. Rostasy K, Mader S, Schanda K, et al. Anti-MOG antibodies in children with optic neuritis. Arch Neurol 2012;69:752–6.

80. Huppke P, Rostasy K, Karenfort M, et al. Acute disseminated encephalomyelitis followed by recurrent or monophasic optic neuritis in pediatric patients. Mult Scler 2013;19:941–6.

81. Miyauchi A, Monden Y, Watanabe M, et al. Persistent presence of the anti-myelin oligodendrocyte glycoprotein autoantibody in a pediatric case of acute disseminated encephalomyelitis followed by optic neuritis. Neuropediatrics 2014;45:196–9.

82. Tenembaum S. Comment on multiphasic disseminated encephalomyelitis followed by optic neuritis in a child with gluten sensitivity. Mult Scler 2015; 21:1212–4.

83. Wingerchuk DM, Banwell B, Bennett JL, et al. International consensus diagnostic criteria for neuromyelitis optica spectrum disorders. Neurology 2015;85: 177–89.

84. Banwell B, Tenembaum S, Lennon VA, et al. Neuromyelitis optica-IgG in childhood inflammatory demyelinating CNS disorders. Neurology 2008;70:344–52.

85. Lotze TE, Northrop JL, Hutton GJ, et al. Spectrum of pediatric neuromyelitis optica. Pediatrics 2008;122: e1039–47.

86. Tenembaum S, Chitnis T, Nakashima I, et al. Neuromyelitis optica spectrum disorders in children and adolescents. Neurology 2016;87(Suppl 2):S59–66.

87. Lennon VA, Wingerchuk DM, Kryzer TJ, et al. A serum autoantibody marker of neuromyelitis optica: distinction from multiple sclerosis. Lancet 2004;364:2106–12.

88. McKeon A, Lennon VA, Lotze T, et al. CNS aquaporin-4 autoimmunity in children. Neurology 2008;71:93–100.

89. Collongues N, Marignier R, Zephir H, et al. Long-term follow-up of neuromyelitis optica with a pediatric onset. Neurology 2010;75:1084–8.

90. Pena JA, Ravelo ME, Mora-La Cruz E, et al. NMO in pediatric patients: brain involvement and clinical expression. Arq Neuropsiquiatr 2011;69:34–8.

91. Kremer L, Mealy M, Jacob A, et al. Brainstem manifestations in neuromyelitis optica: a multicenter study of 258 patients. Mult Scler 2014;20:843–7.

92. Absoud M, Lim MJ, Appleton R, et al. Paediatric neuromyelitis optica: clinical, MRI of the brain and prognostic features. J Neurol Neurosurg Psychiatr 2015;86:470–2.

93. Kim HJ, Paul F, Lana-Peixoto MA, et al. MRI characteristics of neuromyelitis optica spectrum disorder. An international update. Neurology 2015;84:1165–73.

94. Kremer S, Renard F, Achard S, et al. Use of advanced magnetic resonance imaging techniques in neuromyelitis optica spectrum disorder. JAMA Neurol 2015;72:815–22.

95. Rennebohm R, Susac JO, Egan RA, et al. Susac's syndrome—update. J Neurol Sci 2010;299(1–2): 86–91.

96. Wuerfel J, Sinnecker T, Ringelstein EB, et al. Lesion morphology at 7 Tesla MRI differentiates Susac syndrome from multiple sclerosis. Mult Scler 2012;18: 1592–9.

97. Vodopivec I, Prasad S. Treatment of Susac syndrome. Curr Treat Options Neurol 2016;18:3.

Neuromyelitis Optica Spectrum Disorders

Tetsuya Akaishi, MD[a], Ichiro Nakashima, MD[a], Douglas Kazutoshi Sato, MD[a,b,c], Toshiyuki Takahashi, MD[a,d], Kazuo Fujihara, MD[a,b,e],*

KEYWORDS

- Neuromyelitis optica spectrum disorders • Anti-aquaporin-4 antibody
- Anti-myelin oligodendrocyte glycoprotein antibody • MR imaging • Optical coherence tomography

KEY POINTS

- Neuromyelitis optica spectrum disorders (NMOSD) is now divided into anti-aquaporin-4-antibody (anti-AQP4-Ab)-seropositive NMOSD and -seronegative NMOSD (or unknown serostatus).
- In anti-AQP4-Ab-seropositive NMOSD, optic neuritis (ON) is often severe and may involve the optic chiasm, and acute myelitis is longitudinally extensive (>3 vertebral segments) and preferentially involves the central gray matter. Area postrema lesions associated with intractable hiccup, nausea, and vomiting, and other brain syndromes may develop in some patients.
- A fraction of anti-AQP4-Ab-seronegative patients with NMOSD are positive for anti-myelin oligodendrocyte glycoprotein-antibody (anti-MOG-Ab), and anti-MOG-Ab-seropositive NMOSD has some unique features as compared with anti-AQP4-Ab-seropositive NMOSD (fewer relapses and better prognosis, simultaneous bilateral ON, lumbosacral myelitis). Double-seronegative NMOSD might include heterogeneous groups of diseases.
- Optical coherence tomography shows relatively milder neuronal damage in anti-MOG-Ab-seropositive ON than in anti-AQP4-Ab-seropositive ON.
- MR imaging and OCT are powerful tools to diagnose and evaluate both types of autoantibody-associated NMOSD.

INTRODUCTION

Neuromyelitis optica (NMO) is clinically characterized by severe optic neuritis (ON) and transverse myelitis. NMO spectrum disorder (NMOSD) is a newly emerging disease spectrum with or without anti-aquaporin-4-autoantibody (anti-AQP4-Ab) and includes typical NMO. Until recently, ON (often severe and simultaneous bilateral) and acute transverse myelitis (mostly longitudinally extensive, >3 vertebral segments) have been the cardinal clinical symptoms of NMO and were absolutely needed for the diagnosis. Then the term NMOSD was introduced for anti-AQP4-Ab-seropositive cases with

Disclosure Statements: See last page of article.
[a] Department of Neurology, Tohoku University Graduate School of Medicine, 1-1 Seiryomachi, Aobaku, Sendai 980-8574, Japan; [b] Department of Multiple Sclerosis Therapeutics, Tohoku University Graduate School of Medicine, 1-1 Seiryomachi, Aobaku, Sendai 980-8574, Japan; [c] Brain Institute, The Pontifical Catholic University of Rio Grande do Sul, Av. Ipiranga, 6690 - Building 63, Porto Alegre, Rio Grande do Sul 90610-000, Brazil; [d] Department of Neurology, Yonezawa National Hospital, 26100-1 Misawa, Yonezawa 992-1202, Japan; [e] Department of Multiple Sclerosis Therapeutics, Multiple Sclerosis & Neuromyelitis Optica Center, Southern TOHOKU Research Institute for Neuroscience, Fukushima Medical University School of Medicine, 7-115 Yatsuyamada, Koriyama 963-8563, Japan
* Corresponding author: Department of Neurology, Tohoku University Graduate School of Medicine, 1-1 Seiryomachi, Aobaku, Sendai 980-8574, Japan.
E-mail address: fujikazu@med.tohoku.ac.jp

Neuroimag Clin N Am 27 (2017) 251–265
http://dx.doi.org/10.1016/j.nic.2016.12.010
1052-5149/17/© 2017 Elsevier Inc. All rights reserved.

neuroimaging.theclinics.com

typical NMO, ON (recurrent or simultaneous bilateral), longitudinally extensive transverse myelitis (LETM), or ON/LETM with systemic autoimmune diseases or brain lesions typical of NMO (hypothalamic, corpus callosal, periventricular, or brainstem). However, it has been recognized that cerebral and brainstem lesions occasionally develop as the onset events in some anti-AQP4-Ab-seropositive patients. Based on those observations, NMOSD has recently been redefined, and certain types of brain syndromes were also included as core clinical characteristics of NMOSD in the 2015 international consensus diagnostic criteria.[1] The MR imaging findings in AQP4-Ab-seropositive NMOSD are usually distinct from those in typical multiple sclerosis (MS). Differential diagnosis between NMOSD and MS are critically important because such disease-modifying drugs for MS as interferon-β, natalizumab, and fingolimod may aggravate anti-AQP4-Ab-seropositive NMOSD.

Another serum autoantibody called anti-myelin oligodendrocyte glycoprotein-antibody (anti-MOG-Ab) has been detected in a fraction of patients with NMOSD without anti-AQP4-Ab. Patients with anti-AQP4-Ab and those with anti-MOG-Ab seem to have distinct pathophysiologies, although there are some overlaps of their clinical manifestations. Massive astrocytic destruction associated with autoimmunity to AQP4 is a dominant pathology in patients with anti-AQP4-Ab,[2] whereas anti-MOG-Ab-associated NMOSD seems to be an inflammatory demyelinating disease,[3] and immunosuppression is needed in the relapsing form of both antibody-associated NMOSD. Distributions and other features of the MR imaging lesions in cases with anti-AQP4-Ab and anti-MOG-Ab are distinguishable to some extent.

This article presents the clinical manifestations, MR imaging findings, and optical coherence tomography (OCT) findings in the patients with anti-AQP4-Ab-seropositive NMOSD and those with anti-MOG-Ab-seropositive NMOSD. All MR imaging shown here is derived from our own database of NMOSD at Tohoku University Hospital, a center of NMOSD research in Japan. Patients with NMOSD without those two autoantibodies certainly exist, but such a disease entity is heterogeneous and is not mentioned here.

ANTI-AQUAPORIN-4-AUTOANTIBODY-SEROPOSITIVE NEUROMYELITIS OPTICA SPECTRUM DISORDER

More than half of the patients with anti-AQP4-Ab develop typical NMO (ON and LETM), but some of the patients develop LETM or ON alone for unknown reasons. In addition to these conventional central nervous system (CNS) lesions, brainstem lesions including area postrema syndrome and certain types of cerebral lesions have also been recognized as the CNS lesions unique to NMOSD. Patients with anti-AQP4-Ab show high rates of relapses if untreated, and thus soon after the patients develop those CNS lesions and are found to be anti-AQP4-Ab-seropositive, immunosuppressive therapy to prevent relapse should be considered.

MR Imaging Findings

Optic neuritis
Distribution ON lesions in anti-AQP4-Ab-seropositive NMOSD are often longer than half of the optic nerve length and the optic chiasmal involvement is not uncommon. The distribution of T2-ON lesions in the subsegments of optic nerves on orbital MR imaging from 26 ON eyes in 23 patients with anti-AQP4-Ab NMOSD seen at Tohoku University Hospital is shown in **Table 1**. The numbers of affected subsegments in each patient were 2.8 ± 1.5, and thus the sum of the percentages in **Table 1** exceeds 100%. The incidence of ON was the highest in the intraorbital portion, and the chiasmal lesions were seen in about one out of four lesions.

Characteristics in the acute phase Affected optic nerves in the acute phase of ON in patients with anti-AQP4-Ab show on orbital MR imaging long lesions (≥2 subsegments in **Table 1**) and swelling and contrast enhancement.[4] To detect ON, short tau inversion recovery (STIR) and fat-suppressed gadolinium-enhanced T1-weighted image are useful (**Fig. 1**). Axial fast spin echo T2-weighted imaging could also be used in depicting ON lesions with adequate sensitivity.[5]

Characteristics in the chronic phase Affected optic nerves in the chronic phase of ON in patients with anti-AQP4-Ab often show long-segmental atrophy with high signal on T2-weighted images, fluid attenuated inversion recovery, and STIR (**Fig. 2**).

Table 1
Lesion distribution of anti-AQP4-Ab-seropositive optic neuritis in the subsegments of optic nerves

Subsegment	Midorbit	Retro-orbit	Canalicular	Intracranial	Chiasmal	Optic Tract
Incidence (percentage)	17/26 (65.0)	18/26 (69.0)	14/26 (53.8)	13/26 (50.0)	7/26 (26.9)	3/26 (11.5)

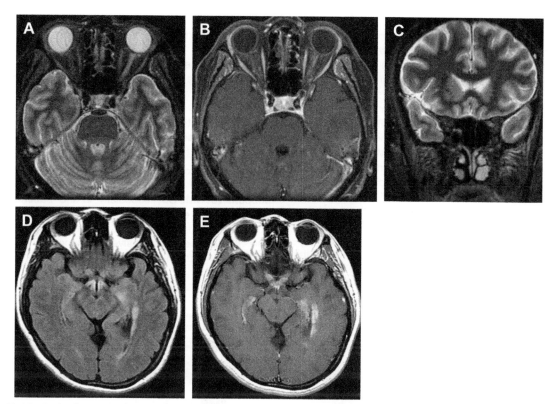

Fig. 1. ON in the acute phase in anti-aquaporin-4-antibody-seropositive patients. (*A–C*) Left ON (intraorbital) in a 55-year-old woman. (*A*) STIR. (*B*) Fat-suppressed T1 with gadolinium enhancement. (*C*) STIR, coronal view (canalicular lesion). (*D, E*) Chiasmal and optic tract lesions in a 44-year-old woman. (*D*) Fluid attenuated inversion recovery. (*E*) T1 with gadolinium-enhancement.

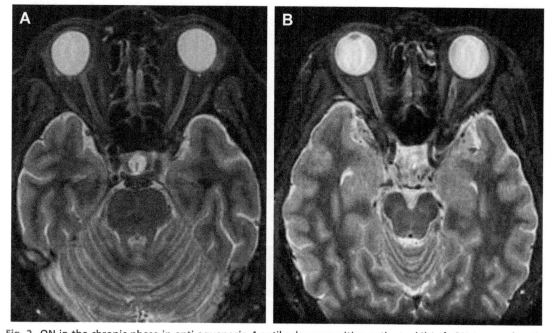

Fig. 2. ON in the chronic phase in anti-aquaporin-4-antibody-seropositive patients. (*A*) Left ON 1 year after the onset (see **Fig.** 1A–C) in a 56-year-old woman, hyperintense lesions persisted on STIR. (*B*) Right ON after 8 years of ON onset in a 57-year-old woman. The hyperintense lesions were still seen and the affected optic nerve that was somewhat atrophic on STIR.

Acute myelitis

Longitudinally extensive transverse myelitis Longitudinally extensive spinal cord lesions extending over more than three contiguous vertebral segments, or LETM (Fig. 3), is one of the most characteristic MR imaging findings in patients with anti-AQP4-Ab, and is atypical for MS.[6] Length of myelitis in anti-AQP4-Ab-seropositive NMOSD has clinical implications, because it correlates with motor disability in the patients.[7] NMOSD myelitis is more often seen in the upper spinal cord (cervical and upper thoracic) than in the lower spinal cord. The spinal lesions in anti-AQP4-Ab-seropositive myelitis often show swelling and gadolinium enhancement in the acute phase (see Fig. 3) and become atrophied in the chronic phase. Anti-AQP4-Ab-seropositive myelitis could involve the entire spinal cord on the sagittal images.

Axial view of longitudinally extensive transverse myelitis LETM in anti-AQP4-Ab-seropositive patients with NMOSD preferentially involves the central gray matter of the spinal cord and could show H-shaped T2-hyperintense lesions in the axial images in some patients (Fig. 4A).[8] This is in contrast to the distribution of myelitis in patients with MS whose spinal cord lesions are likely to appear in such white matters as lateral and posterior funiculi. Myelitis in patients with NMO often spread across the axial plane, resulting in transverse myelitis (see Fig. 4B).

Spinal cord atrophy in the chronic phase In the chronic phase of myelitis in anti-AQP4-Ab-seoporisive NMOSD, especially in the patients with repeated episodes of myelitis,[9] the spinal cord at the levels of LETM is atrophied (Fig. 5). The longitudinally extensive T2-hyperintensity may persist permanently in many patients.

Area postrema lesions and other brainstem lesions

One of the most characteristic brain symptoms in patients with anti-AQP4-Ab is intractable hiccup,

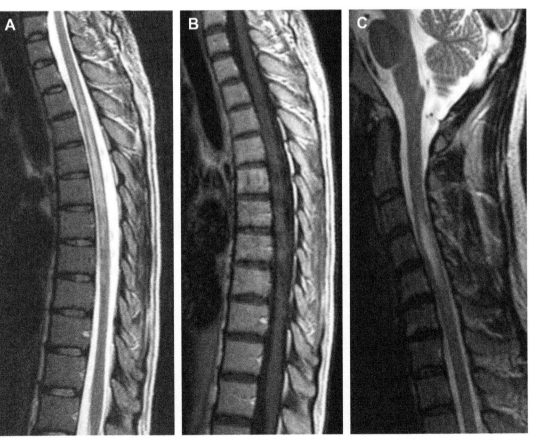

Fig. 3. Sagittal views of acute myelitis in anti-aquaporin-4-antibody-seropositive patients. (A) Longitudinally extensive T2-hyperintense spinal cord lesions (T3-T9) in a 35-year-old woman. (B) diffuse gadolinium enhancement on T1-weighted image in the same patient in A. (C) T2, longitudinally extensive T2-hyperintense cervical cord lesion with mild swelling in a 35-year-old woman.

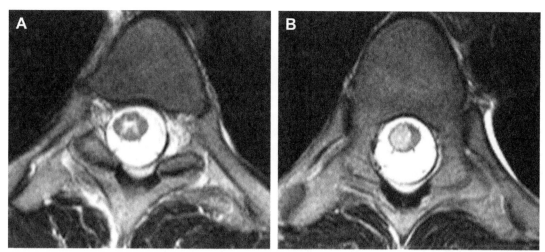

Fig. 4. Axial views of acute myelitis in an anti-aquaporin-4-antibody-seropositive patient. (A) H-shaped T2-hyperintense myelitis at T10 in a 35-year-old woman. (B) Nearly transverse T2-hyperintense lesions at T12 in the same patient.

nausea, and vomiting (IHN), and IHN is often attributable to lesions affecting the chemoreceptor trigger zone located in the medulla oblongata, also known as the vomiting center.[10] In particular, the posterior part of medulla called the area postrema is a well-known region affected in patients with NMO (Fig. 6A). IHN could precede acute exacerbations or relapses of myelitis in some anti-AQP4-Ab-seropositive patients with NMOSD, and thus the patients with IHN must be checked for the presence of the medullary lesions.[11]

Brainstem lesions other than those in the area postrema may be seen in some patients. Such lesions could be seen in any parts of brainstem including the cerebral peduncles (Fig. 6B), cerebellar peduncles (Fig. 6C), and the medulla other than the area postrema (Fig. 6D). Those brainstem lesions are likely to be asymmetrical. Symptoms caused by such brainstem lesions vary depending on the lesion localization, and include hemiplegia, vertigo, dysphagia, respiratory disturbance, and consciousness disturbance.

Diencephalic lesions
Diencephalic lesions, especially those in the hypothalamus, can also develop in a small number of anti-AQP4-Ab-seropositive patients with NMOSD.[12] Such lesions could appear in the regions adjacent to the basilar cistern or the third ventricle (Fig. 7). Diencephalic lesions are likely to appear bilaterally. Various endocrinologic symptoms can develop including syndrome of inappropriate secretion of antidiuretic hormone, narcolepsy, irregular menstruation, and hyperprolactinemia in the patients.

Cerebral lesions
Cerebral lesions other than diencephalic lesions have also been noticed as a part of brain syndromes in anti-AQP4-Ab-seropositive patients with NMOSD. Although the appearance of the lesions is typically different from those in patients with MS,[13] white matter lesions could be seen in roughly half of anti-AQP4-Ab-seropositive patients. These lesions are typically extensive with irregular and indistinct borders (Fig. 8A, B). Although multiple periventricular lesions typically seen in patients with MS are not common in anti-AQP4-Ab-seropositive patients with NMOSD, diffuse periventricular lesions could be seen in some anti-AQP4-Ab-seropositive patients with NMOSD (Fig. 8C).[12] Cerebral lesions in anti-AQP4-Ab-seropositive patients with NMOSD usually appear in the deep and subcortical white matter, but are rare in the cortical gray matter regions.[14] Some patients could show symmetric cerebral lesions (Fig. 8D). Large edematous lesions in the corpus callosum develop in some patients (Fig. 8E), and could cause disconnection syndrome.

Advanced MR Imaging in Patients With Anti-aquaporin-4-Autoantibody

In addition to conventional MR imaging, advanced imaging measures including proton MR spectroscopy, diffusion tensor imaging, magnetization transfer imaging, quantitative MR volumetry, functional MR imaging, and imaging at ultrahigh magnetic field strengths (7-T MR imaging) have been examined in anti-AQP4-Ab-seropositive patients with NMOSD to further clarify the pathology.[15] However, most of those studies were small-scale and each cohort

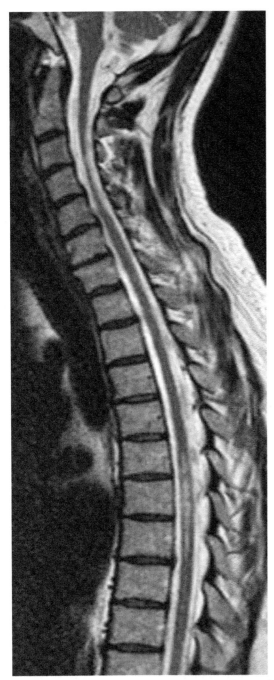

Fig. 5. Spinal cord atrophy in the chronic phase of myelitis in an anti-aquaporin-4-antibody-seropositive patient. T2-weighted image in a 47-year-old woman. Twelve years after myelitis developed at 35 years of age, severe atrophy was seen in the cervical cord. In the thoracic cord, T2-hyperintensity persisted.

included heterogeneous patient groups with respect to anti-AQP4-Ab serostatus. Therefore, the usefulness of advanced MR imaging in NMOSD has not yet been established.

However, some advanced MR imaging measures have been suggested to be promising in considering the pathomechanisms in NMOSD. First, preliminary diffusion tensor imaging and brain quantitative MR volumetry data indicated that the white matter degeneration was greater than gray matter degeneration in patients with NMOSD. These finding were reconfirmed in MR imaging with ultrahigh magnetic field strengths (7-T MR imaging), which showed that nearly 70% of patients with NMOSD had white matter abnormalities. A proton MR spectroscopy study in the upper cervical cord has shown significantly lower *myo*-inositol/creatine values in patients with NMOSD as compared with those in healthy control subjects and patients with MS.[16] *Myo*-inositol is considered to be a biomarker of activity and proliferation of astrocytes. Thus, the decreased level of *myo*-inositol in NMOSD lesions is compatible with severe astrocytic damage in NMOSD proven in the pathologic studies of autopsied cases of NMOSD and remarkably elevated levels of glial fibrillary acidic protein, an astrocyte damage marker, in the cerebrospinal fluids during the acute phase of anti-AQP4-Ab-seropositive NMOSD.

Future studies may increase the significance of advanced MR imaging in patients with NMOSD from the viewpoints of early diagnosis and elucidation of the pathologic processes.

Optical Coherence Tomography Findings in Chronic Phase (>3 Months from Onset)

Circumpapillary retinal nerve fiber layer
Circumpapillary retinal nerve fiber layer (cpRNFL) is the most superficial nerve fiber layer around optic disk. Average thickness of the quadrants (nasal, temporal, superior, and inferior) is usually evaluated. In patients with ON with anti-AQP4-Ab, cpRNFL is often severely thin in the patients with irreversible visual impairment. In the acute phase, cpRNFL is thicker because of inflammation around the optic disk, and thus the value should not be used for statistical analysis. Thinning of cpRNFL in the chronic phase mainly results from irreversible neuronal damage in the optic nerves, and it is used as a biomarker of permanent visual impairment, especially those in the superior and inferior quadrants.[4]

Macular ganglion cell complex
Macular ganglion cell complex (GCC) is a combined thickness of two superficial layers in the macula of retina. Thinning in macular GCC in the chronic phase well correlates with irreversible visual impairment, and thus can be used as another

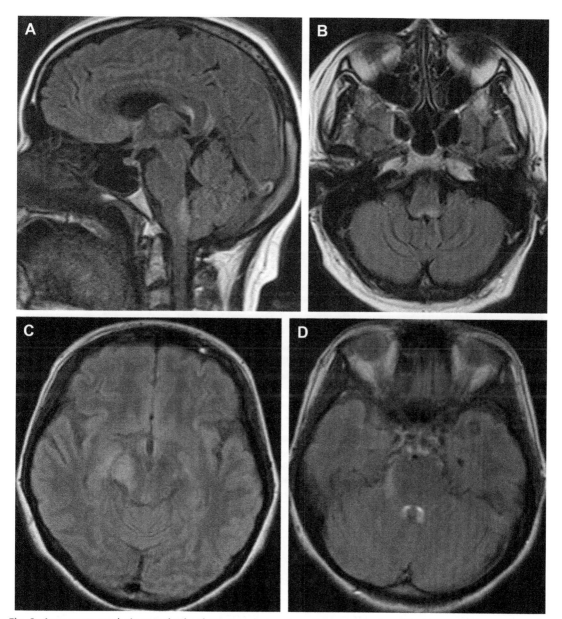

Fig. 6. Area postrema lesions and other brainstem lesions in anti-aquaporin-4-antibody-seropositive patients. (*A*) An area postrema lesion with intractable hiccup, nausea, and vomiting on fluid-attenuated inversion recovery (FLAIR) image in a 44-year-old woman. (*B*) Axial FLAIR in the same 44-year-old patient in *A*. (*C*) FLAIR-hyperintense lesion in the right cerebral peduncle in a 33-year-old woman. (*D*) FLAIR-hyperintense lesion in the pons in the same 33-year-old patient in *C*.

biomarker reflecting irreversible visual impairment. Macular GCC and cpRNFL show a strong correlation in patients with ON with anti-AQP4-Ab. These findings suggest that the thinning of cpRNFL after damages in the optic nerves would soon result in the thinning of macular GCC. Patients with NMOSD with the macular GCC thickness being less than 60 μm are likely to be legally blind (corrected visual acuity ≤20/200).

ANTI-MYELIN OLIGODENDROCYTE GLYCOPROTEIN-AUTOANTIBODY– SEROPOSITIVE NEUROMYELITIS OPTICA SPECTRUM DISORDER

More than 10% of patients with the diagnosis of definite NMO have been known to be seronegative for anti-AQP4-Ab.[17] Recently, in a fraction of the seronegative-patients with NMOSD, serum anti-

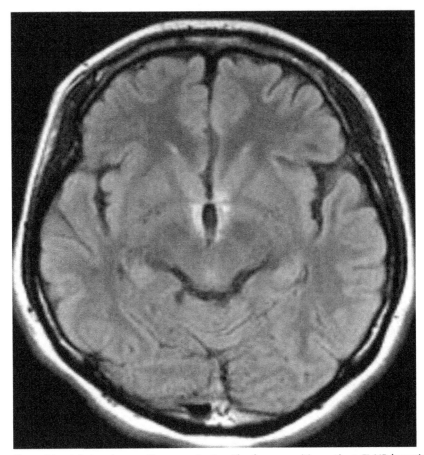

Fig. 7. Bilateral hypothlamic lesions in an anti-aquaporin-4-antibody-seropositive patient. FLAIR-hyperintense lesions were seen in hypothalamic regions in a 32-year-old woman.

MOG-Ab has been detected. As of now, the prevalence of anti-MOG-Ab among seronegative-patients with NMOSD is unclear, because the measurement of serum anti-MOG-Ab by highly sensitive and specific cell-based assays has not yet been widely available. For this reason, the frequency and features of NMOSD truly seronegative for both anti-AQP4-Ab and anti-MOG-Ab are unconcluded. However, clinical, MR imaging, and laboratory features and therapeutic response in patients with NMOSD with serum anti-MOG-Ab have been gradually elucidated.

Anti-MOG-Ab is often proved in serum of children diagnosed with acute disseminated encephalomyelitis, but could be also detected in some patients with NMOSD. The autoantibody injected into the mouse brains caused reversible myelin changes without inflammation, axonal loss, neuronal or astrocytic death,[18] and the changes were independent of complements, which is in contrast to anti-AQP4-Ab complement-dependent cytotoxicity to astrocytes followed by myelin and neuronal damages. In our adult patients seen at Tohoku University Hospital, average onset age in the patients with anti-MOG-Ab is around 30 years old, and is much younger than that in patients with anti-AQP4-Ab (40 years). In the patients with anti-AQP4-Ab, more than 90% are female, but in patients with anti-MOG-Ab, there is no apparent gender difference. In contrast to patients with anti-AQP4-Ab, ON is the most frequent CNS manifestation in patients with anti-MOG-Ab.

The neurologic symptoms seem to be milder in patients with anti-MOG-Ab compared with those with anti-AQP4-Ab. However, if proper treatments were not provided early in the course of the disease, the symptoms of anti-MOG-Ab-seropositive NMOSD could get worse in some patients. Thus, suspecting anti-MOG-Ab-seropositive NMOSD in the early phase would be important for early diagnosis and treatment just like anti-AQP4-Ab-seropositive NMOSD. In this section, we present characteristic MR imaging findings in the acute phase, which would be helpful to doubt the presence of serum anti-MOG-Ab.

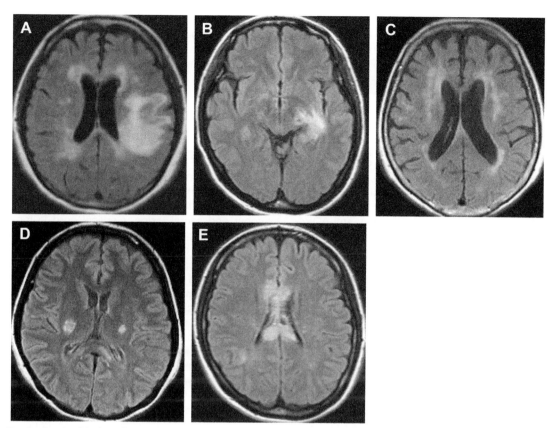

Fig. 8. Cerebral lesions in anti-aquaporin-4-antibody-seropositive patients. (*A*) FLAIR in a 52-year-old woman. Diffuse periventricular lesions were seen and a large lesion in the left brain hemisphere involved the subcortical and deep white matter regions with irregular margins. (*B*) FLAIR-hyperintense lesion in the left deep white matter in a 35-year-old woman. (*C*) FLAIR-hyperintense periventricular lesions in a 75-year-old woman. These lesions are somewhat different from multiple periventricular lesions in typical patients with MS. (*D*) FLAIR-hyperintense lesions affecting the posterior limb of both internal capsules, in a 33-year-old woman. (*E*) FLAIR-hyperintense edematous callosal lesions in a 35-year-old woman.

MR Imaging Findings

Optic nerve lesions

Distribution ON in anti-MOG-Ab-seropositive patients is usually long and severely edematous. In our own patients (16 ON eyes in 12 patients with anti-MOG-Ab), the involvement of the subsegments of optic nerves based on orbital MR imaging is shown in **Table 2** (it should be noted that the optic chiasmal lesions resulted from the intracranial lesions extending into the edge of chiasma and were not the primary ones in any case). Among the 16 patients with ON, 15 patients were without any neurologic episodes other than ON, but one patient showed simultaneous cervical myelitis.

As shown in **Table 2**, the canalicular and intracranial segments were the most frequent involved in ON in patients with anti-MOG-Ab. ON were likely to be longer in patients with anti-MOG-Ab compared with patients with anti-AQP4-Ab, although the visual prognosis was much better in the former group.[4]

Table 2						
Lesion distribution of anti-MOG-Ab-seropositive optic neuritis in the subsegments of optic nerves						
Subsegment	Midorbit	Retro-orbit	Canalicular	Intracranial	Chiasmal	Optic Tract
Incidence (percentage)	13/16 (81.3)	15/16 (93.8)	16/16 (100.0)	16/16 (100.0)	2/16 (12.5)	0/16 (0.0)

The chiasmal lesions were seen only at the edge of chiasma as a result of the intracranial lesions extending into that portion.

A recent report from Australia showed different distributions of ON-lesions in anti-MOG-Ab- and anti-AQP4-Ab-seropositive patients, and the intracranial ON lesions were more frequent in patients with anti-AQP4-Ab than in those with anti-MOG-Ab.[19] The results were a bit different from our data, but the reason is unclear at present.

Optic neuritis lesions in the acute phase As seen in anti-AQP4-Ab-seropositive ON, ON in patients with anti-MOG-Ab often exhibits severe swelling and gadolinium enhancement in the acute phase. One characteristic finding discriminating the anti-MOG-Ab-seropositive ON from anti-AQP4-Ab-seropositive ON is that affected optic nerve becomes tortuous because of severe swelling in anti-MOG-Ab-seropositive ON (**Fig. 9**), which is much less common in patients with anti-AQP4-Ab. All-around contrast enhancement resembling optic perineuritis is also characteristic to ON with anti-MOG-Ab, if present. Frequency of bilateral onset in ON with anti-MOG-Ab is 20% to 40%, which is higher than in ON with anti-AQP4-Ab.

Optic neuritis lesions in the chronic phase Unlike ON with anti-AQP4-Ab, ON with anti-MOG-Ab usually does not cause optic nerve atrophy. Most patients show full recovery in the visual acuity and do not show any abnormal findings in orbital MR imaging in the chronic phase. However, if a patient with anti-MOG-Ab does not receive appropriate treatment, such as high-dose intravenous methylprednisolone therapy in the acute phase, the patients could develop atrophy in the affected optic nerves and irreversible visual impairment. In such cases, affected atrophic optic nerves could show T2 fluid attenuated inversion recovery and STIR-hyperintensity as seen in patients with anti-AQP4-Ab.

Spinal cord lesions
Based on our database, spinal cord lesions were observed in 5 of 16 patients (31.3%) with serum anti-MOG-Ab. All of the five patients showed short myelitis in cervical cord. Two of them also had long-segmental thoracic cord lesions and another patient showed longitudinally extensive lumbar and sacral lesion. Cervical cord lesions were short (**Fig. 10**A, B), but other spinal cord lesions were longitudinally extensive lesions, which could appear at any levels between cervical cord and cauda equine (**Fig. 10**A–D). Because the spinal cord lesions in patients with anti-MOG-Ab also usually lie in the central part of spinal cord in cross section (**Fig. 10**E), they could also present H-shaped lesions, and distinguishing them from longitudinally extensive spinal cord lesions with anti-AQP4-Ab is often difficult.[20] However, spinal cord lesions in patients with anti-MOG-Ab do not usually show severe swelling or strong contrast enhancement, both of which are frequently seen in patients with anti-AQP4-Ab.

Cerebral lesions
Distributions of cerebral lesions vary widely from one patient to another in anti-MOG-Ab-seropositive patient group. Cerebral lesions could appear in any parts of the cortical

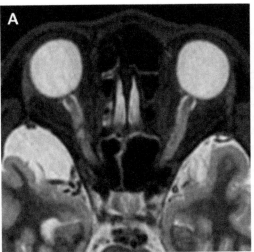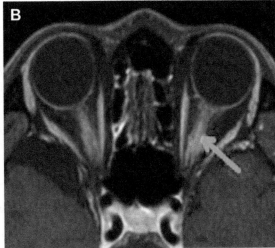

Fig. 9. ON in the acute phase in an anti-myelin oligodendrocyte glycoprotein-antibody–seropositive patient. (*A*) STIR and (*B*) fat-suppressed T1-weighted gadolinium enhancement in a 37-year-old man. Bilateral optic nerves were swollen and tortuous and left optic nerve showed contrast enhancement (*arrow*).

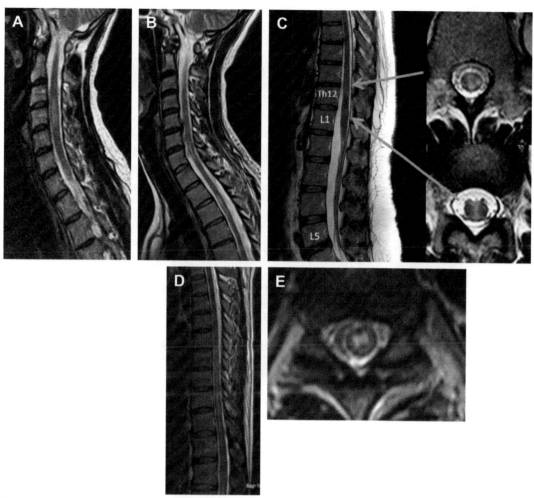

Fig. 10. Spinal cord lesions in anti-myelin oligodendrocyte glycoprotein-antibody–seropositive patients. (*A*) T2-hyperintense lesion at C3-4 with swelling in a 31-year-old man. Distinction between this lesion and antiaquaporin-4-antibody-seropositive myelitis could be difficult. (*B*) Short T2-hyperintense lesion at C7 in a 32-year-old woman. Contrast enhancement was confirmed in this lesion. (*C*) Vague T2-hyperintense lesions in the lower spinal cord in a 29-year-old woman (*arrows*). (*D*) Long T2-hyperintense lesion extending from the lower cervical cord to the distal cord in a 42-year-old woman. Contrast enhancement was not evident. This patient suffered from dysuria in the chronic phase. (*E*) T2-hyperintense lesion at C7 in the axial plane in a 42-year-old woman. In this patient, the spinal cord lesion was centrally located, mimicking the H-shaped central cord lesion seen in patients with antiaquaporin-4-antibody.

gray matter, and in the subcortical and deep white matter areas (Fig. 11A). However, there are some characteristic findings helpful to suspect anti-MOG-Ab-seropositive disease. First, the lesions distributions do not meet Paty's criteria for MS, although some small multiple periventricular lesions could be seen (Fig. 11B). Second, cerebral lesions could develop in the limbic system including the posterior hippocampal region and cingulate gyrus. Pulvinar lesions are also relatively characteristic and were seen in two patients in our series. Most cerebral lesions are asymmetric and ill-demarcated, but some lesions could appear symmetric (Fig. 11C–E).

Brainstem lesions

Brainstem lesions may develop in some patients with serum anti-MOG-Ab. Most brainstem lesions are short and ill-demarcated as compared with brainstem lesions in MS (Fig. 12). Although the brainstem lesions localized at the area postrema are rare, some patients with anti-MOG-Ad develop medullary lesions causing intractable hiccup just like some anti-AQP4-Ab-seropositive patients with NMOSD.

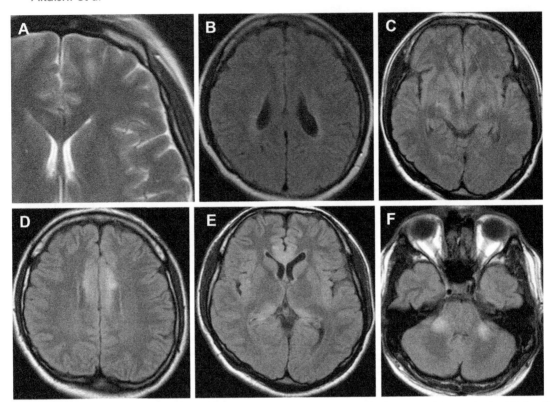

Fig. 11. Cerebral lesions in anti-myelin oligodendrocyte glycoprotein-antibody-seropositive patients. (A) Small subcortical T2-hypereintense lesion in the left frontal pole in a 31-year-old woman. (B) Subtle FLAIR-hyperintense periventricular lesions in a 28-year-old woman. (C) Subtle FLAIR-hyperintense lesions in posterior limb of both internal capsules in a 29-year-old man. (D) FLAIR-hyperintense lesions in bilateral cingulate gyri in the same man. (E) Bilateral FLAIR-hyperintense pulvinar lesions in the same man. (F) Bilateral FLAIR-hyperintense cerebellar peduncular lesions in the same man.

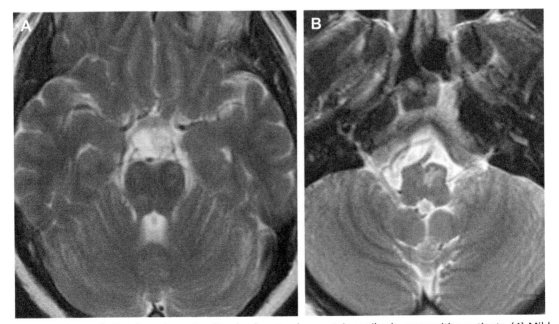

Fig. 12. Brainstem lesions in anti-myelin oligodendrocyte glycoprotein-antibody–seropositive patients. (A) Mild T2-hyperintense lesion in the right dorsal pons in a 28-year-old woman. (B) T2-hyperintense lesion in the left ventral medulla with irregular but relatively clear margins in a 31-year-old woman.

Optical Coherence Tomography Findings in Chronic Phase

Circumpapillary retinal nerve fiber layer

Thickness of the superior and inferior quadrants in cpRNFL tends to be preserved as compared with those in cpRNFL in ON with anti-AQP4-Ab. However, the nasal and temporal quadrants of cpRNFL are thin similar to those in ON with anti-AQP4-Ab.

Macular ganglion cell complex

Macular GCC thickness is relatively preserved (thicker than 50 μm) even in the chronic phase. Thus, the eventual visual acuity is much better in

Table 3
Comparison of the symptomatic episodes between patients with NMOSD with anti-AQP4-Ab and those with anti-MOG-Ab (based on database at Tohoku University Hospital)

	Anti-AQP4-Ab (+)	Anti-MOG-Ab (+)
Total numbers (%) of symptomatic episodes (classified in CNS manifestations)		
Optic nerve	101/360 (28.1)	22/36 (61.1)
Cerebrum	15/360 (4.2)	6/36 (16.7)
Brainstem	43/360 (11.9)	3/36 (8.3)
Spinal cords	201/360 (55.8)	5/36 (13.9)
Optic neuritis		
Sex ratio	Female predominant (>90%)	No difference
Length and distribution	Varied length of ON Intraorbit (>60%) Optic chiasm (>10%–20%)	Much longer Canalicular and intracranial (>90%) Not in optic chiasma
MR imaging appearance in the acute phase	Swelling (+) Contrast enhancement (+)	Swelling (+) Tortuous optic nerves Contrast enhancement (+) in ON lesion and intraorbital fat tissue
MR imaging appearance in the chronic phase	Atrophy (+)	Atrophy (±)
Visual outcome	Poor	Good
OCT	Atrophy (++)	Atrophy (±)
CNS lesions other than ON		
Sex ratio	Female predominant (>90%)	No difference
Onset age	About 40 y on average	In their 3rd or 4th decades
Distribution of myelitis	Cervical–upper thoracic cord Central gray matter	Cervical and/or lower spinal cord (central gray matter?)
Distribution of other CNS lesions	Juxtacortical/subcortical (rare in the cerebral cortex) Hypothalamic Periventricular Basal ganglia Brainstem (area postrema) Corpus callosum Cerebellum	Juxtacortical/subcortical (could involve the cerebral cortex) Pulvinar Paralimbic system Brainstem Cerebellum
MR imaging appearance in the acute phase	Distinct and prominent Contrast enhancement (+) Swelling in spinal cord LETM	Indistinct and vague Contrast enhancement (±) No swelling in spinal cord Varying lengths H-shaped in the cross section
MR imaging appearance in the chronic phase	Spinal cord atrophy (++) MR imaging abnormalities could remain	Spinal cord atrophy (±) MR imaging abnormalities usually shrink
Neurologic disability	Severer (poor prognosis)	Milder (better prognosis)

patients with anti-MOG-Ab than in those with anti-AQP4-Ab.

SUMMARY

Lesion distribution and characteristic clinical and MR imaging findings in patients with NMOSD with anti-AQP4-Ab or anti-MOG-Ab seen at Tohoku University Hospital are summarized in **Table 3** and the findings are essentially similar to the results reported by other investigators. Acute myelitis is the most common neurologic episode in patients with anti-AQP4-Ab, whereas ON was the most frequent one in patients with anti-MOG-Ab. Involvement of both optic nerves is frequent in ON with anti-MOG-Ab, whereas optic chiasmal involvement is common in ON with anti-AQP4-Ab. LETM with severe swelling in the acute phase and severe atrophy in the chronic phase is characteristic in patients with anti-AQP4-Ab. However, myelitis in patients with anti-MOG-Ab is milder with no severe swelling in the acute phase, although they could be longitudinally extensive in some patients. Cervical myelitis is the most frequent spinal cord involvement in both patient groups, but lumbosacral myelitis is common in patients with anti-MOG-Ab. Various brain syndromes can develop in both groups.

The OCT data and ON lesion lengths in both antibody-seropositive patient groups in our cohort are summarized in **Table 4**. OCT data in the chronic phase show the relatively preserved cpRNFL-S and cpRNFL-I in patients with ON with anti-MOG-Ab as compared with those with anti-AQP4-Ab, suggesting the visual prognosis is better in ON with anti-MOG-Ab than ON with anti-AQP4-Ab.

DISCLOSURE STATEMENTS

Dr T. Akaishi reports no disclosures. Dr I. Nakashima has received funding for travel and received speaker honoraria from Mitsubishi Tanabe Pharma Corporation and has received research funding from LSI Medience Corporation and the Grants-in-Aid for Scientific Research from the Ministry of Education, Culture, Sports, Science and Technology of Japan. Dr D.K. Sato has received a scholarship from the Ministry of Education, Culture, Sports, Science and Technology of Japan, a grant-in-aid for scientific research from the Japan Society for the Promotion of Science (KAKENHI 15K19472), research support from CAPES/Brazil (CSF-PAJT—88887.091277/2014-00), and speaker honoraria from Novartis. Dr T. Takahashi reports no disclosures. Prof K. Fujihara serves on scientific advisory boards for Bayer Schering Pharma, Biogen Idec, Mitsubishi Tanabe Pharma Corporation, Novartis Pharma, Chugai Pharmaceutical, Ono Pharmaceutical, Nihon Pharmaceutical, Merck Serono, Alexion Pharmaceuticals, Medimmune, and Medical Review; has received funding for travel and speaker honoraria from Bayer Schering Pharma, Biogen Idec, Eisai Inc, Mitsubishi Tanabe Pharma Corporation, Novartis Pharma, Astellas Pharma Inc, Takeda Pharmaceutical Company Limited, Asahi Kasei Medical Co, Daiichi Sankyo, and Nihon Pharmaceutical; serves as an editorial board member of Clinical and Experimental Neuroimmunology (2009-present) and an advisory board member of Sri Lanka Journal of Neurology; has received research support from Bayer Schering Pharma, Biogen Idec Japan, Asahi Kasei Medical, The Chemo-Sero-Therapeutic Research Institute, Teva Pharmaceutical, Mitsubishi Tanabe Pharma,

Table 4
Comparison of OCT, orbital MR imaging, and the last visual acuity between patients with ON with anti-AQP4-Ab and those with anti-MOG-Ab seen at Tohoku University Hospital

	Anti-AQP4-Ab (+)	Anti-MOG-Ab (+)	P Value
Macular GCC	72.7 ± 16.6 μm	88.6 ± 19.0 μm	.0061
cpRNFL-average	74.4 ± 15.1	100.6 ± 23.8	<.0001
cpRNFL-S	85.9 ± 25.7	123.6 ± 34.7	<.0001
cpRNFL-I	85.3 ± 26.2	131.4 ± 43.5	<.0001
cpRNFL-N	64.4 ± 12.6	80.7 ± 24.4	.0045
cpRNFL-T	62.4 ± 14.8	73.4 ± 20.0	.0288
Number of ON-affected subsegments[a] (mean and range)	2 (0–6)	4 (2–5)	.0199

[a] Optic nerves divided into the following six subsegments: preorbit, retro-orbit, canalicular, intracranial, chiasmal, and optic tract.

Teijin Pharma, Chugai Pharmaceutical, Ono Pharmaceutical, Nihon Pharmaceutical, and Genzyme Japan; and is funded by the Grants-in-Aid for Scientific Research from the Ministry of Education, Culture, Sports, Science and Technology of Japan (#22229008, 2010-2015; #26293205, 2014-2016) and by the Grants-in-Aid for Scientific Research from the Ministry of Health, Welfare and Labor of Japan (2010-present).

REFERENCES

1. Wingerchuk DM, Banwell B, Bennett JL, et al. International consensus diagnostic criteria for neuromyelitis optica spectrum disorders. Neurology 2015; 85(2):177–89.

2. Misu T, Fujihara K, Itoyama Y. Neuromyelitis optica and anti-aquaporin 4 antibody–an overview. Brain Nerve 2008;60(5):527–37 [in Japanese].

3. Ikeda K, Kiyota N, Kuroda H, et al. Severe demyelination but no astrocytopathy in clinically definite neuromyelitis optica with anti-myelin-oligodendrocyte glycoprotein antibody. Mult Scler 2015;21(5):656–9.

4. Akaishi T, Sato DK, Nakashima I, et al. MRI and retinal abnormalities in isolated optic neuritis with myelin oligodendrocyte glycoprotein and aquaporin-4 antibodies: a comparative study. J Neurol Neurosurg Psychiatry 2016;87(4):446–8.

5. Gass A, Moseley IF, Barker GJ, et al. Lesion discrimination in optic neuritis using high-resolution fat-suppressed fast spin-echo MRI. Neuroradiology 1996; 38(4):317–21.

6. Wingerchuk DM, Lennon VA, Pittock SJ, et al. Revised diagnostic criteria for neuromyelitis optica. Neurology 2006;66(10):1485–9.

7. Takano R, Misu T, Takahashi T, et al. Astrocytic damage is far more severe than demyelination in NMO: a clinical CSF biomarker study. Neurology 2010;75(3): 208–16.

8. Nakamura M, Miyazawa I, Fujihara K, et al. Preferential spinal central gray matter involvement in neuromyelitis optica. An MRI study. J Neurol 2008; 255(2):163–70.

9. Hironishi M, Ishimoto S, Sawanishi T, et al. Neuromyelitis optica following thymectomy with severe spinal cord atrophy after frequent relapses for 30 years. Brain Nerve 2012;64(8):951–5 [in Japanese].

10. Misu T, Fujihara K, Nakashima I, et al. Intractable hiccup and nausea with periaqueductal lesions in neuromyelitis optica. Neurology 2005;65(9):1479–82.

11. Takahashi T, Miyazawa I, Misu T, et al. Intractable hiccup and nausea in neuromyelitis optica with anti-aquaporin-4 antibody: a herald of acute exacerbations. J Neurol Neurosurg Psychiatry 2008;79(9): 1075–8.

12. Pittock SJ, Weinshenker BG, Lucchinetti CF, et al. Neuromyelitis optica brain lesions localized at sites of high aquaporin 4 expression. Arch Neurol 2006; 63(7):964–8.

13. Paty DW, Oger JJ, Kastrukoff LF, et al. MRI in the diagnosis of MS: a prospective study with comparison of clinical evaluation, evoked potentials, oligoclonal banding, and CT. Neurology 1988;38(2): 180–5.

14. Popescu BF, Parisi JE, Cabrera-Gomez JA, et al. Absence of cortical demyelination in neuromyelitis optica. Neurology 2010;75(23):2103–9.

15. Kremer S, Renard F, Achard S, et al. Use of advanced magnetic resonance imaging techniques in neuromyelitis optica spectrum disorder. JAMA Neurol 2015;72(7):815–22.

16. Ciccarelli O, Thomas DL, De Vita E, et al. Low myo-inositol indicating astrocytic damage in a case series of neuromyelitis optica. Ann Neurol 2013;74(2):301–5.

17. Jiao Y, Fryer JP, Lennon VA, et al. Updated estimate of AQP4-IgG serostatus and disability outcome in neuromyelitis optica. Neurology 2013;81(14): 1197–204.

18. Saadoun S, Waters P, Owens GP, et al. Neuromyelitis optica MOG-IgG causes reversible lesions in mouse brain. Acta Neuropathol Commun 2014;2:35.

19. Ramanathan S, Prelog K, Barnes EH, et al. Radiological differentiation of optic neuritis with myelin oligodendrocyte glycoprotein antibodies, aquaporin-4 antibodies, and multiple sclerosis. Mult Scler 2015; 22(4):470–82.

20. Amano H, Miyamoto N, Shimura H, et al. Influenza-associated MOG antibody-positive longitudinally extensive transverse myelitis: a case report. BMC Neurol 2014;14:224.

Radiologically Isolated Syndrome

MR Imaging Features Suggestive of Multiple Sclerosis Prior to First Symptom Onset

Darin T. Okuda, MD, MS

KEYWORDS

- Multiple sclerosis • MR imaging • Radiologically isolated syndrome

KEY POINTS

- MR imaging anomalies highly suggestive of inflammatory demyelinating disease may be observed incidentally within the brain and spinal cord.
- Radiologically isolated syndrome (RIS) is established following fulfillment of both clinical and radiological criteria.
- Non-specific white matter lesions are frequently observed as an incidental finding following brain MR imaging and commonly misinterpreted as sequelae from *in situ* demyelination.
- Approximately 1/3 of subjects with radiologically isolated syndrome evolve to experience a first acute or progressive clinical event related to CNS demyelination in 5 years.
- Future scientific efforts in RISH will allow for the development of surveillance guidelines and therapeutic strategies aimed at prevention of symptomatic evolution.

INTRODUCTION

The application of MR imaging within the field of multiple sclerosis (MS) has not only transformed the diagnostic capabilities but also enhanced the clinical management of patients through noninvasive assessments of the optic nerve, brain, brainstem, and spinal cord. In the proper clinical setting, the observation of anomalies within the central nervous system (CNS) may support the diagnosis of MS given the presence of lesions containing distinct radiological features (Fig. 1). In addition, the evaluation of the temporal profile of radiological change may offer insights into the natural history of the disease course or the impact of prescribed agents aimed at modulating disease behavior.

With increased utilization of MR imaging technology throughout the world and improved access by patients, healthy individuals who do not exhibit signs of neurologic dysfunction commonly have brain MR imaging studies performed in the setting of an investigation focused on a medical reason other than for an evaluation for inflammatory demyelinating disease. A disproportionate number of subjects are identified with cryptogenic white matter changes, punctuated by the presence of nonspecific and punctuate hyperintense foci. However, in some cases, the study results reveal lesions highly suggestive of in situ demyelination given their size, location within the CNS, and morphology.

This article focuses on a unique group of individuals who appear to exhibit the first visual manifestation of MS, the radiologically isolated syndrome (RIS). A review of the existing diagnostic criteria, recent scientific advancements pertaining to the study of RIS subjects, challenges faced by health care providers with the interpretation of MR imaging studies containing

Neuroinnovation Program, Multiple Sclerosis and Neuroimmunology Imaging Program, Department of Neurology and Neurotherapeutics, Clinical Center for Multiple Sclerosis, University of Texas Southwestern Medical Center, 5323 Harry Hines Boulevard, Dallas, TX 75390-8806, USA
E-mail address: darin.okuda@utsouthwestern.edu

Neuroimag Clin N Am 27 (2017) 267–275
http://dx.doi.org/10.1016/j.nic.2016.12.008
1052-5149/17/© 2017 Elsevier Inc. All rights reserved.

neuroimaging.theclinics.com

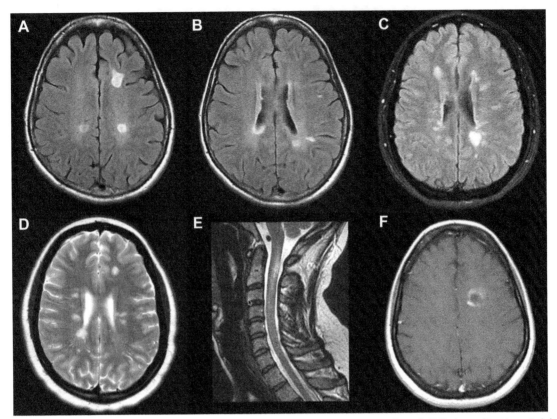

Fig. 1. Incidentally identified anomalies in subjects lacking symptoms suggestive of CNS demyelination. Axial brain MR images (*A–D*) demonstrating multifocal areas of T2-hyperintensity with size and morphology, and with spatial distribution highly suggestive of CNS demyelination. (*E*) Sagittal T2-weighted image demonstrating an asymptomatic focus of high signal intensity at C2-C3. (*F*) Axial post-T1-weighted brain MR image demonstrating an asymptomatic enhancing lesion involving the left frontal lobe.

incidentally observed lesions, and future research opportunities for earlier treatment are discussed.

THE CONCEPT OF PRECLINICAL DISEASE ACTIVITY

Similar to many other chronic conditions, signs of impending disease activity may be appreciated in the months to years preceding a formal diagnosis and, therefore, the observation of incidentally identified structural anomalies suggestive of demyelination within the CNS following MR imaging is expected. Patients clinically evaluated following a seminal neurologic event may demonstrate clear signs of prior disease activity following MR imaging studies of the brain and spinal cord. In addition, the MR imaging study acquired near the time of the presenting first symptom may reveal the presence of contrast-enhancing demyelinating lesions, providing localization for the presenting neurologic complaint, superimposed over a background of nonactive demyelinating foci. To further emphasize features that predate the onset of

disease activity, regional and global brain volume reductions appreciated via conventional imaging techniques may exist, representing features beyond expectations for a stated chronologic age.

Beyond routine experiences among health care practitioners, prior imaging efforts involving asymptomatic relatives of sporadic and familial patients with MS further support the existence of a presymptomatic phase.[1–3] A scientifically beautiful effort involved the use of a mobile 1.0-T MR imaging scanner in Sardinia to assess brain involvement in both first-degree relatives of patients with sporadic and familial MS. Of the 152 asymptomatic first-degree and 88 familial MS individuals studied, focal brain abnormalities with an imaging pattern similar to MS meeting the criteria of Barkhof and colleagues[4] were observed in 4% and 10% of individuals, respectively.[2] Of the 56 healthy control subjects studied, abnormal MR imaging signals were detected in 9 individuals; however, none fulfilled spatial dissemination criteria for MS. The observation of structural changes demonstrating a pattern of distribution indistinguishable from MS supports the existence of preclinical demyelination.

The scientific literature also contains post-mortem data involving large numbers of autopsy cases, highlighting the existence of unanticipated gross and histopathological features supportive of CNS demyelination. Compiling data from 3 large autopsy studies involving more than 34,000 individuals, in which incidental postmortem features consistent with CNS demyelination were identified, a prevalence rate of 0.1% was observed (30/34,194).[5-7] These data indicate a high prevalence rate for those with unanticipated demyelinating abnormality when compared with worldwide prevalence rates of MS.[8] Whether these individuals represent a more "benign" form of MS, or if the extent of inflammation and subsequent axonal compromise within observed lesions is lower as supported by previous observations of higher magnetization transfer ratios[9] and reduced microstructural injury[10] observed in RIS compared with those with relapsing remitting MS (RRMS), or if lesions exist more frequently in noneloquent regions of the brain, is currently unclear.

Overall, data extending from both premortem and postmortem periods affirm the observation of clinically silent disease. However, an acceptable definition and criteria for the identification of such individuals were not available within this era, resulting in greater heterogeneity from described cases. These data are vital when attempting to deconstruct the early events leading to the development of a first lesion within the CNS in addition to identifying differentiating mechanisms for disease behavior between asymptomatic and eventual symptomatic groups.

RADIOLOGICALLY ISOLATED SYNDROME

Specialists involved in the diagnosis and treatment of MS are frequently challenged by requests for consultation for demyelinating disease on subjects with or without neurologic symptoms typical for MS after the detection of unexpected T2 hyperintensities on brain MR imaging. With the expanded use of MR imaging technology in many medical disciplines, the appreciation of incidental anomalies within the CNS is an inevitable consequence of its implementation. Although a disproportionately high number of individuals will be recognized with punctate, nonspecific abnormalities, in some instances, radiological features clearly supportive of MS may be observed when no medical history of neurologic symptoms suggestive of CNS demyelination exists. The serendipitous appreciation of these anomalies is also not limited to adult groups and may be recognized in pediatric cohorts.[11]

The observation of unanticipated structural brain anomalies that appear to be highly suggestive of MS in healthy individuals following a brain MR imaging study is well established within the scientific literature.[12-14] In 2009, the RIS was introduced, and formal criteria were published to better define and characterize a relevant group of individuals who are at risk for future demyelinating events.[14] Included within the diagnostic criteria were requirements for dissemination in space, to increase the specificity for demyelinating lesions within the CNS, and clinical criteria to ensure the proper exclusion of other medical processes that may result in white matter injury. Observed anomalies that were suggestive of MS were greater than 3 mm^2, ovoid in shape, and well circumscribed, with homogeneous signal characteristics within the lesion.[4,15] The observed lesions were also required to be located within distinct regions of the CNS, with placement in the juxtacortical, periventricular, infratentorial regions of the brain, or spinal cord. Clearly defined clinical parameters were also described to ensure a lack of prior clinical symptoms consistent with demyelinating events or the existence of a better medical explanation for the structural anomalies.

The seminal report on RIS reported on 44 healthy individuals who underwent brain MR imaging as a part of a medical workup for headache complaints, trauma, or amenorrhea, or as a control subject for a research study, and so forth.[14] Nearly 60% of subjects were identified as having new or enlarging T2-hyperintensities on repeat MR imaging. In addition, a greater than 3-fold risk of developing more lesions was identified if gadolinium enhancement was observed on the initial brain MR imaging.

Building on the author's previous report, the impact of asymptomatic cervical spinal cord lesions in predicting a first neurologic event was studied.[16] A total of 71 RIS subjects were studied. Over a median time of nearly 2 years, 84% of RIS subjects with at least one cervical spinal cord lesion evolved to experience a first neurologic attack compared with those without cervical spinal cord involvement (7%). An asymptomatic lesion within the cervical spinal cord increased the risk for evolution to a first clinical event related to CNS demyelination (odds ratio: 128, 95% confidence interval 13–1257, $P<.0001$). This work highlighted the clinicoradiologic paradox within the demyelinating field, punctuating the discordance between MR imaging findings and physical function.

Following the proposed formal classification of individuals with incidental anomalies highly suggestive of MS, subsequent imaging studies pertaining to RIS focused on brain volumetric changes,[9,17] cortical involvement,[18] and metabolic differences between symptomatic and asymptomatic groups.[19]

Expanding beyond observations from a single center, a multinational effort was pursued. Retrospectively identified RIS subjects arising from greater than 20 clinical databases from the United States, France, Turkey, Spain, and Italy were included.[20] Of the 451 subjects included in the analysis, the mean age at RIS was identified at 37.2 years (standard deviation [SD]: 11.2 years). The 5-year observed conversion rate to the first clinical events was 34% (standard error = 3%). In the multivariate model, age, sex (male), and lesions within the cervical or thoracic spinal cord were identified as significant predictors for the development of a first clinical event related to CNS demyelination. The risk for first symptom development was more clearly delineated given the presence of any one risk factor or the concomitant presence of multiple risk factors. Another unique observation within those who evolved to a first clinical symptom involved a group of individuals (9.6%) who fulfilled criteria for primary progressive MS (PPMS). The observed findings validated the major premise that a meaningful number of RIS subjects who are asymptomatic for neurologic symptoms typically observed in MS are at risk for a future demyelinating attack while providing evidence of the existence of a subclinical form of PPMS.

Features supportive of early CNS neurodegeneration in RIS are supported by observations from novel imaging studies. In a case-control study involving 63 individuals (21 subjects with RIS and 42 healthy control participants), differences between normalized total gray and white matter volumes were not observed between groups.[21] However, a significant reduction in mean thalamic volumes (0.0045 ± 0.0005 vs 0.0049 ± 0.0004; $P = .004$) was observed in RIS subjects. The reduction in thalamic volumes appears consistent with previous reports in children with MS,[22] those who have experienced a single clinical attack,[23] and relapsing-remitting patients.[24] The demonstrated findings in RIS signify early features of CNS neurodegeneration, even before first symptom manifestation.

Despite advancements in the characterization of RIS subjects,[10,18,19,25] and in the understanding of risk factors for initial symptom development,[16,26] the natural course of such cases and validated risk profiles for a seminal neurologic event, from prospectively acquired data, remain unclear.

RADIOLOGICALLY ISOLATED SYNDROME EVOLVING TO PRIMARY PROGRESSIVE MULTIPLE SCLEROSIS

The observation of a preprogressive phase of MS in which asymptomatic individuals possess incidentally identified anomalies within the CNS that may be indistinguishable from those who eventually present with an acute demyelinating event is intriguing.[20] The development of a clinical symptom, usually a long-tract motor sign, followed by a history of neurologic worsening occurring over a period of at least 12 months with the requisite imaging features is diagnostic of PPMS.[27]

Evaluation of data from a large multinational effort of RIS subjects revealed 153 individuals who experienced a seminal neurologic event within a 5-year period from the first abnormal MR imaging demonstrating unanticipated features supportive of CNS demyelination.[20] Of the individuals who developed symptoms, 15 experienced a first, nonacute, neurologic complaint followed by clinical worsening from symptom incipience.[28] The prevalence of a progressive phenotype was determined to be 11.7%. The mean onset age in these individuals was 49.1 years (SD 12.1 years). Most progressive converters were male patients ($P = .005$) with an older age of symptom onset ($P<.001$) when compared with individuals who experienced acute neurologic demyelinating events. With respect to structural neuroimaging features, a high degree of involvement was observed within the cervical and thoracic spinal cord. All subjects who evolved to PPMS were found to have spinal cord lesions before symptomatic evolution as compared with those who experienced a first clinical event (64%) and those who remained asymptomatic (23%).[28]

The observed incidence of those fulfilling diagnostic criteria for PPMS from RIS appeared to mirror population-based studies.[29] Key clinical markers that differentiated individuals with acute versus progressive phenotypes included a higher rate of abnormal cerebrospinal fluid profiles consistent with CNS demyelination, in addition to presymptomatic involvement of the spinal cord with the observation of gadolinium enhancement before first symptom onset. These data suggest that the MR imaging findings appear similar to imaging profiles in those with relapsing forms of MS before the emergence of secondary progressive MS.

Important questions remain from these findings. Based on the existing data and through future scientific efforts, could those individuals who may be at risk for developing a progressive phenotype of MS from RIS be identified? Would aggressive treatment intervention while individuals are asymptomatic alter the eventual clinical course in any way? Currently, health care providers are faced with unique individuals who present with features supportive of RIS who have profound involvement of the spinal cord (Fig. 2). Despite the degree of involvement within the spinal cord parenchyma, these individuals possess a history devoid of neurologic symptoms related to MS or identifiable abnormalities on neurologic examination. Future scientific initiatives focused on better understanding the mechanisms involved in progression and the development of targeted therapeutics beyond the broad targeting of adaptive immune responses outside the CNS may

transform the approach to the management of these individuals.

COGNITIVE FUNCTION IN RADIOLOGICALLY ISOLATED SYNDROME

The current diagnostic criteria for MS clearly describe both the requisite number and the location of structural anomalies within the CNS following symptoms consistent with CNS inflammatory demyelinating disease.[27] Although clear signs of cognitive dysfunction may be observed in patients with early or long-standing MS, the presence of cortical injury and onset of symptoms may occur even before a first definable neurologic event, highlighting the complexity of symptom

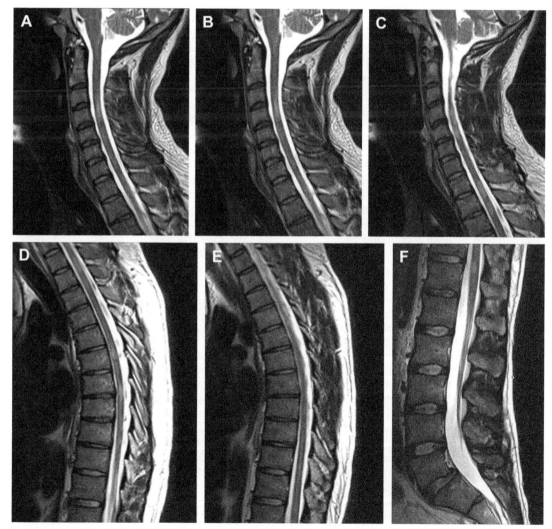

Fig. 2. Sagittal T2-weighted MR images of the cervical (A–C), thoracic (D–E), and lumbar spine (F) from a 37-year-old healthy man with RIS who initially underwent imaging of the brain as part of a medical evaluation for infertility. Multifocal T2-hyperintensities, highly suggestive of CNS demyelination, throughout the spinal cord parenchyma that were not associated with clinical symptoms or deficiencies on neurologic examination.

association with in situ demyelination and influences of potential effect modification.[18]

Lebrun and colleagues[30] reported cognitive performance data on 26 RIS subjects from France. Cognitive performance was assessed, using a French adaptation of the Brief Repeatable Battery, between an equal amount of MS and healthy individuals that were matched for age, sex, and level of education. Cognitive performance was identified to be significantly lower in the RIS and MS groups when compared with healthy controls. Performance deficiencies were identified in the Paced Auditory Serial Addition Test (PASAT-3), phonemic fluencies, digit symbol subtest of the WAIS-R (Wechsler Adult Intelligence Scale-Revised), direct and indirect digit span tests, cross-tapping, and Go-No-Go tests. These findings appeared to be independent of clinical, biological, and features on MR imaging.

Similar results were observed in a subsequent study performed by Amato and colleagues[17] in their study of cognitive changes and relationships between quantitative MR imaging metrics in RIS, RRMS patients, and healthy control subjects. Cognitive performance between 29 RIS subjects, 26 patients with RRMS, and 21 healthy control subjects was performed. In subjects with RIS, 27.6% demonstrated deficiencies in cognition with reduced performance on the PASAT-2 and Word List Generation Test. These cognitive limitations were unrecognized by both RIS subjects along with their family members. In addition, high T1 lesion volumes and low cortical volumes were associated with declines in performance.

THE CLINICAL MANAGEMENT OF RADIOLOGICALLY ISOLATED SYNDROME SUBJECTS

Despite the seemingly obvious health-related concerns of the autoimmune consequences of clinically incongruent CNS anomalies suggestive of MS, the understanding of these findings remains incomplete because of the lack of systematically acquired data within the scientific literature defining risk factors for evolution from RIS to a first demyelinating event. In addition, the knowledge regarding the appropriate recommendations for clinical and radiological surveillance remains deficient, and many patients are managed based on existing practices for those with MS. It is unclear if the frequency of repeat MR imaging studies should mirror the current MS management style or if a more, or less, frequent approach to repeat imaging should be followed. Individualized approaches to treatment would be expected based on the recognition of

significant risk factors alone, or in combination, for future demyelinating events.

A significant number of RIS subjects are being exposed to approved disease-modifying therapies (DMTs) before the development of a first clinical episode despite the lack of scientific data supporting the use of these agents.[20] A substantial body of evidence exists regarding the positive impact of early treatment in relation to clinical outcomes in MS, and intuitively, treating RIS subjects appears to represent a rational approach; however, data pertaining to reductions in disease activity following treatment are unknown.[31–34]

Treatment data from the largest published RIS cohort demonstrated that 16.2% of individuals were exposed to approved DMTs. Insights into the decision-making process and attitudes by both referring health care providers and patients, along with their family members, were unclear.[20] Formalized, well-structured studies designed for breaking new therapeutic ground by assessing the impact of DMTs in individuals with RIS may transform the understanding of the impact of early treatment. Based on the available data, earlier interventions in RIS that may increase the magnitude of improving disability outcomes appear highly promising.

Until clearly defined data pertaining to treatment outcomes in RIS are available, continued clinical and radiological surveillance and efforts to identify a better reason for the observed structural anomalies are recommended. Recommendations may be refined based on a family history for MS, features on imaging, or findings on paraclinical laboratory, eye, electrophysiological studies, or the temporal profile of radiological evolution.

RISK OF INACCURATE CLASSIFICATION

The unfortunate consequence of the high sensitivity of current MR imaging technology is the potential for incidentally observed anomalies to be inaccurately classified as being related to in situ demyelination. Following a referral for MR imaging features possibly consistent with CNS inflammatory disease and after a review of historical elements and diagnostic test data, only a modest proportion of subjects fulfills criteria for RIS because a disproportionately high number of individuals possess features consistent with nonspecific white matter disease[35] (Fig. 3).

Technology aimed to differentiate between demyelinating T2-hyperintensities from other medical conditions (ie, migraine headaches, hypertension) that may be easily incorporated into

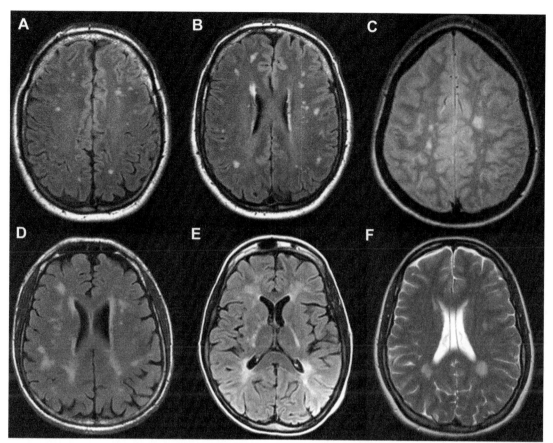

Fig. 3. Axial brain MR images featuring incidentally identified, asymmetric white matter T2-hyperintensities involving the subcortical and deep white matter (*A–D*) and structural anomalies with symmetric characteristics with periventricular and paraventricular involvement (*E–F*). Note that the observed structural features, including the spatial distribution, appear highly nonspecific for CNS inflammatory disease.

MR imaging protocols used daily for clinical application would be of remarkable benefit to health care providers. For now, clinicians are faced with the daily challenges of searching for the cause of the T2-hyperintensities observed when the presenting scan is equivocal or inconsistent with demyelinating features, with knowledge that in 30% to 40% of cases, an associated disorder causative for the observed anomalies may not be identified.[36] A sound and practical clinical approach involving repeat MR imaging investigations along with continued neurologic assessments is of great importance in efficiently optimizing medical management.[37]

It is estimated that a significant number of RIS subjects are being exposed to costly MS therapies that are recommended by their health care providers or from individuals aggressively seeking treatment following research online. These common observations emphasize the need to increase scientific knowledge within the field of RIS, and MS, by improving the specificity for

characterization through an in-depth understanding of the presence of specific MR imaging features, including the extent of involvement within the brain and spinal cord along with the prevalence of baseline demographic and paraclinical laboratory features.

SUMMARY

Future research efforts in RIS relating to the verification of previously identified risk factors and the discovery of other demographic, clinical, radiologic, genetic, or environmentally linked risk factors for a first neurologic attack would significantly impact the day-to-day management of subjects with RIS by reducing the amount of overdiagnosed individuals and exposure to unnecessary tests and exposure to approved DMTs and their associated high costs and risks. In addition, these data will positively impact medical counseling by reducing psychological harm that may occur following discussions around disease classification and potential outcomes. The generation of peer-adopted clinical surveillance and medical follow-up recommendations would also have a direct impact on the clinical care of such individuals. Additional knowledge may further challenge the existing treatment paradigms, providing compelling support for the earlier use of DMTs to prevent onset of a seminal neurologic attack or to prevent the onset of symptoms consistent with PPMS, matching medical approaches to common chronic conditions (ie, hypertension, hypercholesterolemia, diabetes mellitus).

In a time when the knowledge pertaining to clinical and radiological features in the early symptomatic forms of MS have been explored in great detail, the next phase of scientific exploration in MS will focus on those individuals at risk for a first clinical event related to CNS demyelination, symptom development prevention strategies, better radiological classification profiles for demyelinating disease, and scientific efforts pertaining to significant early lifetime events that may be responsible for disease incipience. Dynamic collaborations involving interdisciplinary teams throughout the world will be highly relevant in changing the existing approach to the future management of MS.

REFERENCES

1. Tienari PJ, Salonen O, Wikstrom J, et al. Familial multiple sclerosis: MRI findings in clinically affected and unaffected siblings. J Neurol Neurosurg Psychiatry 1992;55:883–6.
2. De Stefano N, Cocco E, Lai M, et al. Imaging brain damage in first-degree relatives of sporadic and familial multiple sclerosis. Ann Neurol 2006;59:634–9.
3. Lynch SG, Rose JW, Smoker W, et al. MRI in familial multiple sclerosis. Neurology 1990;40:900–3.
4. Barkhof F, Filippi M, Miller DH, et al. Comparison of MRI criteria at first presentation to predict conversion to clinically definite multiple sclerosis. Brain 1997;120(Pt 11):2059–69.
5. Georgi W. Multiple sclerosis. Anatomopathological findings of multiple sclerosis in diseases not clinically diagnosed. Schweiz Med Wochenschr 1961; 91:605–7 [in German].
6. Gilbert JJ, Sadler M. Unsuspected multiple sclerosis. Arch Neurol 1983;40:533–6.
7. Engell T. A clinical patho-anatomical study of clinically silent multiple sclerosis. Acta Neurol Scand 1989;79:428–30.
8. Koch-Henriksen N, Sorensen PS. The changing demographic pattern of multiple sclerosis epidemiology. Lancet Neurol 2010;9:520–32.
9. De Stefano N, Stromillo ML, Rossi F, et al. Improving the characterization of radiologically isolated syndrome suggestive of multiple sclerosis. PLoS One 2011;6:e19452.
10. Giorgio A, Stromillo ML, De Leucio A, et al. Appraisal of brain connectivity in radiologically isolated syndrome by modeling imaging measures. J Neurosci 2015;35:550–8.
11. George IC, DeStefano K, Makhani N. Radiologically isolated syndrome in a pediatric patient. Pediatr Neurol 2016;56:86–7.
12. Lebrun C, Bensa C, Debouverie M, et al. Unexpected multiple sclerosis: follow-up of 30 patients with magnetic resonance imaging and clinical conversion profile. J Neurol Neurosurg Psychiatry 2008;79:195–8.
13. Siva A, Saip S, Altintas A, et al. Multiple sclerosis risk in radiologically uncovered asymptomatic possible inflammatory-demyelinating disease. Mult Scler 2009;15:918–27.
14. Okuda DT, Mowry EM, Beheshtian A, et al. Incidental MRI anomalies suggestive of multiple sclerosis: the radiologically isolated syndrome. Neurology 2009; 72:800–5.
15. Waubant E, Chabas D, Okuda DT, et al. Difference in disease burden and activity in pediatric patients on brain magnetic resonance imaging at time of multiple sclerosis onset vs adults. Arch Neurol 2009;66: 967–71.
16. Okuda DT, Mowry EM, Cree BA, et al. Asymptomatic spinal cord lesions predict disease progression in radiologically isolated syndrome. Neurology 2011; 76:686–92.
17. Amato MP, Hakiki B, Goretti B, et al. Association of MRI metrics and cognitive impairment in radiologically isolated syndromes. Neurology 2012;78: 309–14.
18. Giorgio A, Stromillo ML, Rossi F, et al. Cortical lesions in radiologically isolated syndrome. Neurology 2011;77:1896–9.
19. Stromillo ML, Giorgio A, Rossi F, et al. Brain metabolic changes suggestive of axonal damage in radiologically isolated syndrome. Neurology 2013; 80:2090–4.
20. Okuda DT, Siva A, Kantarci O, et al. Radiologically isolated syndrome: 5-year risk for an initial clinical event. PLoS One 2014;9:e90509.
21. Azevedo CJ, Overton E, Khadka S, et al. Early CNS neurodegeneration in radiologically isolated syndrome. Neurol Neuroimmunol Neuroinflamm 2015; 2:e102.
22. Aubert-Broche B, Fonov V, Ghassemi R, et al. Regional brain atrophy in children with multiple sclerosis. Neuroimage 2011;58:409–15.
23. Henry RG, Shieh M, Okuda DT, et al. Regional grey matter atrophy in clinically isolated syndromes at presentation. J Neurol Neurosurg Psychiatry 2008; 79:1236–44.
24. Wylezinska M, Cifelli A, Jezzard P, et al. Thalamic neurodegeneration in relapsing-remitting multiple sclerosis. Neurology 2003;60:1949–54.

25. Gabelic T, Radmilovic M, Posavec V, et al. Differences in oligoclonal bands and visual evoked potentials in patients with radiologically and clinically isolated syndrome. Acta Neurol Belg 2013; 113(1):13–7.

26. Lebrun C, Le Page E, Kantarci O, et al. Impact of pregnancy on conversion to clinically isolated syndrome in a radiologically isolated syndrome cohort. Mult Scler 2012;18:1297–302.

27. Polman CH, Reingold SC, Banwell B, et al. Diagnostic criteria for multiple sclerosis: 2010 revisions to the McDonald criteria. Ann Neurol 2011; 69:292–302.

28. Kantarci OH, Lebrun C, Siva A, et al. Primary progressive multiple sclerosis evolving from radiologically isolated syndrome. Ann Neurol 2016;79: 288–94.

29. Tutuncu M, Tang J, Zeid NA, et al. Onset of progressive phase is an age-dependent clinical milestone in multiple sclerosis. Mult Scler 2013;19: 188–98.

30. Lebrun C, Blanc F, Brassat D, et al, CFSEP. Cognitive function in radiologically isolated syndrome. Mult Scler 2010;16:919–25.

31. Jacobs LD, Beck RW, Simon JH, et al. Intramuscular interferon beta-1a therapy initiated during a first demyelinating event in multiple sclerosis.

CHAMPS Study Group. N Engl J Med 2000;343: 898–904.

32. Comi G, Filippi M, Barkhof F, et al. Effect of early interferon treatment on conversion to definite multiple sclerosis: a randomised study. Lancet 2001; 357:1576–82.

33. Kappos L, Freedman MS, Polman CH, et al. Effect of early versus delayed interferon beta-1b treatment on disability after a first clinical event suggestive of multiple sclerosis: a 3-year follow-up analysis of the BENEFIT study. Lancet 2007;370:389–97.

34. Comi G, Martinelli V, Rodegher M, et al. Effect of glatiramer acetate on conversion to clinically definite multiple sclerosis in patients with clinically isolated syndrome (PreCISe study): a randomised, double-blind, placebo-controlled trial. Lancet 2009;374: 1503–11.

35. Lebrun C, Cohen M, Chaussenot A, et al. A prospective study of patients with brain MRI showing incidental t2 hyperintensities addressed as multiple sclerosis: a lot of work to do before treating. Neurol Ther 2014;3:123–32.

36. Schiffmann R, van der Knaap MS. Invited article: an MRI-based approach to the diagnosis of white matter disorders. Neurology 2009;72:750–9.

37. Okuda DT. Incidental lesions suggesting multiple sclerosis. Continuum (Minneap Minn) 2016;22: 730–43.

MR Imaging in Monitoring and Predicting Treatment Response in Multiple Sclerosis

Jordi Río, MD[a],*, Cristina Auger, MD[b,c], Àlex Rovira, MD[b,c]

KEYWORDS

- Multiple sclerosis • MR imaging • Interferon • Patient assessment
- Relapsing-remitting multiple sclerosis • Scoring system • Treatment response

KEY POINTS

- Conventional MR imaging measures have been established as a promising tool for predicting and monitoring treatment response, mainly if combined with clinical measures (relapses and disability progression).
- Baseline brain MR imaging scans are required in any patient starting a disease-modifying treatment. Timing of this reference scan should consider the precise onset of treatment and the mechanism of action of the drug that is being evaluated.
- There is a need for additional and alternative MR imaging markers for disease and treatment monitoring leading to an individualized therapeutic approach, including new targets of immune modulation/suppression, neuroprotection, and remyelination.
- MR imaging studies should be performed with at least 1.5-T field strength magnets, using a standardized protocol, and following the technical recommendations suggested in recently published guidelines.
- The data currently available are not sufficient to support the use of volume measures of brain or spinal cord to monitor treatment response.

INTRODUCTION

Multiple sclerosis (MS) is a chronic disorder of the central nervous system in which autoreactive immune cell activation causes a focal and diffuse inflammation, demyelination, and axonal loss.

MR imaging is the most sensitive tool for the identification of lesions that characterize MS, as detected in more than 97% of patients with clinically definite MS. As a result of this high sensitivity, MR imaging has become an essential technique not only in the diagnosis of MS but also as a prognostic marker in the initial phase of the disease, both in relation to the prediction of clinical relapses and the severity of future disability, and contributing to the understanding of its natural history.[1]

[a] Department of Neurology/Neuroimmunology, Centre d'Esclerosi Múltiple de Catalunya (Cemcat), Hospital Universitari Vall d'Hebron, Universitat Autònoma de Barcelona, Passeig Vall d'Hebron 119-129, Barcelona 08035, Spain; [b] Neuroradiology Unit, Department of Radiology (IDI), Hospital Universitari Vall d'Hebron, Universitat Autònoma de Barcelona, Passeig Vall d'Hebron 119-129, Barcelona 08035, Spain; [c] Magnetic Resonance Unit, Department of Radiology (IDI), Hospital Universitari Vall d'Hebron, Universitat Autònoma de Barcelona, Passeig Vall d'Hebron 119-129, Barcelona 08035, Spain
* Corresponding author.
E-mail address: jrio@cem-cat.org

Neuroimag Clin N Am 27 (2017) 277–287
http://dx.doi.org/10.1016/j.nic.2017.01.001
1052-5149/17/© 2017 Elsevier Inc. All rights reserved.

With the approval of a new generation of disease modifying drugs (DMD) for MS, MR imaging is acquiring an important role in monitoring and predicting the efficacy of these treatments, as well as in the detection of opportunistic infections and paradoxic reactions.

MR IMAGING MEASURES
Conventional Techniques

In the study of MS, T2-weighted sequences (T2 conventional, fast T2, T2-fluid-attenuated inversion recovery [FLAIR]), and contrast-enhanced T1-weighted sequences, are considered conventional MR imaging techniques. Despite its limited specificity in determining the pathologic substrate of focal MS lesions, T2-weighted sequences are useful in the study of the natural history of MS. Thus, longitudinal studies have revealed that new lesions appear 5 to 10 times more frequently than clinical relapses, indicating that MS is a dynamic disease even in phases of clinical remission (**Fig. 1**).[2] This progression can be quantified from the number of new or enlarged T2 lesions, or by calculating their volume (lesion load) using semi-automated or fully automated segmentation techniques. These measures commonly are used as a surrogate marker in assessing the effectiveness of new treatments in phase III clinical trials. The increase of this lesion volume ranges from 5% to 10% annually. DMD have shown a significant and sustained reduction in the degree of this increase[3,4] (**Table 1**).

Natural history studies of MS using contrast-enhanced T1-weighted sequences also show that the activity and progression of the disease still exist in phases of clinical stability. Active lesions that enhance gadolinium are more frequent than clinical relapses.[2] A significant decrease in the number of lesions with inflammatory activity has also been observed in clinical trials in patients receiving DMD,[3] and nowadays this measure is used in the monitoring of inflammatory activity in patients receiving these treatments[5] (see **Table 1**).

Brain Atrophy

From all MR imaging techniques that have been used to measure the neurodegenerative component of MS, cerebral volume as an atrophy marker has been proved to be the most robust and feasible for use in clinical studies.[6]

Interest in using brain volume as a marker of neurodegeneration has increased in recent years with the development of new treatments with a potential neuroprotective effect. Brain volume measures are used routinely as surrogate markers of efficacy in clinical trials, in order to analyze the potential protective effect of treatments on the progression of brain atrophy.[7] Brain atrophy, which is detectable even in the early stages of disease, correlates not only with the irreversible disability but also with fatigue and cognitive impairment.[8,9] Global or regional brain atrophy Is currently considered a clinically relevant measure in relation to the progression of the disease.[10] In addition, brain volumetric measures have proved to be robust and sensitive to longitudinal changes, and are also good predictors of patients who develop significant disability progression. The progressive decline in brain volume occurs in patients with MS more rapidly than in healthy persons (**Fig. 2**). It has been reported that the annual rate of decline in brain volume is approximately 0.5% to 1.3% in patients with MS, which is higher than in young adults (18–50 years old), which ranges from 0.1% to 0.3%.[11]

Different studies have shown that the degree of progression of brain atrophy in short periods of time (1–2 years) is a good predictor of the degree of disability in the medium term (8–10 years).[12] In addition, brain atrophy occurs in the earliest stages of the disease. It has been reported that during the first 9 months after a clinically isolated syndrome (CIS) a significant decrease in brain volume occurs in patients who experienced a second clinical episode and thus converted to clinically definite MS (CDMS).[8] In contrast, other reports showed that the progression of brain atrophy

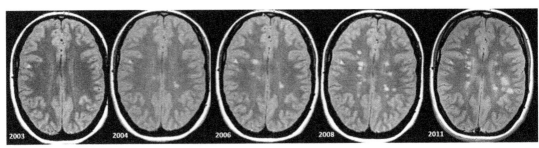

Fig. 1. Proton density-weighted sequences. Serial study for 8 years in a patient with MS showing the progression in the number and volume of focal demyelinating lesions affecting the white matter of the cerebral hemispheres.

Table 1
Clinical and MR imaging results from different phase III clinical trials

Drug	Name of Trial	Number of Patients	Relapses (%)	Disability Progression (%)	Gadolinium Enhancing Lesions (%)	T2 Lesions (%)
Natalizumab (vs placebo)	AFFIRM	942	68	42	92	83
Fingolimod (vs placebo)	FREEDOMS	1272	54–60	31	82	74
BG-12 BID (vs placebo)	DEFINE	1200	53	38	90	85
BG-12 BID (vs placebo, GA)	CONFIRM	1200	44	Nonsignificant	74	71
Teriflunomide (7–14 mg vs placebo)	TEMSO	1088	31	30	80	69
Laquinimod (vs placebo)	ALLEGRO	1106	23	49	37	30
Alemtuzumab (vs IFN-β1a 44 µg)	CAREMS-I	581	54	Nonsignificant	63	17
Alemtuzumab (vs IFN-β1a 44 µg)	CAREMS-II	840	49	42	61	32
Ocrelizumab 600 mg (vs IFN-β1a 44 µg)	OPERA I	821	46	40	94	77
Ocrelizumab 600 mg (vs IFN-β1a 44 µg)	OPERA II	835	47	40	95	83
Daclizumab 150 mg (vs IFN-β1a)	DECIDE	835	45	25–27	65	54

Abbreviations: BID, twice a day; IFN, interferon.

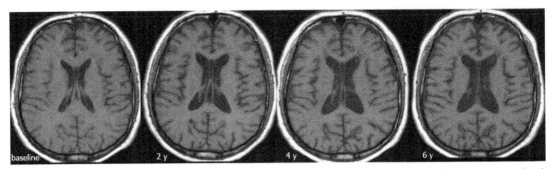

Fig. 2. Unenhanced T1-weighted sequences. Serial study for 6 years in a patient with MS showing progression in the degree of brain atrophy (ventricular and cortical sulci enlargement).

was similar in the different clinical phenotypes of the disease, when these values are normalized based on baseline brain volume.[13]

The regional analysis (white matter and gray matter) of the brain volume has clear clinical implications. In this sense, different studies have shown that selective atrophy of gray matter (cortical and subcortical) has particular clinical relevance, showing a better correlation and predictive value with clinical parameters (development of disability and cognitive impairment)[14] in cross-sectional studies than atrophy of the white matter.

Furthermore, atrophy measures of the gray matter are not influenced by changes in the distribution of brain water produced by the antiinflammatory effect of DMD (pseudoatrophy effect),[15] which makes it especially attractive for analyzing volumetric changes produced in short time intervals. However, these atrophy measures are technically more complex and less robust than global measures of brain volume, especially when used in longitudinal studies, making it difficult to implement in clinical trials.[6]

Brain volume measures could be considered as markers of treatment effect on disability, as revealed in a recent meta-analysis showing that the effect of immunomodulatory drugs on disability can be predicted through the effect produced on the progression of brain atrophy and development of new focal lesions.[16]

PROGNOSTIC VALUE OF BASELINE MR IMAGING

Conventional MR imaging measures, such as T2 lesion volume/number, do not fully correlate with clinical measures of disability in patients with MS, but there is growing evidence that MR imaging at the onset of the disease may serve as a prognostic marker of disability accumulation.[17]

A follow-up study of 20 years showed that the presence of T2 lesions in the baseline MR imaging

studies obtained in patients with a CIS was associated with conversion to CDMS, whereas 79% of patients with CIS and normal baseline brain MR imaging did not convert after 20 years of follow-up.[18] This study also showed that the number of lesions in T2 at baseline was associated, although weakly, with the progression of disability, whereas this relationship was stronger when the increase in lesion volume during the first years after the CIS was considered.[18] Subsequent studies showed that, in patients with CIS, it is not only the number of lesions detected that has prognostic relevance but also its topography. Thus, infratentorial lesions are significant, because the presence of at least 1 cerebellar lesion is related to a higher rate of conversion to CDMS, and the presence of at least 1 lesion in the brainstem correlates with an increased risk of conversion and also disability progression.[19] Another study also suggests that the presence of at least 2 infratentorial lesions in patients with CIS has a high value in predicting disability in the long term.[20]

Histopathologic and MR imaging studies have established that cortical lesions in MS are frequent in all disease phenotypes, especially in progressive MS, and have clinical relevance, because their presence and increase not only predict the risk of conversion in patients with an isolated neurologic syndrome[21] but are correlated with the degree and progression of neurologic and cognitive impairment.[22–25] Despite the diagnostic and prognostic relevance of the detection of cortical lesions, the MR imaging techniques that are currently available are not sufficiently precise for its recognition. The recognition of cortical lesions is still low even with the use of sequences such as double inversion recovery or phase-sensitive inversion recovery.[26–28] Moreover, their interpretation is subject to great variability, limiting their use in clinical practice, especially in the analysis of new cortical lesions in longitudinal studies.[29]

In the same way, the presence of spinal cord lesions, in addition to infratentorial and gadolinium-enhancing lesions, predicts the level of disability in patients who converted to CDMS after 6 years of follow-up.[30] Another study in patients with CIS who had a spinal cord syndrome showed that a large number of spinal lesions at the baseline predicts poor clinical outcome.[31] More recently, another article reported that patients with early relapsing-remitting forms of MS (RRMS) that showed a diffuse pattern of injury in the spinal cord reached high disability levels compared with patients without this pattern.[32] All these studies indicate that the presence and extent of lesions detected with MR imaging in the spinal cord in the early stages of the disease confer a poor outcome.

Different studies have shown the presence of cervical spinal cord atrophy in MS, even in the early stages of disease[33] (Fig. 3). This finding, which reflects demyelination and axonal loss, has a strong relationship with neurologic disability.[34] At present, there are tools that automatically quantify the degree of atrophy of the cervical cord and are also able to detect changes in this area. Moreover, these changes in spinal cord progress faster than brain changes.[13,35] The cervical spinal cord atrophy is starting to be used as a marker in clinical trials testing the efficacy of new treatments, and as a measure to monitor the progression of the disease.

EVALUATION OF TREATMENT RESPONSE

Patients with MS who continue to experience clinical or radiological disease activity despite being under DMD treatment are classified as nonresponders.[36–39] Early identification of nonresponders allows an immediate change to a more effective treatment. However, identifying the patients who will not respond to these treatments, and to what extent, it is still an unresolved challenge.

Early Prediction

Some evidence suggests that certain demographic variables at baseline, such as age at treatment onset, clinical activity (including duration of the disease at treatment onset and relapse rate before treatment), and radiological activity (lesion volume at baseline and number of new T2 lesions or gadolinium-enhancing lesions), can help to identify the patients who will benefit from early treatment, and who will have a poor response.[36,40] However, studies that have analyzed cohorts who received different formulations of beta-interferons (IFN-β) have not produced consistent results, and have failed to predict adequately the response to treatment in daily clinical practice.

Another approach for predicting response to treatment is to analyze the clinical and radiological variables that occur after initiation of treatment. Several studies have attempted to define criteria and strategies for early identification of suboptimal response in patients through a combination of clinical and MR imaging measures during the first 6 to 12 months after the start of treatment.[37,38,41–45] These criteria are partially or fully based on detecting clinical activity (relapses and/or progression)

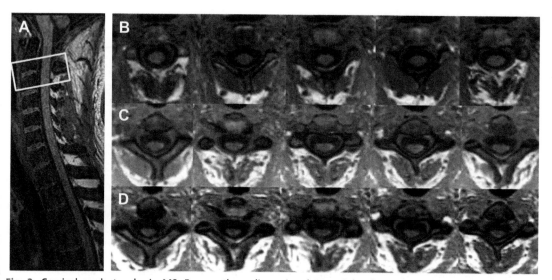

Fig. 3. Cervical cord atrophy in MS. From a three-dimensional T1-weighted sequence obtained in the sagittal plane (A), reformatted transverse images centered at C2-C3 level (*yellow rectangle*) were obtained and used to measure the cross-sectional area. Note a normal area in a healthy patient (B), and reduced area in patients with MS and moderate (C) or marked (D) disability.

and/or radiological activity defined as enhancing T1, or new/enlarged T2 lesions compared with a previous study usually obtained immediately before the start treatment (Table 2). Active lesions (enhancing or new/enlarged T2) are grouped into a single measure. These 2 radiological variables have significant differences. The contrast-enhancing lesions are considered as markers of blood-brain barrier impairment, which has been associated with the presence of perivascular inflammation in patients with MS. The new T2 lesions just reflect the irreversible imprint of a focal inflammatory lesion that developed in the interval between 2 MR imaging scans. Therefore, 2 important factors must be taken into account when interpreting the finding of new T2 lesions: the time point when the baseline scan (pretreatment) was performed, and the mechanism of action of the drug evaluated. In this sense, note that some drugs, such as glatiramer acetate, require up to 6 months to be effective. Therefore, the presence of new T2 lesions in studies with a follow-up of 6 to 12 months does not necessarily reflect a suboptimal response because it could only reflect the activity of the disease during the period before the treatment became effective. This effect could explain the results of a recent study in which patients who presented new T2 lesions in the first months of treatment with glatiramer acetate without clinical relapses or progression did not experience a significant risk of new clinical activity

in the ensuing years.[46] Therefore, in assessing clinical response to therapies other than IFN-β, the significance of the appearance of new lesions on T2 imaging may be related to its mechanism of action. Consequently, therapeutic algorithms on treatment response in patients receiving IFN-β are not necessarily able to be extrapolated to patients receiving other drugs. Thus, some experts have proposed that the reference MR imaging scan should be done 3 to 6 months after the onset of treatment to avoid a bias related to the mechanisms of action of the different drugs.[44,46]

Monitoring Treatment Response

Current immunomodulatory treatments are only partially effective, so detection of active lesions in follow-up studies is an expected outcome in patients who are on treatment.

The identification of gadolinium-enhancing lesions is simpler and more reproducible than the new T2 lesions, and is also less dependent on technical factors, such as the acquisition parameters and anatomic repositioning of serial MR imaging studies. In addition, some new T2 lesions can be visually detected only after being identified on T1-weighted sequences after gadolinium administration, because of their small size or their location in areas with lesional confluence. However, detection of active lesions is not exclusively based on the detection of enhancing lesions because the

Table 2
MR imaging criteria to predict treatment response

Criterion	Outcome Measure	Result
Three or more active lesions in 1 y[42]	Disability progression over 3 y	OR 8.3 71% sensitivity 71% specificity
3 or more active and ≥1 relapse of ≥1 point confirmed EDSS score increase in 1 y (Rio score ≥2)[26]	Relapse rates and/or disability progression over 3 y	OR 3.3–9.8 for relapses OR 6.5–7.1 for progression
Modified Rio score ≥2 y, >5 new T2 lesions plus 1 relapse; or >1 relapse[31]	Relapse rates and/or disability progression over 4 y	24% sensitivity 97% specificity
≥1 relapse and ≥9 T2 lesions or ≥1 enhancing lesion[32]	Relapse rates and/or disability progression over 4 y	34% sensitivity 90% specificity
≥1 relapse or ≥1 enhancing lesion[32]	Relapse rates and/or disability progression over 4 y	68% sensitivity 80% specificity
≥1 enhancing lesion or ≥2 new T2 lesions[32]	Relapse rates and/or disability progression over 4 y	61% sensitivity 83% specificity

All included patients were treated with IFN-β.
Abbreviations: EDSS, Expanded Disability Status Scale; OR, odds ratio.

enhancement lasts approximately 3 weeks,[47] and, considering that the intervals in which serial MR imaging studies are performed are longer (often obtained on an annual basis in clinical practice), most of them are not detected. Therefore, the combination of gadolinium-enhancing lesions and new or enlarged T2 lesions is the more sensitive strategy for detecting MR imaging disease activity.

Detection of active T2 lesions may also be limited by interobserver variability.[48] Techniques of coregistration and subtraction in MR imaging studies obtained twice can minimize this limitation (**Fig. 4**), and although recent data have shown that this automated identification of new T2 lesions is robust, accurate, and sensitive, supporting its use to evaluate treatment efficacy in clinical trials,[49] it is a technique that is not yet available for use in clinical practice.

The predictive value of MR imaging activity in the long term is more robust in patients with RRMS under treatment than in those who are not. A recent study showed that the number of enhancing lesions in patients treated with IFN-β was the best predictor of disability increase measured by the Expanded Disability Status Scale (EDSS).[50] During the first year of treatment with IFN-β, the presence of enhancing T1 or new T2 lesions was significantly associated with an increased risk of relapses and progression of disability.[37,42,43] It has been estimated that the risk of progression of EDSS is higher in those patients who develop a higher number of new T2 lesions during the first year of treatment. Likewise, after 15 years of follow-up of the patients enrolled in the pivotal trial with intramuscular IFN-β, the activity of the disease in the first 2 years of treatment was strongly associated with a more severe long-term disability (odds ratio 8.96 for 2 or more lesions with gadolinium enhancement, 2.90 for more than 2 new T2 lesions, and 4.44 for the presence of more than 1 relapse).[50] Also, a recent systematic review showed that the activity of the disease in the first 6 to 24 months of treatment with IFN-β defined by 2 or more new T2 lesions or enhancing lesions was predictive of treatment failure and progression of the disability.[51]

Obviously, the accumulation of new T2 lesions during treatment is not desirable. However, several published studies differ in determining the number of active lesions detected by MR imaging required for defining substantial disease activity. This cutoff is frequently subjective in clinical practice. The available data, based on a 2-year placebo-controlled trial, set the cutoff for MR imaging lesions as the median in the placebo group, which is 3 or more new T2 lesions during the trial.[52] Thus, minor changes (<3 new T2 lesions) did not seem to be clearly associated with a poor prognosis in the short and long term. This same cutoff was also used in a recent study that analyzed a large data set of patients with RRMS on IFN-β treatment to define substantial MR imaging activity.[53] Substantial MR imaging activity, particularly if in combination with clinical relapses, during the first year of treatment with IFN-β indicates significant risk of treatment failure and EDSS worsening in the short term.

In a recent systematic review analyzing the role of MR imaging in the evaluation of response to treatment with IFN-β, the pooled data of new T2 lesions showed no statistical significance for patients who accumulate only 1 new T2 lesion.[51] However, there is increasing evidence about the relationship between the number of new T2 lesions during the first months of treatment and an increased risk of treatment failure.[43]

Given the increasing therapeutic options for MS in recent years, and considering that the presence of disease activity may be associated with poor

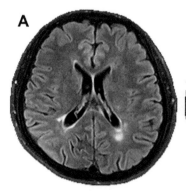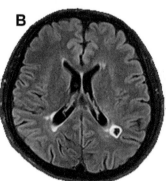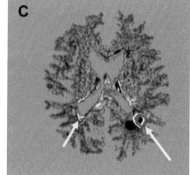

Fig. 4. Automated identification of new T2 lesions. Two T2-FLAIR images obtained at different time points (*A, B*) were coregistered and subtracted to facilitate the identification of new lesions (*arrows* in *C*).

long-term prognosis, it is desirable to maintain patients completely free of activity. However, there is insufficient evidence to establish the minimum number of new T2 lesions during treatment that confers a risk of poor long-term prognosis. In addition, this number may vary depending on the type of treatment used in the patient, and also by the MR imaging technique and the time intervals used in the MR imaging acquisition.

Scoring Systems

Different scoring methods based on the combination of clinical and radiological measures for identifying patients with suboptimal response to DMD have been proposed. Moreover, these criteria have been developed almost exclusively in patients treated with IFN-β and there are limited data in patients treated with other drugs (Table 3).

Initially, the Canadian MS Working Group (CMSWG) proposed the combined use of different parameters of disease activity for predicting response to treatment.[44] The CMSWG describe a model based on different levels of disability progression, the presence of relapses, and MR imaging activity during treatment, which are classified with different levels of concern. Although this method does not provide quantitative principles for treatment changes, it was able to identify groups of nonresponders.

In a later study, based on patients who were treated with IFN-β for longer than 1 year, the investigators proposed a more quantitative version of the response to treatment.[37] This scoring system was based on the presence of clinical relapses, EDSS worsening, and active lesions on MR imaging after 1 year of treatment. Patients who were positive for at least 2 out of the 3 criteria analyzed (presence of at least 1 relapse, increase of at least 1 EDSS point, and the presence of at least 3 active lesions) after the first year of treatment with IFN-β had a significant risk of experiencing further progression of disability or new relapses during the next 2 years. Patients at risk were therefore candidates to modify treatment. This scoring system was named the Rio score (RS). A later study proposed a simplified version of the RS (the Modified Rio score [MRS]).[42] This new scale was based on an analysis of the treatment groups in the Prevention of Relapses and Disability by Interferon Beta-1a Subcutaneously in Multiple Sclerosis (PRISMS) study involving 365 patients with RRMS who were treated with 2 doses of subcutaneous IFN-β1a. Based on this analysis, the investigators found that new T2 lesions and relapses during the first year of treatment were able to explain the overall effect of the treatment on the progression of disability in the ensuing years. Cutoff values for the number of relapses and the number of new T2 lesions during the first year of treatment were established by statistical modeling (see Table 3). The results of this analysis were validated in a separate data set, which was used for the development of the scale of the original RS. The MRS also categorizes patients into 3 risk categories. The probability of disability progression was 24% in the low-risk group, 33% in the medium-risk group, and 65% in the high-risk group.

With the introduction of more effective treatments, there has been a change in expectations in the response to treatment. Nowadays, there is an idea based on the absolute absence of evident disease activity (no evidence of disease activity [NEDA]) as the response criterion that is the new target of treatments.[45] However, the clinical significance of NEDA, defined as no clinical activity (relapses, disability progression) and MR imaging activity (active lesions), remains to be elucidated, because the proportion of patients maintaining a state of NEDA in the medium term is low, even

Table 3
Rio score and Modified Rio score

Rio Score[26]		Modified Rio Score[31]	
Criterion	Change in First Year	Criterion	Change in First Year
Criterion MR imaging = 0	≤2 active lesions	Criterion MR imaging = 0	≤5 new T2 lesions
Criterion MR imaging = 1	>2 active lesions	Criterion MR imaging = 1	>4 new T2 lesions
Criterion relapse = 0	No relapses	Criterion relapse = 0	No relapses
Criterion relapse = 1	≥1 relapse	Criterion relapse = 1	1 relapse
		Criterion relapse = 2	≥2 relapses
Criterion EDSS = 0	<1 EDSS point	Criterion EDSS = 0	Not included
Criterion EDSS = 1	≥1 EDSS point	Criterion EDSS = 1	

Active lesions = new T2 lesions and/or enhancing lesions.

with the use of the most effective drugs.[5] Therefore, although NEDA seems to be a good marker of efficacy in clinical trials, it does not seem to be a realistic goal in clinical practice.

Advantages and Limitations of Scoring Systems

In clinical practice, neurologists should decide on the best therapeutic approach for the particular patient. In MS, these decisions are based primarily on the presence of clinical and MR imaging activity, although, as mentioned earlier, scientific evidence that sustains treatment decisions is still weak in treated patients. The main importance of scoring systems is to provide quantitative decision rules based on evidence, in which different parameters of disease activity are integrated.

Different scoring systems show acceptable specificity but have a poor sensitivity. Also, although the negative predictive value is high, the positive predictive value is low. These data allow clinicians to predict the patients who will have adequate response, but it is still difficult to fully identify patients who will have suboptimal responses.

Based on these data, the use of scoring systems in MS must be open to improvement through the integration of new and more specific components of the disease. The incorporation of other measures, such as MR imaging brain volume measurement, and other clinical measures, such as fatigue, cognition, and quality of life, could improve the predictive value of these scoring systems.

RECOMMENDATIONS

Baseline measures of brain MR imaging do not predict satisfactorily the response to treatment in clinical practice, but the detection of active lesions in the first months after initiation of treatment does seem to predict treatment response in patients receiving IFN-β or glatiramer acetate.

During follow-up, brain MR imaging should be performed 12 months after starting treatment and compared with that obtained in the first months after starting treatment (reference study) to determine the presence and number of active lesions. The timing of this reference scan is based on the onset of treatment and mechanism of action of the drug used; 3 to 6 months is probably the most appropriate time.

MR imaging studies should be performed in at least 1.5-T field strength magnets, using a standardized protocol including at least T2 and contrast T1-weighted sequences, following the technical recommendations suggested in recently published guidelines.[54,55] In this sense, it is essential that follow-up studies are conducted using the same standardized technique used at baseline studies, and if possible with the same equipment.

The count of active lesions on MR imaging studies should be performed by observers with enough experience to minimize interobserver variability. The use of automated tools improves accuracy and sensitivity in the identification of active lesions, and decreases the variability, although validation studies and technical improvements are needed before these tools can be incorporated into clinical practice.

The data currently available are not sufficient to support the use of volume measures of brain or spinal cord to predict individual response to treatment.

FUTURE PROSPECTS

The role of MR imaging in monitoring MS is becoming more relevant not only in research but also in clinical practice. Different options and therapeutic strategies for patients with MS are moving toward an individualized approach that includes conventional targets of immunomodulation and immunosuppression, and new goals, such as neuroprotection and remyelination. Therefore, they will require new MR imaging biomarkers that allow analysis of the neurodegenerative disease component, being measures of brain atrophy that have proved to be more robust and feasible to use in clinical practice.

However, there is still a need for improvements in both acquisition and analysis of MR imaging studies, in order to increase the sensitivity in detecting cortical lesions and reduce variability in detecting new lesions on longitudinal studies (through automated tools). In the same way, automated tools that are easy to implement and that robustly detect variations in global and regional measures of brain volume should be developed for use in clinical practice. In addition, studies analyzing the possible contribution of spinal MR imaging measures (focal lesions, atrophy) in monitoring the disease should be performed. These strategies in the near future would allow the incorporation of different MR parameters considered clinically relevant for predicting the course of the disease and response to different treatments. Only in this way can MR imaging be considered a true biomarker for monitoring and predicting treatment response in MS.

REFERENCES

1. Miller DH, Filippi M, Fazekas F, et al. Role of magnetic resonance imaging within diagnostic criteria for multiple sclerosis. Ann Neurol 2004;56:273–8.

2. Miller DH. Magnetic resonance in monitoring the treatment of multiple sclerosis. Ann Neurol 1994; 36(Suppl):S91–4.

3. Nixon R, Bergvall N, Tomic D, et al. No evidence of disease activity: indirect comparisons of oral therapies for the treatment of relapsing-remitting multiple sclerosis. Adv Ther 2014;31:1134–54.

4. Sormani MD, Bruzzi P. MRI lesions as a surrogate for relapses in multiple sclerosis: a meta-analysis of randomised trials. Lancet Neurol 2013;12:669–76.

5. Rotstein DL, Healy BC, Malik MT, et al. Evaluation of no evidence of disease activity in a 7-year longitudinal multiple sclerosis cohort. JAMA Neurol 2015;72:152–8.

6. De Stefano N, Airas L, Grigoriadis N, et al. Clinical relevance of brain volume measures in multiple sclerosis. CNS Drugs 2014;28:147–56.

7. Vidal-Jordana A, Sastre-Garriga J, Rovira A, et al. Treating relapsing-remitting multiple sclerosis: therapy effects on brain atrophy. J Neurol 2015;262:2617–26.

8. Pérez-Miralles F, Sastre-Garriga J, Tintoré M, et al. Clinical impact of early brain atrophy in clinically isolated syndromes. Mult Scler 2013;19:1878–86.

9. Radue EW, Barkhof F, Kappos L, et al. Correlation between brain volume loss and clinical and MRI outcomes in multiple sclerosis. Neurology 2015;84:784–93.

10. Filippi M, Rocca MA. MR imaging of gray matter involvement in multiple sclerosis: implications for understanding disease pathophysiology and monitoring treatment efficacy. AJNR Am J Neuroradiol 2010;31:1171–7.

11. De Stefano N, Stromillo ML, Giorgio A, et al. Establishing pathological cut-offs of brain atrophy rates in multiple sclerosis. J Neurol Neurosurg Psychiatry 2015;87:93–9.

12. Fisher E, Rudick RA, Simon JH, et al. Eight-year follow-up study of brain atrophy in patients with MS. Neurology 2002;59:1412–20.

13. De Stefano N, Giorgio A, Battaglini M, et al. Assessing brain atrophy rates in a large population of untreated multiple sclerosis subtypes. Neurology 2010;74:1868–76.

14. Lavorgna L, Bonavita S, Ippolito D, et al. Clinical and magnetic resonance imaging predictors of disease progression in multiple sclerosis: a nine-year follow-up study. Mult Scler 2014;20:220–6.

15. Vidal-Jordana A, Sastre-Garriga J, Pérez-Miralles F, et al. Early brain pseudoatrophy while on natalizumab therapy is due to white matter volume changes. Mult Scler 2013;19:1175–81.

16. Sormani MP, Arnold DL, De Stefano N. Treatment effect on brain atrophy correlates with treatment effect on disability in multiple sclerosis. Ann Neurol 2014;75:43–9.

17. Tintore M, Rovira À, Río J, et al. Defining high, medium and low impact prognostic factors for developing multiple sclerosis. Brain 2015;138:1863–74.

18. Fisniku LK, Brex PA, Altmann DR, et al. Disability and T2 MRI lesions: a 20-year follow-up of patients with relapse onset of multiple sclerosis. Brain 2008;131:808–17.

19. Tintore M, Rovira A, Arrambide G, et al. Brainstem lesions in clinically isolated syndromes. Neurology 2010;75:1933–8.

20. Minneboo A, Barkhof F, Polman CH, et al. Infratentorial lesions predict long-term disability in patients with initial findings suggestive of multiple sclerosis. Arch Neurol 2004;61:217–21.

21. Filippi M, Rocca MA, Calabrese M, et al. Intracortical lesions: relevance for new MRI diagnostic criteria for multiple sclerosis. Neurology 2010;75:1988–94.

22. Calabrese M, Poretto V, Favaretto A, et al. Cortical lesion load associates with progression of disability in multiple sclerosis. Brain 2012;135:2952–61.

23. Roosendaal SD, Moraal B, Pouwels PJ, et al. Accumulation of cortical lesions in MS: relation with cognitive impairment. Mult Scler 2009;15:708–14.

24. Filippi M, Preziosa P, Copetti M, et al. Gray matter damage predicts the accumulation of disability 13 years later in MS. Neurology 2013;81:1759–67.

25. Calabrese M, Rocca MA, Atzori M, et al. A 3-year magnetic resonance imaging study of cortical lesions in relapse-onset multiple sclerosis. Ann Neurol 2010;67:376–83.

26. Geurts JJ, Pouwels PJ, Uitdehaag BM, et al. Intracortical lesions in multiple sclerosis: improved detection with 3D double inversion-recovery MR imaging. Radiology 2005;236:254–60.

27. Sethi V, Yousry TA, Muhlert N, et al. Improved detection of cortical MS lesions with phase-sensitive inversion recovery MRI. J Neurol Neurosurg Psychiatry 2012;83:877–82.

28. Simon B, Schmidt S, Lukas C, et al. Improved in vivo detection of cortical lesions in multiple sclerosis using double inversion recovery MR imaging at 3 Tesla. Eur Radiol 2010;20:1675–83.

29. Sethi V, Muhlert N, Ron M, et al. MS cortical lesions on DIR: not quite what they seem? PLoS One 2013;8:e78879.

30. Swanton JK, Fernando KT, Dalton CM, et al. Early MRI in optic neuritis: the risk for disability. Neurology 2009;72:542–50.

31. Cordonnier C, de Seze J, Breteau G, et al. Prospective study of patients presenting with acute partial transverse myelopathy. J Neurol 2003;250:1447–52.

32. Coret F, Bosca I, Landete L, et al. Early diffuse demyelinating lesion in the cervical spinal cord predicts a worse prognosis in relapsing-remitting multiple sclerosis. Mult Scler 2010;16:935–41.

33. Biberacher V, Boucard CC, Schmidt P, et al. Atrophy and structural variability of the upper cervical cord in early multiple sclerosis. Mult Scler 2015;21:875–84.

34. Daams M, Weiler F, Steenwijk MD, et al. Mean upper cervical cord area (MUCCA) measurement in long-standing multiple sclerosis: relation to brain findings and clinical disability. Mult Scler 2014;20:1860–5.

35. Lukas C, Knol DL, Sombekke MH, et al. Cervical spinal cord volume loss is related to clinical disability progression in multiple sclerosis. J Neurol Neurosurg Psychiatry 2015;86:410–8.

36. Río J, Nos C, Tintoré M, et al. Defining the response to interferon-β in relapsing-remitting multiple sclerosis patients. Ann Neurol 2006;59:344–52.

37. Río J, Castilló J, Rovira A, et al. Measures in the first year of therapy predict the response to interferon β in MS. Mult Scler 2009;15:848–53.

38. Río J, Rovira A, Tintoré M, et al. Relationship between MRI lesion activity and response to IFN-β in relapsing-remitting multiple sclerosis patients. Mult Scler 2008;14:479–84.

39. Río J, Comabella M, Montalban X. Predicting responders to therapies for multiple sclerosis. Nat Rev Neurol 2009;5:553–60.

40. Signori A, Schiavetti I, Gallo F, et al. Subgroups of multiple sclerosis patients with larger treatment benefits: a meta-analysis of randomized trials. Eur J Neurol 2015;22:960–6.

41. Sormani MP, De Stefano N. Defining and scoring response to IFN-β in multiple sclerosis. Nat Rev Neurol 2013;9:504–12.

42. Sormani MP, Rio J, Tintorè M, et al. Scoring treatment response in patients with relapsing multiple sclerosis. Mult Scler 2013;19:605–12.

43. Prosperini L, Mancinelli CR, De Giglio L, et al. Interferon beta failure predicted by EMA criteria or isolated MRI activity in multiple sclerosis. Mult Scler 2014;20:566–76.

44. Freedman MS, Selchen D, Arnold DL, et al. Treatment optimization in MS: Canadian MS Working Group updated recommendations. Can J Neurol Sci 2013;40:307–23.

45. Stangel M, Penner IK, Kallmann BA, et al. Towards the implementation of 'no evidence of disease activity' in multiple sclerosis treatment: the multiple sclerosis decision model. Ther Adv Neurol Disord 2014;8:3–13.

46. Río J, Rovira A, Tintoré M, et al. Evaluating the response to glatiramer acetate in relapsing-remitting multiple sclerosis (RRMS) patients. Mult Scler 2014;20:1602–8.

47. Cotton F, Weiner HL, Jolesz FA, et al. MRI contrast uptake in new lesions in relapsing-remitting MS followed at weekly intervals. Neurology 2003;60:640–6.

48. Erbayat Altay E, Fisher E, Jones SE, et al. Reliability of classifying multiple sclerosis disease activity using magnetic resonance imaging in a multiple sclerosis clinic. JAMA Neurol 2013;70:338–44.

49. Battaglini M, Rossi F, Grove RA, et al. Automated identification of brain new lesions in multiple sclerosis using subtraction images. J Magn Reson Imaging 2014;39:1543–9.

50. Bermel RA, You X, Foulds P, et al. Predictors of long-term outcome in multiple sclerosis patients treated with interferon beta. Ann Neurol 2013;73:95–103.

51. Dobson R, Rudick RA, Turner B, et al. Assessing treatment response to interferon-β: is there a role for MRI? Neurology 2014;82:248–54.

52. Rudick RA, Lee JC, Simon J, et al. Defining interferon β response status in multiple sclerosis patients. Ann Neurol 2004;56:548–55.

53. Sormani MP, Gasperini C, Romeo M, et al. Assessing response to interferon-b in a multicenter dataset of patients with MS. Neurology 2016;87:1–7.

54. Rovira À, Wattjes MP, Tintoré M, et al. Evidence-based guidelines: MAGNIMS consensus guidelines on the use of MRI in multiple sclerosis-clinical implementation in the diagnostic process. Nat Rev Neurol 2015;11:471–82.

55. Wattjes MP, Rovira À, Miller D, et al. Evidence-based guidelines: MAGNIMS consensus guidelines on the use of MRI in multiple sclerosis-establishing disease prognosis and monitoring patients. Nat Rev Neurol 2015;11:597–606.

Brain Atrophy in Multiple Sclerosis
Clinical Relevance and Technical Aspects

 CrossMark

Jaume Sastre-Garriga, MD, PhD[a],*, Deborah Pareto, PhD[b,c],
Àlex Rovira, MD[b,c]

KEYWORDS

- Multiple sclerosis • MR imaging • Brain atrophy • Gray matter • Biological confounding factors
- Disability

KEY POINTS

- Brain volume decreases can be observed in patients with all disease phenotypes, and seem to proceed at a faster pace in gray matter than in white matter.
- Brain volume measurements are associated with the clinical status of patients and are independently predictive of their clinical evolution.
- Progressive loss of whole or regional brain volume can be detected in vivo in a sensitive and reproducible manner by MR imaging, mainly with the use of quantitative measures acquired by automated techniques.
- Several physiologic and multiple sclerosis–related confounding factors and sources of error related to image acquisition and processing can affect brain volume measurements.
- In spite of encouraging evidence in favor of the use of brain volume measurement as a treatment monitoring tool, confirmatory studies at the patient level are still needed before this can become clinical practice.

INTRODUCTION

The neurodegenerative nature of multiple sclerosis (MS) was reappraised in 2 studies published in the late 1990s, in which an immediate connection between the inflammatory process and axonal loss was confirmed,[1,2] providing a strong rationale for the use of the antiinflammatory therapies that had been widely shown to affect clinical outcomes in MS trials. Axonal loss, and as a consequence brain tissue loss, had previously been considered mostly as the final outcome of the long-standing inflammatory damage to myelin and, therefore, a pathologic process that could only be seen and measured at the very late stages of MS. In parallel, the first MR imaging studies performed in patients with MS to measure the magnitude of brain atrophy already showed significant atrophy evolution over short periods of time and clinical correlations of atrophy changes.[3] Altogether, brain atrophy became attractive from the clinical point of view and measurable from the technical perspective and so research interest in this area increased exponentially. In consequence, in the last 20 years, a growing number of studies have further increased the knowledge of the neurodegenerative phenomenon in MS through MR imaging

[a] Department of Neurology/Neuroimmunology, Centre d'Esclerosi Múltiple de Catalunya (Cemcat), Hospital Universitari Vall d'Hebron, Universitat Autònoma de Barcelona, Passeig Vall d'Hebron 119-129, Barcelona 08035, Spain; [b] Neuroradiology Unit, Department of Radiology (IDI), Hospital Universitari Vall d'Hebron, Universitat Autònoma de Barcelona, Passeig Vall d'Hebron 119-129, Barcelona 08035, Spain; [c] Magnetic Resonance Unit, Department of Radiology (IDI), Hospital Universitari Vall d'Hebron, Universitat Autònoma de Barcelona, Passeig Vall d'Hebron 119-129, Barcelona 08035, Spain
* Corresponding author.
E-mail address: jsastre-garriga@cem-cat.org

Neuroimag Clin N Am 27 (2017) 289–300
http://dx.doi.org/10.1016/j.nic.2017.01.002

volumetric techniques; a succinct summary of the evidence gathered to date is presented later.

BRAIN ATROPHY IN MULTIPLE SCLEROSIS: A PATHOLOGIC PROCESS

Even though brain volume loss occurs naturally in healthy people and it is regionally variable,[4] pathologic changes well beyond what is seen in controls have been observed in many studies in patients with MS of different phenotypes.[5–8] In those studies it was early observed that not only white but also gray matter was also importantly affected, thus challenging the earlier concept of MS being fundamentally a white matter disease and in accordance with contemporaneous pathology work.[9] Posterior studies have shown,[10,11] using different methods, that such changes seem to be more relevant in certain gray matter areas, including the basal ganglia bilaterally, the precentral and postcentral regions bilaterally, and the cingulate bilaterally.[10] Overall, it has been well established that pathologic brain volume decreases can be observed in patients with MS, of all disease phenotypes, and that those losses are not uniformly widespread but mostly caused by tissue damage in particular gray matter regions.

NATURAL HISTORY OF BRAIN ATROPHY IN MULTIPLE SCLEROSIS

In accordance with cross-sectional research, many studies have shown that the rate of brain volume loss is also higher in patients with MS compared with healthy controls[12] soon after disease onset.[13–15] In this regard, a large study[16] indicated that brain volume loss seems to proceed at a similar pace in patients with clinically isolated syndromes compared with those with progressive (primary and secondary) forms of MS, challenging the view that brain tissue loss only occurred as a late neurodegenerative phenomenon in this disease and in accordance with the pathologic studies mentioned before.[1,2] Longitudinal studies have also shown, in all clinical subtypes of MS, that measurable tissue loss seems to proceed at a faster pace in gray matter compared with white matter.[13–15,17] In these studies it was also shown that the degree of inflammation affects white matter volume measurements in a way that increased inflammation produces spurious increases in white matter volume and that gray matter volume changes seem to be independent of the amount of white matter lesions and of changes in their volume.

A recent study has tried to obtain a cutoff for the rate of brain tissue loss that may be useful to differentiate patients with MS from healthy individuals.[18] In this study, 207 patients with different clinical phenotypes (relapsing-remitting, secondary, and primary progressive) showed an annualized percentage brain volume change of −0.57% compared with −0.27% in healthy controls. The cutoff point to maximize discrimination between both groups was −0.37%, with a sensitivity of 67% and a specificity of 80%. However, application of such cutoff at an individual level remains challenging.

CLINICAL RELEVANCE OF BRAIN ATROPHY IN MULTIPLE SCLEROSIS: CONCURRENT AND PREDICTIVE VALUE

From the early studies, clinical associations of brain volume measurements were evident.[3] Losseff and colleagues[3] described, in a group of 26 patients with relapsing-remitting and secondary progressive MS, a significant difference in brain volume loss between those with definite disability progression, measured with the Expanded Disability Status Scale (EDSS), and those without, favoring the latter. Posterior studies have shown this to be applicable to all disease phenotypes, early from disease course and for different clinically relevant disease end points. Early in the disease evolution, Pérez-Miralles and colleagues[19] showed that brain volume loss in the first 9 months after a first attack of MS is associated with the presence of a second attack in the short to medium term and Di Filippo and colleagues[20] showed that brain volume loss in the first year after a first attack was associated with disability after 6 years. Note that the role of gray matter volume loss seems to be central for these correlations, as was shown by Dalton and colleagues,[13] and more recently by Pérez-Miralles and colleagues.[19] Even before any clinical symptom has appeared, recent evidence suggests that brain volume may already be associated with cognitive performance on formal neuropsychological testing, as shown by Amato and colleagues[21]; this study also showed a significant decrease in the brain volumes in this group of extremely early patients compared with healthy individuals. Significant associations between clinical findings and brain volume changes both globally and for gray matter have been shown in many studies not only for global quantitative measures but also using regionally specific techniques.[10]

From a clinical point of view, it is of utmost importance to show whether brain volumetry techniques may predict disease evolution. This importance has been shown by several studies from early in the disease course[19] but, most importantly, their added predictive value to other clinical and radiological parameters has also been confirmed in natural history studies. In particular, Popescu and colleagues,[22] using a large, multicenter, longitudinal, clinical-radiological data set, showed that brain volume loss and lesion volume changes over 1 year were predictive of EDSS status 10 years later. Another large multicenter data set of patients with primary progressive MS also showed the complementary value of lesion parameters and whole-brain volume changes to predict EDSS status after 5[23] and 10[24] years of follow-up.

In summary, brain volume measurements, namely gray matter volume estimates, are associated with the clinical status of patients with MS. The clinical relevance of this association is enhanced by brain volume estimates being independently predictive of clinical evolution when considered together with lesion volume parameters.

BRAIN ATROPHY MEASURES AS A TREATMENT MONITORING TOOL

The effect of disease-modifying therapies for MS on brain volume measurements has been tested for virtually all approved drugs.[25] Interferon-beta and glatiramer acetate initially had mostly negative results, but later studies showed a hint of efficacy and, most importantly, an association between clinical evolution on therapy and decreased rates of brain volume loss.[26,27] More recent drugs have also reported brain volume outcomes in almost all placebo-controlled trials, with diverging results, maybe suggesting a differential effect of some drugs on the neurodegenerative phenomenon in MS. Although some drugs have been convincingly shown to decrease the rate of brain volume loss (eg, fingolimod or alemtuzumab), others have shown mixed results (eg, dimethyl-fumarate or teriflunomide) or even negative results (eg, natalizumab).[25] Against this background, the association between brain volume, lesion counts, and disability changes at a trial level has been proved in a meta-analysis including 13 recently performed trials,[28] suggesting that the observed treatment effects on disability progression are better explained when the effects on focal lesions and brain volume are jointly considered. Although technically feasible, the validity of these quantitative measures as surrogate end points for treatment efficacy in clinical practice needs confirmation at an individual level (Fig. 1).

At a patient level, the presence of pseudoatrophy (fluid shifts that result in brain volume reduction with no associated loss of cell structures) is thought by some investigators to be one of the big hurdles to be overcome by brain volume measurements before moving into clinical practice as a useful drug efficacy monitoring tool.[29] The well-known pseudoatrophy phenomenon induced by the antiinflammatory effect of disease-modifying therapies[30,31] has been held responsible for some of the negative findings in clinical trials (eg, interferon-beta or natalizumab), but other drugs have managed to obtain positive results in spite of also showing superiority compared with placebo or interferon-beta in antiinflammatory properties (eg, alemtuzumab or fingolimod). Notwithstanding this phenomenon, a few studies have already suggested the validity of brain volume measurements at the individual level using data from patients treated with fingolimod[32] and interferon.[33,34] Results from these studies again suggest a complementary role of lesion and brain volume monitoring to predict disability status on therapy. At this point, an appropriate threshold for brain volume changes to be considered suggestive of disease breakthrough should be defined for use in routine clinical settings. A similar debate has been going on in determining the best cutoff for new lesion development, with some investigators suggesting that a few new lesions should be accepted[35] and others proposing a zero-tolerance scheme.[36] In line with the zero-tolerance strategy and within the overarching concept of no evidence of disease activity (NEDA), a threshold for brain volume loss has been set at -0.4% per year in treated patients based on research performed mostly in fingolimod-treated patients.[37] In patients treated with interferon-beta[34] a more lenient cutoff has been proposed at -0.86%, allowing for some pseudoatrophy to take place before a consideration of treatment failure is in place. As shown by De Stefano and colleagues,[18] the -0.4% per year cutoff provides a high specificity and good sensitivity to discriminate presence or absence of pathologic brain volume loss, but may not be easily extrapolated to other measurement tools and clinical settings (patients initiating a range of different antiinflammatory drugs).

In summary, in spite of encouraging evidence in favor of the use of brain volume measurements together with lesion counts as treatment monitoring tools, confirmatory studies at the patient level are still needed, including drugs other than fingolimod and interferon, before this can become clinical practice. In addition, studies are needed of the outstanding technical and methodological issues affecting brain volume measurements.

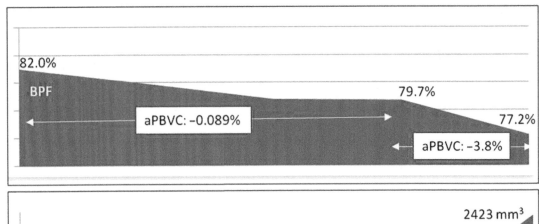

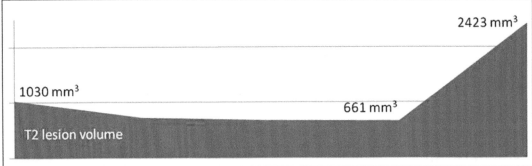

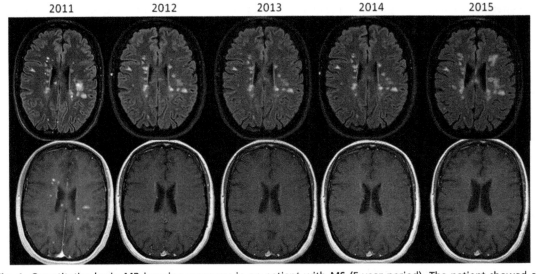

Fig. 1. Quantitative brain MR imaging measures in an patient with MS (5-year period). The patient showed a moderate T2 lesion load and high inflammatory activity at initial diagnosis in 2011. The patient initiated a disease-modifying treatment that halted disease activity and minimized brain volume loss (annualized percentage of brain volume change of −0.089% between 2011 and 2014). In 2014 the patient discontinued the treatment, and follow-up MR imaging in 2015 showed marked increase in T2 lesion volume (from 661 mm³ to 2423 mm³), and acceleration of brain volume loss (annualized percentage of brain volume change of −3.8% in the last year). aPBVC, annualized percentage of brain volume change; BPF, brain parenchymal fraction.

BRAIN VOLUME MEASUREMENTS
Technical Aspects

Progressive loss of whole or regional brain volume can be detected in vivo in a sensitive and reproducible manner by MR imaging, mainly with the use of quantitative measures acquired by automated techniques. These techniques can be classified into 2 broad categories: segmentation-based techniques and registration-based techniques. Segmentation-based techniques enable measurement of whole or regional (eg, gray matter) brain volume at a single time point (Fig. 2), whereas registration-based techniques are able to measure changes in whole-brain volume over time by comparing 2 sets of MR imaging scans acquired at different time points (Fig. 3).

Segmentation-based techniques provide heterogeneous results and are influenced by the quality of T1-weighted images; hence, they are not recommended for longitudinal studies. In contrast, registration-based techniques are sensitive to changes over time and are more robust and less dependent on the quality of MR imaging acquisitions, and therefore are recommended for longitudinal studies. Whole-brain volume changes are now commonly used as a secondary outcome measure in randomized clinical trials investigating the effect of certain drugs on preventing diffuse irreversible tissue damage. However, these registration-based measures are not designed to analyze regional volume changes over time. All these MR imaging–based measures can be affected by different confounding factors related to image acquisition and processing, and to different MS-related and non–MS-related pathophysiologic changes.

CONFOUNDING FACTORS RELATED TO IMAGE ACQUISITION
Head Motion During Image Acquisition

The absence of movement during image acquisition is mandatory for any kind of quantification approach. This requisite still needs to be verified visually, by an experienced observer. A study performed by Reuters and colleagues[38] reproduced, in a controlled way, different degrees of movement and quantified the effect on brain volume and cortical thickness measurements. Lower cortical thickness and brain volumes were found as the displacement increased. The analysis was repeated after removing the scanners that an expert would not consider good enough, because of the movement artifacts, and the association was then no longer significant. Most of the commercial scanners include on-line movement correction strategies, which work only for small displacements. Thus, visual verification of the image quality and presence of artifacts is still required and images that do not reach the standard should not be further analyzed.

Magnet System Upgrade

Stability of image acquisition is regarded as essential for reliability of brain volume measures, with each individual ideally being scanned in the same scanner, using the same software revision and pulse sequence. This approach may be impractical in chronic progressive diseases such as MS, because system upgrades, implying sequence innovations and hardware improvements, are inevitable. Even if the same image acquisition parameters are used, image contrast might change because of hardware improvements. In an attempt to ensure the consistency of the image contrast after a system upgrade, a group of healthy people can be scanned before and after the upgrade so that the parameters can be adjusted and calibrated. Controversial results

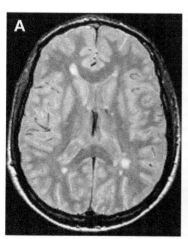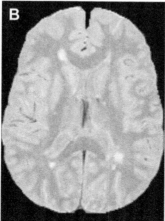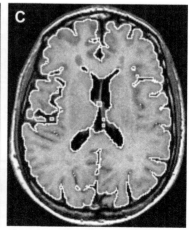

Fig. 2. Brain volume determined from a single scan using contoured surfaces. In this automated pipeline a proton density–weighted sequence (A) was used to segment the total intracranial volume (B) and a T1-weighted sequence to calculate total brain parenchymal tissue using contoured surfaces (C). From these 2 measures, the BPF can be calculated, defined as the ratio of brain parenchymal tissue volume to the total intracranial volume (brain tissue volume plus cerebrospinal fluid).

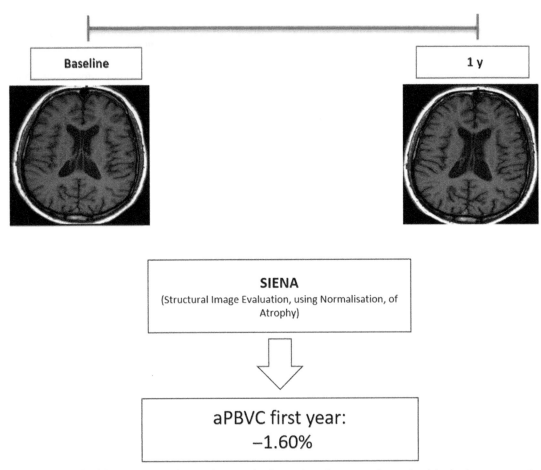

Fig. 3. Longitudinal brain volume change from multiple MR imaging scans determined by brain segmentation and registration. The automated algorithm (SIENA) extracts brain from nonbrain tissue at 2 time points and estimates the outer skull surface at both time points. The registered segmented brain images are used to find local atrophy, measured from the movement of edges between images.

had been reported on transversal studies: some publications concluded that a variable to account for the system upgrade should still be included in the statistical analysis,[39] whereas others concluded that the upgrade did not have a significant effect.[40,41] The effect of the system upgrade has not been assessed in longitudinal studies and may hamper the estimation of individual brain volume changes.

Acquisition Protocols

Some quantification methods are more independent than others of the sequence of choice,[41,42] although differences are less than the intersubject variability. Regarding the choice of the acquisition parameters, great efforts have been made in Alzheimer disease since the Alzheimer's Disease Neuroimaging Initiative (ADNI).[43] ADNI has helped to homogenize MR imaging protocols and has become a reference. Similar initiatives in MS are

needed because the imaging population is different from that of ADNI.

Gradient Distortion

In longitudinal studies, special care should be taken in repositioning the patient in the scanner, to keep the same position relative to the isocenter. A controlled displacement from the isocenter in one study results in an (artifactual) increase in the calculated percentage brain volume change measured between 2 consecutive studies, which was not measured after correcting for gradient distortion.[44] Thus, spending extra time trying to reposition the patient is worthwhile, especially if longitudinal changes need to be assessed.

Scan-Rescan Variability

Even when both technical and physiologic conditions are controlled, there is an inherent variability that affects MR imaging–derived measurements, independently of the method used.[45,46] Studies that estimate the variability error have been performed with FreeSurfer4.[40,47] Within-session reproducibility errors are less than 2.5% for thalamus, hippocampus, basal ganglia, and lateral ventricles, and less than 10.5% for smaller structures (amygdala, pallidum, and inferior lateral ventricles). For more global measurements such as the brain parenchymal fraction, errors less than 1% were found.[48] As a consequence, differences and changes that are smaller than these estimated errors cannot be measured reliably.

CONFOUNDING FACTORS RELATED TO MEASUREMENT METHODS
Brain Volume Measures

Total brain volume estimations can be obtained after applying a segmentation algorithm, based on the calculated image histogram, with or without the help of predefined atlases. These methods are not fully automated and require the adjustment of some parameters. The goal is to estimate the gray and white matter, the cerebrospinal fluid, and the total intracranial volume as the sum of the 3 compartments. Transversal comparisons cannot be performed directly with absolute volumes because of the interindividual variations in head size; instead, fractions such as the gray matter fraction (GMF) and white matter fraction (WMF) can be obtained after dividing by the total intracranial volume. In MS, the brain parenchymal fraction (BPF) has traditionally been used.[49] BPF is fairly robust and less prone to segmentation errors than GMF and WMF. Nevertheless, the insight obtained from estimating GMF and WMF is much more specific than with a global BPF.

Deep Gray Matter Regions

The thalamus is a structure that experiences a prominent volume loss and in MS has been linked to cognition.[50] Methods such as FIRST (FMRIB's [functional MRI of the brain] integrated registration & segmentation tool)[51] and FreeSurfer[52] allow estimation of the volume of the thalamus, among other structures. Both methods are based on the same atlas and results are comparable.[53]

Brain Volume Longitudinal Changes

A very common setting in MS is the need to quantify the brain volume changes between a baseline and a follow-up study, as a way to monitor atrophy progression. One approach is to calculate the differences in the corresponding fractions between the two time points. Another approach is to

use registration-based methods, such as SIENA (Structural Image Evaluation using Normalization of Atrophy),[54] an FSL (FMRIB software library) tool that calculates the percentage brain volume change between 2 time points. The reported error in SIENA is 0.2%, which is in the range of the expected change in healthy people over a 1-year period. The point in MS is that, at the early stages, patients are young and many of them do not differ from healthy persons in terms of brain volume loss. Thus, estimation of changes in short periods of time (6 months' follow-up) is not recommended.

Voxel-Based Morphometry

Both transversal and longitudinal comparisons can also be performed at a voxel level, using the methodology implemented in statistical parametric mapping.[55] The main point is the use of an atlas, to which all studies are referred. In this context, small and systematical differences between 2 groups can be more easily detected, which are not significant at a global level. In contrast, voxel-based morphometry (VBM) assesses volumetric differences based on an atlas, and image segmentation depends on the image intensity values, which in MS may differ from healthy individuals. Whether or not this has an effect on VBM results has not been tested yet.

Cortical Thickness

Changes in brain volume are the result of changes in cortical folding, surface area, and thickness. Specific methods have been developed that just measure cortical thickness.[52,56,57] The measures of cortical thickness are time consuming, besides manual corrections being required in order to get accurate measurements.

NON–MULTIPLE SCLEROSIS–RELATED BIOLOGICAL CONFOUNDING FACTORS
Age

It has been largely known that, after adolescence, gray matter volume starts to decline in a linear way (−0.09%/y), whereas white matter starts this decline after midlife, and at a higher rate (−0.2%/y).[58] Hedman and colleagues[59] did a complete review of the published studies. Regarding cortical thickness, at midlife a global thinning was apparent, spreading over several cortical regions.[60] The decline in the thickness measured was around 0.016 mm per decade. Both volumetric and cortical thickness age-associated changes have been described, implying that age is a variable that should be considered.

Gender and Brain Size

Men had larger gray and white matter volumes compared with women, although differences disappeared after adjusting for total intracranial volume.[58] Regarding cortical thickness, men showed slightly larger cortical thickness compared with women only at midlife, and the rate of progressive thinning was similar for both groups.[60] A more recent study reported that cortical thickness was associated with total intracranial volume, but not with gender.[61] Because gender and total intracranial volume are highly correlated, it is a matter of debate whether 1 or both variables should be considered.[39,62]

Diurnal Fluctuations

When large data sets are analyzed, a (reversible) linear decrease in the BPF during the day has been found,[63] which could have a significant impact on volumetric MR imaging studies of brain. Although a clear explanation for this time-related reversible brain volume fluctuation has not been established, it seems to be associated with brain hydration status.

To minimize this potential confounding effect, it has been recommended, particularly in small studies, to scan all patients in the same time period.

Hydration State

Fluid loss and fluid intake affect body volume and also brain volume. Experimental studies that used an extreme hyperhydration-dehydration paradigm[64,65] have shown that hydration status induces significant ventricular volume changes. Nevertheless, this paradigm is not a real clinical scenario because these extreme conditions rarely occur. In contrast, the percentage of brain volume loss in MS, even at the early stages of the disease, seems to be higher than the changes caused by hydration changes.[66] Despite the marginal effect of hydration status on brain volume measures, it has been recommended, particularly in small longitudinal studies, to scan the patients under similar hydration conditions.

Cardiovascular Risk Factors

Alcohol, diabetes, cardiac left ventricular hypertrophy, smoking, and obesity are associated with an increased number of brain white matter signal abnormalities and decreased whole-brain and gray matter volumes in the MS population.[67] All these factors, or at least some of them, should be considered as covariates in the interpretation of volumetric measures in clinical studies, although it is difficult to account for the influence of all of them when measuring brain volume in patients with MS.[68]

Genetic and Environmental Confounding Factors

Different genetic and environmental factors have been associated with a decreased brain volume.[68] African Americans have higher rates of brain atrophy, which might be linked to their inherent increased cardiovascular risk. Higher apolipoprotein E levels are associated with deep gray matter atrophy in high-risk patients with clinically isolated syndrome. In addition, more advanced whole-brain and cortical atrophy have also been described associated with a humoral response to anti–Epstein-Barr virus and the presence of different autoimmune diseases (psoriasis, thyroid disease, and type 2 diabetes mellitus).

MULTIPLE SCLEROSIS–RELATED BIOLOGICAL CONFOUNDING FACTORS
White Matter Focal Lesions

Focal white matter brain lesions are a typical feature in patients with MS. Some of these lesions are seen as isointense to hypointense compared with gray matter on T1-weighted images, being erroneously considered gray matter by most of the automated segmentation tools. This error leads to an overestimation in the estimated GMF. Different approaches, such as automated T1 lesion mask and filling, have been developed to avoid this contribution[69,70] and significant reductions in the GMF have been found, even in patients with low lesion load.[71] The effect of these approaches on VBM studies should be further investigated.

Pseudoatrophy Effect

Disease-modifying drugs and steroids used for the treatment of MS have often been associated with an acceleration of brain volume loss, because of their antiinflammatory effect (Fig. 4). This phenomenon, referred to as pseudoatrophy, is generally assumed to be caused by the resolution of edema, and mostly targets white matter during the first months after therapy initiation.[30,31] This phenomenon complicates the interpretation of treatment effects on brain volume in clinical studies, particularly in patients with a significant degree of baseline inflammatory activity, because it counteracts the expected treatment effect. various strategies have been proposed to minimize this pseudoatrophy

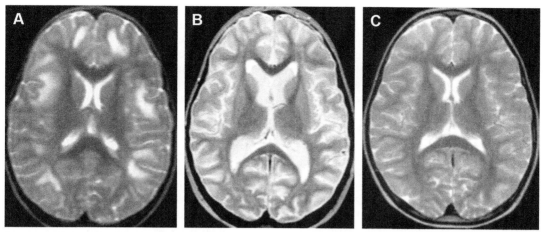

Fig. 4. Pseudoatrophy effect induced by steroids. An 11-year old boy diagnosed with acute disseminated encephalomyelitis, showing at baseline multiple large subcortical white matter lesions (*A*). Follow-up brain MR imaging 3 months later (*B*) shows marked increase in ventricular size and cortical sulci, reflecting brain volume loss, which completely resolved 9 months later (*C*).

effect, such as analyzing gray matter volume changes or considering as baseline volumetric measures those obtained on scans acquired at least 6 to 12 months after therapy initiation.[68]

SUMMARY

Although MS is typically characterized by focal areas of demyelination and inflammation, significant brain atrophy mainly involving the gray matter, which is a measure of the most destructive pathologic process in MS, is also observed and may lead to irreversible neurologic and cognitive impairment. Whole and regional (gray matter) brain atrophy have emerged as clinically relevant components of disease progression, and many studies have shown that this MR imaging–based parameter correlates with and predicts subsequent development of disability and cognitive impairment better than focal lesions, and is probably the most feasible and robust measure of the neurodegenerative nature of MS.

Because the control of this neurodegenerative component, in addition to inflammation, represents an important target for treatment, measures of brain volume have been used in randomized clinical trials to monitor treatment effect on brain volume of most disease-modifying therapies, and could probably be incorporated, in the near future, as a marker of disease progression and treatment response in individual patients.

However, several technical and biological factors can generate notable variability in brain atrophy assessments, complicating the interpretation of the measures obtained, particularly at individual levels. For this reason, the authors believe that the

use of longitudinal brain volume assessment as a marker of disease progression in individual patients cannot be considered to be reliable at present. Future studies are needed to establish normative values for brain volume changes (both in healthy individuals and in patients with MS) that take the various potential confounding factors into account.

REFERENCES

1. Trapp BD, Peterson J, Ransohoff RM, et al. Axonal transection in the lesions of multiple sclerosis. N Engl J Med 1998;338:278–85.
2. Ferguson B, Matyszak MK, Esiri MM, et al. Axonal damage in acute multiple sclerosis lesions. Brain 1997;120:393–9.
3. Losseff NA, Wang L, Lai HM, et al. Progressive cerebral atrophy in multiple sclerosis. A serial MRI study. Brain 1996;119:2009–19.
4. Raz N, Lindenberger U, Rodrigue KM, et al. Regional brain changes in aging healthy adults: general trends, individual differences and modifiers. Cereb Cortex 2005;15:1676–89.
5. Chard DT, Griffin CM, Parker GJ, et al. Brain atrophy in clinically early relapsing-remitting multiple sclerosis. Brain 2002;125:327–37.
6. Sastre-Garriga J, Ingle GT, Chard DT, et al. Grey and white matter atrophy in early clinical stages of primary progressive multiple sclerosis. Neuroimage 2004;22:353–9.
7. Kalkers NF, Bergers E, Castelijns JA, et al. Optimizing the association between disability and biological markers in MS. Neurology 2001;57:1253–8.
8. De Stefano N, Matthews PM, Filippi M, et al. Evidence of early cortical atrophy in MS: relevance to

white matter changes and disability. Neurology 2003;60:1157–62.

9. Calabrese M, Magliozzi R, Ciccarelli O, et al. Exploring the origins of grey matter damage in multiple sclerosis. Nat Rev Neurosci 2015;16:147–58.

10. Lansley J, Mataix-Cols D, Grau M, et al. Localized grey matter atrophy in multiple sclerosis: a meta-analysis of voxel-based morphometry studies and associations with functional disability. Neurosci Biobehav Rev 2013;37:819–30.

11. Narayana PA, Govindarajan KA, Goel P, et al, The CombiRx Investigators Group. Regional cortical thickness in relapsing remitting multiple sclerosis: a multi-center study. Neuroimage Clin 2012;2:120–31.

12. Fox NC, Jenkins R, Leary SM, et al. Progressive cerebral atrophy in MS: a serial study using registered, volumetric MRI. Neurology 2000;54:807–12.

13. Dalton CM, Chard DT, Davies GR, et al. Early development of multiple sclerosis is associated with progressive grey matter atrophy in patients presenting with clinically isolated syndromes. Brain 2004;127:1101–7.

14. Tiberio M, Chard DT, Altmann DR, et al. Gray and white matter volume changes in early RRMS: a 2-year longitudinal study. Neurology 2005;64:1001–7.

15. Sastre-Garriga J, Ingle GT, Chard DT, et al. Grey and white matter volume changes in early primary progressive multiple sclerosis: a longitudinal study. Brain 2005;128:1454–60.

16. De Stefano N, Giorgio A, Battaglini M, et al. Assessing brain atrophy rates in a large population of untreated multiple sclerosis subtypes. Neurology 2010;74:1868–76.

17. Valsasina P, Benedetti B, Rovaris M, et al. Evidence for progressive gray matter loss in patients with relapsing-remitting MS. Neurology 2005;65:1126–8.

18. De Stefano N, Stromillo ML, Giorgio A, et al. Establishing pathological cut-offs of brain atrophy rates in multiple sclerosis. J Neurol Neurosurg Psychiatry 2016;87:93–9.

19. Pérez-Miralles F, Sastre-Garriga J, Tintoré M, et al. Clinical impact of early brain atrophy in clinically isolated syndromes. Mult Scler 2013;19:1878–86.

20. Di Filippo M, Anderson VM, Altmann DR, et al. Brain atrophy and lesion load measures over 1 year relate to clinical status after 6 years in patients with clinically isolated syndromes. J Neurol Neurosurg Psychiatry 2010;81:204–8.

21. Amato MP, Hakiki B, Goretti B, et al, Italian RIS/MS Study Group. Association of MRI metrics and cognitive impairment in radiologically isolated syndromes. Neurology 2012;78:309–14.

22. Popescu V, Agosta F, Hulst HE, et al, MAGNIMS Study Group. Brain atrophy and lesion load predict long term disability in multiple sclerosis. J Neurol Neurosurg Psychiatry 2013;84:1082–91.

23. Sastre-Garriga J, Ingle GT, Rovaris M, et al. Long-term clinical outcome of primary progressive MS:

predictive value of clinical and MRI data. Neurology 2005;65:633–5.

24. Khaleeli Z, Ciccarelli O, Manfredonia F, et al. Predicting progression in primary progressive multiple sclerosis: a 10-year multicenter study. Ann Neurol 2008;63:790–3.

25. Vidal-Jordana A, Sastre-Garriga J, Rovira A, et al. Treating relapsing-remitting multiple sclerosis: therapy effects on brain atrophy. J Neurol 2015;262:2617–26.

26. Kappos L, Traboulsee A, Constantinescu C, et al. Long-term subcutaneous interferon beta-1a therapy in patients with relapsing-remitting MS. Neurology 2006;67:944–53.

27. Fisher E, Rudick RA, Simon JH, et al. Eight-year follow-up study of brain atrophy in patients with MS. Neurology 2002;59:1412–20.

28. Sormani MP, Arnold DL, De Stefano N. Treatment effect on brain atrophy correlates with treatment effect on disability in multiple sclerosis. Ann Neurol 2014;75:43–9.

29. Filippi M, Rocca MA. Preventing brain atrophy should be the gold standard of effective theraphy in MS (after the first year of treatment): No. Mult Scler 2013;19:1005–6.

30. Vidal-Jordana A, Sastre-Garriga J, Pérez-Miralles F, et al. Early brain pseudoatrophy while on natalizumab therapy is due to white matter volume changes. Mult Scler 2013;19:1175–81.

31. Vidal-Jordana A, Sastre-Garriga J, Pérez-Miralles F, et al. Brain volume loss during the first year of interferon-beta treatment in multiple sclerosis: baseline inflammation and regional brain volume dynamics. J Neuroimaging 2016;26:532–8.

32. Sormani MP, De Stefano N, Francis G, et al. Fingolimod effect on brain volume loss independently contributes to its effect on disability. Mult Scler 2015;21:916–24.

33. Rojas JI, Patrucco L, Miguez J, et al. Brain atrophy as a non-response predictor to interferon-beta in relapsing-remitting multiple sclerosis. Neurol Res 2014;36:615–8.

34. Pérez-Miralles FC, Sastre-Garriga J, Vidal-Jordana A, et al. Predictive value of early brain atrophy on response in patients treated with interferon β. Neurol Neuroimmunol Neuroinflamm 2015;2:e132.

35. Río J. Any evident MRI T2 lesion activity should guide change of therapy in multiple sclerosis: no. Mult Scler 2015;21:132–3.

36. Giovannoni G. Any evident MRI T2-lesion activity should guide change of therapy in multiple sclerosis: yes. Mult Scler 2015;21:134–6.

37. Kappos L, De Stefano N, Freedman MS, et al. Inclusion of brain volume loss in a revised measure of 'no evidence of disease activity' (NEDA-4) in relapsing-remitting multiple sclerosis. Mult Scler 2016;22:1297–305.

38. Reuter M, Tisdall MD, Qureshi A, et al. Head motion during MRI acquisition reduces gray matter volume and thickness estimates. Neuroimage 2015;107: 107–15.

39. Barnes J, Ridgway GR, Bartlett J, et al. Head size, age and gender adjustment in MRI studies: a necessary nuisance? Neuroimage 2010;53:1244–55.

40. Han X, Jovicich J, Salat D, et al. Reliability of MRI-derived measurements of human cerebral cortical thickness: the effects of field strength, scanner upgrade and manufacturer. Neuroimage 2006;32: 180–94.

41. Jovicich J, Czanner S, Han X, et al. MRI-derived measurements of human subcortical, ventricular and intracranial brain volumes: reliability effects of scan sessions, acquisition sequences, data analyses, scanner upgrade, scanner vendors and field strengths. Neuroimage 2009;46: 177–92.

42. Tardif CL, Collins DL, Pike GB. Sensitivity of voxel-based morphometry analysis to choice of imaging protocol at 3 T. Neuroimage 2009;44:827–38.

43. Available at: http://www.adni-info.org/. Accessed on February 7, 2017.

44. Caramanos Z, Fonov VS, Francis SJ, et al. Gradient distortions in MRI: characterizing and correcting for their effects on SIENA-generated measures of brain volume change. Neuroimage 2010;49:1601–11.

45. Morey RA, Selgrade ES, Wagner HR 2nd, et al. Scan-rescan reliability of subcortical brain volumes derived from automated segmentation. Hum Brain Mapp 2010;31:1751–62.

46. Maclaren J, Han Z, Vos SB, et al. Reliability of brain volume measurements: a test-retest dataset. Sci Data 2014;14(1):140037.

47. Yang CY, Liu HM, Chen SK, et al. Reproducibility of brain morphometry from short-term repeat clinical MRI examinations: a retrospective study. PLoS One 2016;11:e0146913.

48. Sampat MP, Healy BC, Meier DS, et al. Disease modeling in multiple sclerosis: assessment and quantification of sources of variability in brain parenchymal fraction measurements. Neuroimage 2010; 52:1367–73.

49. Rudick RA, Fisher E, Lee JC. Simon use of the brain parenchymal fraction to measure whole brain atrophy in relapsing-remitting MS. Multiple Sclerosis Collaborative Research Group. Neurology 1999;53: 1698–704.

50. Houtchens MK, Benedict RH, Killiany R, et al. Thalamic atrophy and cognition in multiple sclerosis. Neurology 2007;69:1213–23.

51. Patenaude B, Smith SM, Kennedy D, et al. A bayesian model of shape and appearance for subcortical brain. Neuroimage 2011;56:907–22.

52. Fischl B, Dale AM. Measuring the thickness of the human cerebral cortex from magnetic resonance images. Proc Natl Acad Sci U S A 2000;97:11050–5.

53. Derakhshan M, Caramanos Z, Giacomini PS, et al. Evaluation of automated techniques for the quantification of grey matter atrophy in patients with multiple sclerosis. Neuroimage 2010;52:1261–7.

54. Smith SM, Zhang Y, Jenkinson M, et al. Accurate, robust, and automated longitudinal and cross-sectional brain change analysis. Neuroimage 2002; 17:479–89.

55. Ashburner J, Friston KJ. Voxel-based morphometry–the methods. Neuroimage 2000;11:805–21.

56. Hutton C, De Vita E, Ashburner J, et al. Voxel-based cortical thickness measurements in MRI. Neuroimage 2008;40:1701–10.

57. Nakamura K, Fox R, Fisher E. CLADA: cortical longitudinal atrophy detection algorithm. Neuroimage 2011;54:278–89.

58. Ge Y, Grossman RI, Babb JS, et al. Age-related total gray matter and white matter changes in normal adult brain. Part I: volumetric MR imaging analysis. AJNR Am J Neuroradiol 2002;23:1327–33.

59. Hedman AM, van Haren NEM, Schnack HG, et al. Human brain changes across the life span: a review of 56 longitudinal magnetic resonance imaging studies. Hum Brain Mapp 2012;33:1987–2002.

60. Salat DH, Buckner RL, Snyder AZ, et al. Thinning of the cerebral cortex in aging. Cereb Cortex 2004;14: 721–30.

61. Im K, Lee JM, Lyttelton O, et al. Brain size and cortical structure in the adult human brain. Cereb Cortex 2008;18:2181–91.

62. Pell GS, Briellmann RS, Chan CH, et al. Selection of the control group for VBM analysis: influence of covariates, matching and sample size. Neuroimage 2008;41:1324–35.

63. Nakamura K, Brown RA, Narayanan S, et al. Diurnal fluctuations in brain volume: statistical analyses of MRI from large populations. Neuroimage 2015;118: 126–32.

64. Nakamura K, Brown RA, Araujo D, et al. Correlation between brain volume change and T2 relaxation time induced by dehydration and rehydration: implications for monitoring atrophy in clinical studies. Neuroimage Clin 2014;6:166–70.

65. Streitbürger DP, Möller HE, Tittgemeyer M, et al. Investigating structural brain changes of dehydration using voxel-based morphometry. PLoS One 2012;7:e44195.

66. Dalton CM, Miszkiel KA, O'Connor PW, et al. Ventricular enlargement in MS: one-year change at various stages of disease. Neurology 2006;66:693–8.

67. Srinivasa RN, Rossetti HC, Gupta MK, et al. Cardiovascular risk factors associated with smaller brain volumes in regions identified as early predictors of cognitive decline. Radiology 2015;278: 198–204.

68. Zivadinov R, Jakimovski D, Gandhi S, et al. Clinical relevance of brain atrophy assessment in multiple sclerosis. Implications for its use in a clinical routine. Expert Rev Neurother 2016;16:777–93.

69. Schmidt P, Gaser C, Arsic M, et al. An automated tool for detection of FLAIR-hyperintense white-matter lesions in multiple sclerosis. Neuroimage 2012;59: 3774–83.

70. Roura E, Oliver A, Cabezas M, et al. A toolbox for multiple sclerosis lesion segmentation. Neuroradiology 2015;57:1031–43.

71. Pareto D, Sastre-Garriga J, Aymerich FX, et al. Lesion filling effect in regional brain volume estimations: a study in multiple sclerosis patients with low lesion load. Neuroradiology 2016;58: 467–74.

Cortical Gray Matter MR Imaging in Multiple Sclerosis

 CrossMark

Massimiliano Calabrese, MD[a],*, Marco Castellaro, PhD[b]

KEYWORDS

- Multiple sclerosis • Gray matter damage • Cortical lesions • Normal-appearing gray matter
- MR imaging

KEY POINTS

- Gray matter damage is a frequent phenomenon in patients with multiple sclerosis since the early phase of the disease. Unfortunately, it is almost undetectable by conventional MR imaging.
- Focal cortical lesions are hallmark of the gray matter damage but also the so-called normal-appearing gray matter is not spared by the pathologic process.
- Several new unconventional MR imaging sequences have been developed to identify cortical lesions and to quantify the damage of the normal-appearing gray matter, but their application in routine clinical practice is far from being standardized.

INTRODUCTION

Multiple sclerosis (MS) is a chronic, disabling, and unpredictable disease of the human central nervous system (CNS), histologically characterized by multifocal areas of inflammatory demyelination. Because MS lesions are macroscopically visible in the white matter (WM), MS has been classically regarded as a "white matter disease." Moreover, with the advent of the diagnostic MR imaging methodology for CNS diseases (namely, T2/fluid-attenuated inversion recovery (FLAIR) -weighted images and contrast-enhanced T1-weighted images), the concept of MS as a disease "almost exclusively" affecting the subcortical myelin was strengthened. However, although the WM abnormality is undoubtedly of major importance in contributing to focal clinical deficits in the relapsing remitting (RR) phase, substantial immunopathologic and imaging evidence has confirmed that tissue damage within the gray matter (GM) is a key component of the demyelination process since early phases of the disease and provides the best correlate of the disability accumulation.[1–4]

The aim of this review is to summarize the most recent and innovative MR imaging techniques developed to identify the GM damage and to monitor its evolution during the disease course.

FOCAL GRAY MATTER ABNORMALITY
The Cortical Lesions

Neuropathologic studies have consistently described several "demyelinating" lesions within the cortical and deep GM of MS brain, when postmortem tissue specimens were stained with histochemical myelin stainings. Peterson and colleagues[5] observed 112 cortical lesions (CLs) in 110 tissue blocks from 50 patients with MS and identified 3 types of cortical demyelination: *Type I* lesions were contiguous with subcortical WM lesions (mixed cortical/leukocortical lesions)

Disclosure Statement: The authors have nothing to disclose.
[a] Neurology B, Department of Neurosciences, Biomedicine and Movement Sciences, University of Verona, Policlinico GB Rossi, Piazzale LA Scuro 10, Verona 37134, Italy; [b] Department of Information Engineering, University of Padova, Via G. Gradenigo 6/a, Padova 35135, Italy
* Corresponding author.
E-mail address: massimiliano.calabrese@univr.it

neuroimaging.theclinics.com

(Fig. 1); *type II* lesions were small, entirely confined within the cortex, and often perivascular (Fig. 2); and *type III* lesions extended from the pial surface to cortical layer 3 or 4. The relevance of cortical demyelination was confirmed by several later pathologic studies that recognized that cortical damage can be extensive, as seen in the analysis of double hemispheric sections, affecting up to 68% of the total forebrain cortical area in some extreme examples.[1,6]

A significant regional variation in the extent of cortical demyelination has been reported. Indeed, the most extensive cortical demyelination was demonstrated in the cingulate gyrus (up to 44%) and in the temporal and frontal cortices (up to 28%), with a lower proportion of demyelinated area in other cortical areas, including the paracentral lobule (11.5%), occipital lobe (8%), and primary motor cortex (3.5%).[7,8] Interestingly, the percentage of demyelinated area was found quite high in the cerebellar cortex.[7,9] Extensive demyelination was also detected in the hippocampus of patients with MS.[10,11] Finally, in spinal cord, the percentage of demyelinated area in the GM was significantly higher than that observed in the WM (33% vs 20%) and was similar in all cord levels. Although most spinal cord lesions were combined WM/GM lesions, pure GM demyelinating lesions were noticed.[12]

Although the above described pathologic data suggest a widespread cortical involvement, especially in patients with long-lasting disease duration, the contribution of cortical abnormality to clinical MS symptoms in vivo was underestimated for a long time. This underestimation is mainly due to the fact that routinely available MR imaging techniques, especially T1-weighted and T2-weighted MR imaging, only rarely detect purely intra-CL. Indeed, among the 3 types of CL described by pathologists, T2-FLAIR sequence can only demonstrate type I (leukocortical) lesions, located at the interface between cortex and WM. Several factors hamper the possibility of demonstrating CL by means of conventional T2-FLAIR sequences: the less inflammatory cell infiltration, the absence of significant blood-brain barrier damage, the low myelin density in upper cortical layers, as well as technical constraints, such as partial volume effects resulting from the proximity of CLs to the cerebrospinal fluid (CSF).[13–17] In a study comparing the number of CL detected by histopathology and postmortem MR imaging, applying dual-echo T2-weighted spin-echo (SE) images and 3-dimensional (3D) T2-FLAIR, the detection rates of T2-FLAIR images were only 5% for pure intracortical lesions and 41% for leukocortical lesions.[18]

Imaging Cortical Lesions by MR Imaging

A significant improvement in the detection rate of CLs and in the delineation of GM structures was obtained by applying 3D double-inversion recovery (DIR) sequences. The use of DIR imaging showed an average increase of 152% and 500% in CLs detection per patient when compared with the 3D T2-FLAIR and the T2-weighted SE, respectively[19,20] (see Figs. 1 and 2). Using such a sequence, CLs have been demonstrated consistently not only in

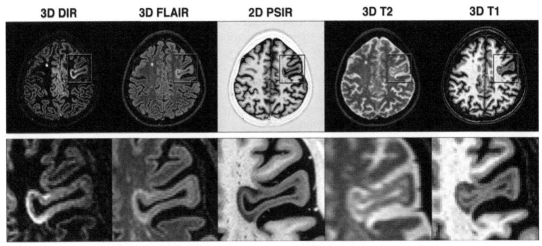

Fig. 1. A big mixed WM and GM MS lesion demonstrated with different MR imaging sequences (upper row): 3D DIR; 3D FLAIR; 2-dimensional (2D) PSIR; 3D T2-weighted turbo spin echo (3D T2); and 3D T1 magnetization prepared recalled gradient echo (3D T1). A red square shows the same lesion zoomed in the lower row. The lesion follows an entire gyrus of the cortex and is mixed with the subcortical WM. The parameters of the sequences used in this protocol are reported in Table 1.

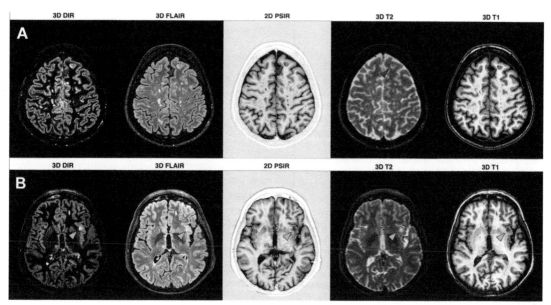

Fig. 2. (A) An intracortical MS lesion (*blue arrows*) shown in different MR imaging sequences. 3D DIR shows a unique tissue contrast relative to GM. The lesions could be easily detected as hyperintense. 3D FLAIR shows signal coming from GM. PSIR shows a T1 contrast. The lesion could be efficiently detected and is shown as hypointense. Conventional 3D T2-weighted turbo spin echo (3D T2) does not show the lesion. 3D T1 magnetization prepared recalled gradient echo (MPRAGE) shows the lesion as hypointense. The parameters of the sequences used in this protocol are reported in Table 1. (B) A mixed WM and GM MS lesion (*green arrows*). 3D DIR shows the lesions as hyperintense. In this case, the lesion is difficult to be detected with the 3D FLAIR. PSIR shows a hypointensity in correspondence to the lesion. Conventional 3D T2-weighted turbo spin echo (3D T2) shows the lesion as hyperintense. 3D T1 MPRAGE shows the lesion as hypointense. The parameters of the sequences used in this protocol are reported in Table 1.

patients with the progressive phenotypes but also in those with RRMS, even at clinical onset[21]; a significant relationship between CL load and physical[22] and cognitive[23] disability has been observed, and the presence of at least 1 CL in patients with clinical isolated syndrome has been considered helpful in the identification of those patients at high risk for conversion to clinical definite MS.[24] Unfortunately, even by the application of DIR sequence, the identification of CLs at 1.5-T MR imaging is still challenging, and several neuropathologic studies have shown that only a small part of the total cortical damage can be observed at this field strength.[25] On the contrary, brain MR imaging scans at 3 T can substantially improve the sensitivity of the DIR sequence in the detection of even small CLs compared with the standard magnetic field strength of 1.5 T.[26,27] As previously described,[25] MR imaging visualization of CL depends mostly on CL size ("tip-of-the-iceberg" effect), and intensity and sensitivity of the sequence. Thus, a larger lesion size would be necessary for detection on DIR, and this could lead to a delay in identification of CL with this sequence.

The combination of DIR with new MR imaging sequences as T1-weighted 3D spoiled gradient-recalled echo[28] or phase sensitive inversion recovery (PSIR; see **Figs. 1** and **2**)[29,30] may allow a better segmentation of CLs, and, therefore, may represent a new tool for a more accurate and reliable analysis of the normal-appearing gray matter (NAGM). In particular, a recent study on CLs revealed that the combination of DIR and PSIR sequences improves the accuracy of CLs classification. Compared with DIR, PSIR detected a greater number of CL and leucocortical lesions and allowed separation of leucocortical lesions and juxtacortical lesions.[31]

THE DIFFUSE GRAY MATTER DAMAGE
The Normal-Appearing Gray Matter

In addition to discrete CLs, expression of a focal damage, several MR imaging studies have also shown the presence of a diffuse pathologic process involving the entire cortical and deep GM (**Box 1**), a process that appears to occur since the early phases of MS.[32–34] In the last 15 years, advances in the use of new nonconventional MR imaging sequences allowed the detection of more subtle GM alterations, which were usually

Recent MR imaging studies have shown that pathologic changes in the deep GM (dGM), particularly in the caudate nucleus and in the thalamus, frequently occur in patients with MS. The main features of dGM abnormality (demyelination, inflammation, and neuronal, axonal, and synaptic abnormality) have recently been described.[88] As expected, the inflammatory process in these nuclei was characterized by a low number of lymphocytes, a preponderance of activated microglia, scarce myelin-laden macrophages, and a low degree of blood-brain barrier disruption. Interestingly, neuronal loss was observed not only in demyelinated dGM but also in the non-demyelinated dGM. Thus, the histologic picture of dGM inflammation is quite similar to that of CLs.

Several studies have evaluated the dGM damage using different MR imaging techniques. In particular, the atrophy of caudate nucleus[89,90] and thalamus[59,91] has been consistently observed since the earliest disease stages and preceded the loss of volume of other GM structures.[46] Selective thalamic atrophy with conservation of cortical GM and other dGM nuclei is a very early phenomenon[46] and has also been described in pediatric-onset MS.[92] Significantly lower levels of NAA have been described in the thalamus.[91] More recently also, DTI metrics from 3-T MR imaging were assessed in the caudate, putamen, and thalamus of 30 patients with MS and 10 controls. FA of the caudate and putamen was higher in patients with MS compared with controls and correlated with neurologic disability (EDSS and ambulation index), whereas putamen and thalamus FA correlated with deficits in memory tests.[94] Finally, iron increase has been observed in dGM of CIS and is associated with worsened clinical status.[77,93] This suggests that the neurodegenerative damage of dGM occurs early in the disease course and plays a key role in disability progression.

undetected by conventional MR imaging. These observations confirmed that GM damage was not exclusive to the progressive stage, but began early during the disease process,[35,36] sometimes already at clinical onset and even preceding the appearance of WM lesions.[21,32]

Moreover, preliminary studies suggested that diffuse GM damage was correlated with physical and cognitive disability[23,37] and could be also used to predict future physical and cognitive disability.[22,38–40] As a consequence, new innovative techniques have been developed and implemented for the quantitative analysis of the brain cortex, allowing the evaluation of the integrity of the so-called NAGM.

Imaging the Normal-Appearing Gray Matter

Conventional T2-weighted MR imaging sequences (included the inversion recovery sequences, FLAIR and DIR), although very sensitive for the detection of MS lesions, have important limitations. First, they lack specificity with regard to the heterogeneous pathologic components of lesions. Indeed, edema, inflammation, demyelination, remyelination, gliosis, and axonal loss all lead to a similar appearance of hyperintensity on T2-weighted images. Second, T2-weighted images do not delineate tissue damage occurring in normal-appearing white matter (NAWM) and NAGM, which usually represents a large portion of the brain tissue in patients with MS and which is known to be damaged. As a consequence, several studies have focused on measuring MR imaging changes in the NAGM by applying nonconventional techniques, such as magnetization transfer ratio (MTR) imaging, relaxation time measurements, proton magnetic resonance spectroscopy (^{1}H-MRS), diffusion tensor imaging (DTI) with several variants, and perfusion imaging.

Global and regional analysis of cortical atrophy

When going beyond the assessment of focal GM abnormality, the measurement of cortical atrophy may provide information about the severity of irreversible neuronal and axonal loss. A progressive reduction of the cortical volume, having a significant impact on clinical disability, was demonstrated to occur quite early in both relapsing remitting MS (RRMS) and primary progressive MS.[33] Dalton and colleagues[34] observed progressive GM but not WM volume loss in people who developed MS within 3 years from clinical onset, with only a minority of GM atrophy seemingly related to WM lesion accrual (about 20% shared variability). More recently, new techniques were developed for the image reconstruction of the brain cortex and the assessment of regional cortical atrophy,[32,41–43] and their application further confirmed that cortical atrophy is associated with disability with a stronger magnitude than conventional MR imaging–derived measures of disease burden in the WM. Consistent with this, clinically isolated syndrome (CIS) patients who have been clinically silent for a follow-up period of 1 year did not show a significant trend in the reduction of cortical thickness compared with healthy volunteers, while a significant reduction in cortical thickness was observed in patients with possible MS at onset (having the criterion of dissemination in space of lesion according to 2010 McDonald

Table 1
Suggested parameters for 3-T Philips System Cortical Pathology Protocol

Sequence	Parameters	Resolution (mm)	Purpose
3D T1-weighted fast field echo	TR/TE = 8.4/3.7 ms	1 × 1 × 1	Cortical atrophy
3D T2-FLAIR turbo spin echo	TR/TE = 5500/292 ms, TI = 1650 ms	1 × 1 × 1	WM lesions
3D DIR turbo spin echo	TR/TE = 5500/292 ms, TI1/TI2 = 525 ms/2530 ms	1 × 1 × 1	GM lesions
2D T1 PSIR	TR/TE = 7300/13 ms, TI = 400 ms	0.5 × 0.5 × 2	GM lesions
3D T2-weighted turbo spin echo	TR/TE = 2600/268	1.7 × 1.7 × 1.7	T2 lesions
2D DTI echo planar imaging	TR/TE = 12,500/109 ms b-value of 700 s/mm^2 (32 directions) and 2000 s/mm^2 (64 directions)	2 × 2 × 2	DTI and NODDI
3D multi-echo gradient echo	TR = 51 ms; 8 echoes, TE1 = 8.15, ΔTE = 4.5	0.5 × 0.5 × 2	QSM and T$_2$*
3D SWI echo planar imaging	TR/TE = 51/29 ms	0.55 × 0.55 × 0.55	QSM

Abbreviations: SWI, susceptibility weighted imaging; TE, echo time; TI, inversion time; TR, repetition time.

criteria for MS[44]) who developed MS. Furthermore, the analysis of the regional distribution of GM atrophy disclosed that the extent of the pathologic process taking place in the cortex is not homogeneous, and that some cortical areas are more susceptible to volume loss than others.[32,41,42,45] Although regional predilections for early GM atrophy have been reported, their exact mapping remains to be clarified. In a 4-month follow-up of patients presenting with CIS and using a voxel-based morphometry (VBM) to look for regions with consistent atrophy, Henry and colleagues[46] found that abnormalities were particularly evident in the thalamus and basal ganglia (ie, deep GM structures) and correlated with T1-weighted lesion loads. Ceccarelli and colleagues,[47] however, were not able to confirm these findings in CIS patients recruited within 3 months from clinical presentation, whereas they confirmed it in patients with clinically established MS. Moreover, VBM analysis of patients with RRMS with a very short disease duration (3 years) confirmed a consistent thalamic atrophy,[45] thus confirming previous data.[48] Finally, a selective left temporal and prefrontal cortical atrophy was observed in a patient studied within 3 years from clinically established MS diagnosis and a mean of 5 years from the first clinical symptoms.[49] Possible explanations for the above reported differences in regional atrophy can be a selective focal pathologic process involving the GM in subgroups of patients, individual local GM susceptibility, a secondary effect consequent to WM tract damage, or even a combination of all of these.

A 20-year longitudinal study has allowed an exploration of the associations and role as predictors of MR imaging measures, tissue-specific (GM and WM) atrophy, and WM lesion load, with clinical phenotype and disability.[3] In this cohort of patients, both GM and WM atrophy were seen in patients with MS compared with healthy subjects, but the extent of GM atrophy was greater than that of WM atrophy. Furthermore, there was significantly more GM, but not WM, atrophy in secondary progressive (SP) MS versus RRMS, and in RRMS versus those remaining CIS. Finally, GM, but not WM volume measurements, correlated with clinical disability. Although T2 lesion load correlated significantly with disability, grey matter fraction (GMF) was a better predictor of disability when included in the regression models.[3] In a recent study,[50] the authors observed that the distribution of GM damage is not homogeneous across different disease subtypes and, in turn, different disease durations. Both focal and diffuse GM damage seem to affect in the earliest phases of the disease (CIS and early RRMS), the fronto-temporal regions, especially hippocampal/parahippocampal gyri, insula, and cingulate, while they become more widespread, involving also precentral, postcentral gyri, and cerebellum, later in the disease course (late RRMS and SPMS). Only in CIS and early RRMS, the authors have found a strong correlation between the appearance of CLs and the cortical thickness change, suggesting that, at least at the beginning of the disease, the early focal cortical abnormality plays a relevant role in the development of brain atrophy.

Proton magnetic resonance spectroscopy

The tissue concentration of a variety of brain metabolites can be measured by ^{1}H-MRS. This technique constitutes a bridge between tissue microstructure and cellular metabolic function. N-acetyl-aspartate (NAA) is predominantly found in neurons and their axonal projections, and its reduction is thought to reflect both neuroaxonal loss and neuronal dysfunction.[51] In WM lesions, reduced NAA has been correlated with a reduced axonal density,[52] thus providing evidence of early neurodegeneration. However, reversible NAA reductions were also observed in WM lesions,[53] suggesting that a transient dysfunction of neurons that does not inevitably lead to their irreparable loss may occur in MS. Creatine (linked to energy flux in the brain[54] and considered a marker of cellular density and metabolic activity), choline-containing compounds (thought to reflect cell membrane turnover), myoinositol (associated with myelin damage and repair), and glutamate and glutamine (that form a cycle between astrocytes and neurons)[55] can be measured by ^{1}H-MRS in the brain of patients with MS.[56] As mentioned above, NAA peaks are thought to represent axonal and neuronal integrity. Whole-brain NAA was, on average, 22% lower (range: 8%–63%) in 71 patients with RRMS as compared with control subjects and appeared to be dependent on GM damage.[57]

A longitudinal study of GM in RRMS showed periodic peaks consistent with the breakdown of myelin-associated macromolecules.[58] These abnormal ^{1}H-MRS peaks had a time course similar to that of evolving WM lesions, but no association with modification in choline and NAA was found. This pattern may reflect the histologic finding that CLs are characterized by demyelination and microglial activation. Reduced NAA that parallels neuronal loss and atrophy has also been documented in deep central gray matter structures.[59] Despite the pathologic specificity of ^{1}H-MRS and the relatively large number of clinical ^{1}H-MRS studies on patients with MS, measures provided by this MR imaging technique are not used routinely for assessing and monitoring patients with MS.

Magnetization transfer MR imaging

Among the quantitative MR imaging techniques, magnetization transfer, based on the movement of protons in tissues, is likely to contribute to a more complete picture of the complex pathologic features of MS occurring not only in brain T2-visible lesions but also in the normal-appearing brain tissues. Proton motion is restricted in cell membranes and increases when the water content in the tissue increases. The degree of signal loss depends on the density of the macromolecules in a given tissue. Thus, low MTR indicates a reduced capacity of the macromolecules in brain tissue to exchange magnetization with the surrounding water molecules, reflecting damage to myelin or to the axonal membrane. In other words, a reduction of the MTR is related to the percentage of residual axons and the degree of demyelination. Similarly, dynamic changes of MTR values in MS lesions have been found to be consistent with demyelination and remyelination.

In a postmortem study,[60] the MTR of MS lesions and NAWM was found to be strongly associated with the degree of myelin and axon loss. In patients with MS, average MTR of lesions correlates better with physical disability than does the T2 lesion volume.[61] In NAGM and NAWM as well as in overt lesions, the MTR is typically decreased. Such decreases are seen in patients at the earliest stage of disease, including in both cortical and subcortical GM areas.[62,63] It has been observed that outer cortical quantitative MR imaging (qMR imaging) (MTR and T_2^*) is different in patients with MS than controls, with a more pronounced MTR reduction in SPMS than in patients with RRMS.[64,65] A study based on 7-T postmortem MR imaging looked at the capacity to distinguish NAGM from subpial lesions with qMR imaging techniques and found lower mean MTR and qR2* in histopathologic verified subpial lesions compared with myelin density-matched NAGM.[66] This observation also supports the notion that lower MTR in the outer cortex of patients is (at least partially) related to demyelination and could reflect the frequently overlooked subpial lesions (type III CLs).[64,67]

The relationship between MTR alterations of the NAGM and the clinical disability gave conflicting results. In a long-term perspective study of a large cohort of patients, disease duration, baseline expanded disability status scale (EDSS), T2 lesion volume, GMF, average GM MTR, and histogram peak height, as well as the 12-month percentage change of average lesion MTR, were all associated with the long-term worsening of disability at the univariate logistic regression analysis. However, when the multivariate model was applied, it retained only GM MTR histogram peak height and average lesion MTR percentage change after 12 months as independent predictors of such an evolution.[68] More recently, a study found that NAGM (more than lesional) MTR was consistently associated with physical and cognitive outcome measures.[61] However, another recent study found that CLs rather than NAGM were related to physical and cognitive outcome measures.[69]

Diffusion-weighted MR imaging

Diffusion-weighted MR imaging is based on the possibility of measuring diffusional motion of water molecules and, as a consequence the interactions between tissue water and cellular structures, providing information about the orientation, size, and geometry of brain structures.[70] In biological systems, molecules are generally confined in restricted regions of space by partially permeable barriers that hinder diffusion and lead to a situation where the diffusion coefficient is always lower than that of free water and is, therefore, called the apparent diffusion coefficient (ADC). Because some cellular structures, such as axons, are aligned on the scale of an image pixel, ADC is also dependent on the measurement direction. A full characterization of diffusion can be achieved in terms of a tensor, a 3×3 matrix that accounts for the correlation existing in anisotropic media between molecular displacement along one direction, and the displacement along orthogonal directions. From the tensor, it is possible to derive some indices that are invariant to changes of the frame of references. These indices include the mean diffusivity (MD = 1/3 of the trace of the tensor) and the fractional anisotropy (FA).[71] The second represents the most robust measure of anisotropy.

Changes in FA of the brain tissue may result either from a decrease of "restricting" barriers, that increases diffusivity, or by microglia activation and loss of neuronal ramification, that increases FA.

When DTI was applied to study the GM damage in patients with MS, FA was significantly increased in CLs and NAGM of patients with RRMS as compared with normal controls. This study confirmed that the involvement of GM in MS was marked and diffuse beyond the focal lesions and indicated that DTI might be a useful tool in analyzing GM abnormality.[72] A recent study compared mean MD, FA, and MTR in CLs (detected using PSIR) and extralesional cortical GM and assessed associations with disability in relapse-onset MS. The abnormalities identified in lesional and extralesional cortical GM were greater in SPMS than in RRMS. Changes in extralesional compared with lesional cortical GM were more consistently associated with disability.[73]

Although DTI has great potential in MS research, the interpretation of diffusion data is not straightforward (Fig. 3). Concomitant factors determine changes of DTI-derived metrics, and it is difficult to relate such changes to the pathologic processes responsible for clinical impairment. In addition, the complexities of the underlying axonal

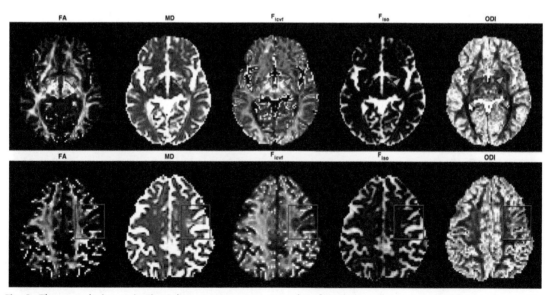

Fig. 3. The same lesion as in **Fig. 2** (upper row, *green arrowhead*) and **Fig. 1** (lower row, *red box*) is shown. The first 2 maps shown are the FA and MD obtained with a classic diffusion-tensor imaging acquisition (32 directions at a b value of 700 s/mm²). It is difficult to delineate the lesion in the FA map of the upper row. However, FA shows a decrement in the mixed lesion (bottom row). MD is increased in both lesions. The other 3 maps are obtained with the NODDI. The intraneurite fraction (F_{icvf}) shows a reduced density of neurite. The isotropic fraction (F_{iso}), which represents the cerebrospinal-like fraction of the voxel, on the contrary, shows an augmented isotropic fraction on both lesions. The ODI, which shows the coherence of orientation of fibers in the voxel, shows a decreased value compared with the surrounding NAGM.

architecture, even without the disease-related structural damage, play an important role in determining the diffusion characteristics. Despite these limitations, DTI appears to offer improved pathologic specificity over conventional MR imaging for assessing the degree of structural damage in individual MS lesions, and its quantitative nature allows an assessment of the more widespread tissue damage occurring outside such lesions. Nevertheless, the application of conventional DTI in GM is limited to the relevant partial volume effect and the intrinsic microstructure of GM, which is not well represented by anisotropic Gaussian diffusion. Novel models such as the neurite orientation dispersion and density imaging (NODDI; see Fig. 3) or the spherical mean technique (SMT)[74] could be used to assess the microstructure of the GM and its damage. NODDI is a nonlinear model that relies on a multicompartment mathematical description of the signal that exploits the additional information provided by multishell acquisitions to obtain several quantitative maps that, unlike classic DTI, are meaningful also in GM regions.[75] NODDI provides the assessment of the contribution of 3 diffusion compartments in each voxel: the compartments identified are CSF-like (F_{ISO} [unitless]), extraneurite, and intraneurite (F_{ICVF} [unitless]), which are characterized by isotropic, anisotropic Gaussian, and anisotropic non-Gaussian diffusion, respectively. A further parameter called orientation dispersion index (ODI) provides the grade of coherence of neurite direction. NODDI has been applied successfully to distinguish between patients with MS with and without concurrent epilepsy showing

significant statistically differences in hippocampus, lateral temporal lobe, cingulate, and insula.[76] Although NODDI have been already applied successfully to MS, SMT remains a novel model, with potential development to produce new biomarkers.

Susceptibility-weighted imaging

Susceptibility-weighted imaging and the novel quantitative susceptibility mapping (QSM; Fig. 4) technique showed the potential of characterizing the iron accumulation in tissues of patients with MS. QSM has been applied successfully both to deep GM structures[77,78] and to characterize focal CLs at high field strength.[79] Quantitative susceptibility can be estimated from phase images of multiecho gradient echo sequences or with novel technique based on total generalized variation and also from single-echo segmented 3D Echo Planar Imaging (EPI).[80] Using the magnitude of a multi-echo acquisition, it is possible to estimate T_2^* relaxation that could be used as a marker of demyelination and iron loss. Moreover, using a surface-based approach and T_2^* mapping, Louapre and colleagues[81] showed that cortical damage is spread beyond visible CLs: nearby lesions in RRMS and more scattered in SPMS. Moreover, another study (measuring the T_2^* at different laminar level of the cortex) showed a gradient in the degree of cortical abnormality throughout stages of MS, that might explain a cortical pathologic process driven from the pial surface.[67] Although only preliminary, results so far available on the application of this sequence in MS suggest that susceptibility-weighted imaging could be a

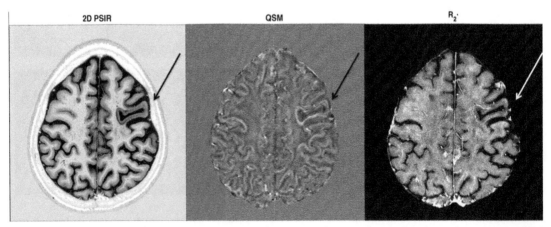

Fig. 4. The same big mixed WM and GM MS lesion of Fig. 1 and Fig. 3 is shown (black or white arrow). PSIR is reported to provide a good anatomic reference. The QSM is obtained from a single-echo flow compensated 3D Echo planar imaging and elaborated with a novel total generalized variation algorithm.[77] The lesion shows a hyperintensity profile. The third image represents the R2* = 1/T_2^* quantified from a 3D multi-echo gradient echo sequence. The lesion in the R2* map shows a less evident hyperintensity than the QSM map. The parameters of the sequence used are reported in Table 1.

helpful tool in the study of GM damage since the early phase of the disease.

Perfusion imaging

GM abnormality in patients with MS could also be related to metabolic deficits that can be measured with perfusion MR imaging.[82] Perfusion-based measures obtained with dynamic susceptibility contrast-MR imaging such as cerebral blood flow (CBF) or cerebral blood volume (CBV) could assess the healthiness of tissues and has been applied to MS in several studies. Reductions in CBF and CBV compared with the NAGM have been consistently described in CLs[83] and in the NAGM in patients with MS.[84] In more recent studies, similar findings were identified in an early cohort of patients with MS,[85] using arterial spin labeling (ASL). This technique can be used also to measure CBF at both normocapnia and hypercapnia to assess the cerebrovascular reactivity that reported a dis-regulation in patients with MS.[86] Endothelial dysfunction caused by oxidative stress and inflammatory activity combined with augmented resistance in venules or reduced stiffness in arterioles could lead to vascular disregulation in MS. These aspects of metabolic and hemodynamic function could also be monitored with a further parameter estimated with ASL: arterial arrival time, which has been shown to be prolonged in deep GM.[87]

SUMMARY

GM damage is a frequent phenomenon in patients with MS since the early phase of the disease and has demonstrated to be clinically relevant. Unfortunately, conventional MR imaging techniques are highly insensitive in the detection of focal or diffuse cortical GM damage. In the last few years, great effort has been made in order to overcome this limitation by developing and implementing advanced and quantitative MR imaging techniques, which have the potential not only of increasing the sensitivity of MR imaging in detecting focal lesions but also of quantifying the type and extension of diffuse GM damage. However, limited availability of these techniques, together with some technical challenges, limits their application to the research field.

REFERENCES

1. Kutzelnigg A, Lucchinetti CF, Stadelmann C, et al. Cortical demyelination and diffuse white matter injury in multiple sclerosis. Brain 2005;128(Pt 11): 2705–12.
2. Wegner C, Esiri MM, Chance SA, et al. Neocortical neuronal, synaptic, and glial loss in multiple sclerosis. Neurology 2006;67(6):960–7.
3. Fisniku LK, Chard DT, Jackson JS, et al. Gray matter atrophy is related to long-term disability in multiple sclerosis. Ann Neurol 2008;64(3):247–54.
4. Frischer JM, Bramow S, Dal-Bianco A, et al. The relation between inflammation and neurodegeneration in multiple sclerosis brains. Brain 2009; 132(Pt 5):1175–89.
5. Peterson JW, Bö L, Mörk S, et al. Transected neurites, apoptotic neurons, and reduced inflammation in cortical multiple sclerosis lesions. Ann Neurol 2001;50(3):389–400.
6. Vercellino M, Plano F, Votta B, et al. Grey matter pathology in multiple sclerosis. J Neuropathol Exp Neurol 2005;64(12):1101–7.
7. Gilmore CP, Donaldson I, Bo L, et al. Regional variations in the extent and pattern of grey matter demyelination in multiple sclerosis: a comparison between the cerebral cortex, cerebellar cortex, deep grey matter nuclei and the spinal cord. J Neurol Neurosurg Psychiatry 2009;80(2):182–7.
8. Albert M, Antel J, Brück W, et al. Extensive cortical remyelination in patients with chronic multiple sclerosis. Brain Pathol 2007;17(2):129–38.
9. Kutzelnigg A, Faber-rod JC, Bauer J, et al. Widespread demyelination in the cerebellar cortex in multiple sclerosis. Brain Pathol 2007;17(1):38–44.
10. Geurts JJG, Bö L, Roosendaal SD, et al. Extensive hippocampal demyelination in multiple sclerosis. J Neuropathol Exp Neurol 2007;66(9):819–27.
11. Papadopoulos D, Dukes S, Patel R, et al. Substantial archaeocortical atrophy and neuronal loss in multiple sclerosis. Brain Pathol 2009;19(51): 238–53.
12. Gilmore CP, Bö L, Owens T, et al. Spinal cord gray matter demyelination in multiple sclerosis—a novel pattern of residual plaque morphology. Brain Pathol 2006;16(3):202–8.
13. Boggild MD, Williams R, Haq N, et al. Cortical plaques visualised by fluid-attenuated inversion recovery imaging in relapsing multiple sclerosis. Neuroradiology 1996;38(Suppl 1):S10–3.
14. Filippi M, Yousry T, Baratti C, et al. Quantitative assessment of MRI lesion load in multiple sclerosis. A comparison of conventional spin-echo with fast fluid-attenuated inversion recovery. Brain 1996; 119(Pt 4):1349–55.
15. Gawne-Cain ML, O'Riordan JI, Thompson AJ, et al. Multiple sclerosis lesion detection in the brain: a comparison of fast fluid-attenuated inversion recovery and conventional T2-weighted dual spin echo. Neurology 1997;49(2):364–70.
16. Rovaris M, Filippi M, Minicucci L, et al. Cortical/subcortical disease burden and cognitive impairment in patients with multiple sclerosis. AJNR Am J Neuroradiol 2000;21(2):402–8.
17. Bakshi R, Ariyaratana S, Benedict RH, et al. Fluid-attenuated inversion recovery magnetic resonance

imaging detects cortical and juxtacortical multiple sclerosis lesions. Arch Neurol 2001;58(5):742–8.

18. Geurts JJG, Bo L, Pouwels PJW, et al. Cortical lesions in multiple sclerosis : combined postmortem MR imaging and histopathology. AJNR Am J Neuroradiol 2005;26(3):572–7.

19. Geurts JJG, Pouwels PJW, Uitdehaag BMJ, et al. Intracortical lesions in multiple sclerosis: improved detection with 3D double inversion-recovery MR imaging. Radiology 2005;236(1):254–60.

20. Pouwels PJW, Kuijer JPA, Mugler JP, et al. Human gray matter: feasibility of single-slab 3D double inversion-recovery high-spatial-resolution MR imaging. Radiology 2006;241(3):873–9.

21. Calabrese M, Gallo P. Magnetic resonance evidence of cortical onset of multiple sclerosis. Mult Scler 2009;15(8):933–41.

22. Calabrese M, Poretto V, Favaretto A, et al. Cortical lesion load associates with progression of disability in multiple sclerosis. Brain 2012;135(Pt 10):2952–61.

23. Calabrese M, Agosta F, Rinaldi F, et al. Cortical lesions and atrophy associated with cognitive impairment in relapsing-remitting multiple sclerosis. Arch Neurol 2009;66(9):1144–50.

24. Filippi M, Rocca MA, Calabrese M, et al. Intracortical lesions: relevance for new MRI diagnostic criteria for multiple sclerosis. Neurology 2010; 75(22):1988–94.

25. Seewann A, Vrenken H, Kooi E-J, et al. Imaging the tip of the iceberg: visualization of cortical lesions in multiple sclerosis. Mult Scler 2011;17(10):1202–10.

26. Mike A, Glanz BI, Hildenbrand P, et al. Identification and clinical impact of multiple sclerosis cortical lesions as assessed by routine 3T MR imaging. AJNR Am J Neuroradiol 2011;32(3):515–21.

27. Simon B, Schmidt S, Lukas C, et al. Improved in vivo detection of cortical lesions in multiple sclerosis using double inversion recovery MR imaging at 3 tesla. Eur Radiol 2010;20(7):1675–83.

28. Bagnato F, Butman JA, Gupta S, et al. In vivo detection of cortical plaques by MR imaging in patients with multiple sclerosis. AJNR Am J Neuroradiol 2006;27(10):2161–7.

29. Sethi V, Yousry TA, Muhlert N, et al. Improved detection of cortical MS lesions with phase-sensitive inversion recovery MRI. J Neurol Neurosurg Psychiatry 2012;83(9):877–82.

30. Nelson F, Poonawalla AH, Hou P, et al. Improved identification of intracortical lesions in multiple sclerosis with phase-sensitive inversion recovery in combination with fast double inversion recovery MR imaging. AJNR Am J Neuroradiol 2007;28(9): 1645–9.

31. Harel A, Ceccarelli A, Farrell C, et al. Phase-sensitive inversion-recovery MRI improves longitudinal cortical lesion detection in progressive MS. PLoS One 2016;11(3):e0152180.

32. Calabrese M, Rinaldi L, Mcauliffe MJM. Cortical atrophy is relevant in multiple sclerosis at clinical onset. J Neurol 2007;254(9):1212–20.

33. Sastre-garriga J, Ingle GT, Chard DT, et al. Grey and white matter volume changes in early primary progressive multiple sclerosis : a longitudinal study. Brain 2005;128(Pt 6):1454–60.

34. Dalton CM, Chard DT, Davies GR, et al. Early development of multiple sclerosis is associated with progressive grey matter atrophy in patients presenting with clinically isolated syndromes. Brain 2004; 127(5):1101–7.

35. De Stefano N, Matthews PM, Filippi M, et al. Evidence of early cortical atrophy in MS: relevance to white matter changes and disability. Neurology 2003;60(7):1157–62. Available at: http://www.ncbi. nlm.nih.gov/pubmed/12682324. Accessed July 15, 2015.

36. Chard D, Miller D. Grey matter pathology in clinically early multiple sclerosis: evidence from magnetic resonance imaging. J Neurol Sci 2009;282(1–2):5–11.

37. De Stefano N, Guidi L, Stromillo ML, et al. Imaging neuronal and axonal degeneration in multiple sclerosis. Neurol Sci 2003;24(Suppl 5):S283–6.

38. Filippi M, Inglese M, Rovaris M, et al. Magnetization transfer imaging to monitor the evolution of MS A 1-year follow-up study. Neurology 2000;55(7):940–6.

39. Filippi M, Preziosa P, Copetti M, et al. Gray matter damage predicts the accumulation of disability 13 years later in MS. Neurology 2013;81(20):1759–67.

40. Giorgio A, De Stefano N. Cognition in multiple sclerosis: relevance of lesions, brain atrophy and proton MR spectroscopy. Neurol Sci 2010;31(Suppl 2): S245–8.

41. Chen JT, Narayanan S, Collins DL, et al. Relating neocortical pathology to disability progression in multiple sclerosis using MRI. Neuroimage 2004; 23(3):1168–75.

42. Sailer M, Fischl B, Salat D, et al. Focal thinning of the cerebral cortex in multiple sclerosis. Brain 2003; 126(8):1734–44.

43. Charil A, Dagher A, Lerch JP, et al. Focal cortical atrophy in multiple sclerosis: relation to lesion load and disability. Neuroimage 2007;34:509–17.

44. Polman CH, Reingold SC, Banwell B, et al. Diagnostic criteria for multiple sclerosis: 2010 revisions to the McDonald criteria. Ann Neurol 2011;69(2): 292–302.

45. Audoin B, Davies GR, Finisku L, et al. Localization of grey matter atrophy in early RRMS: A longitudinal study. J Neurol 2006;253(11):1495–501.

46. Henry RG, Shieh M, Okuda DT, et al. Regional grey matter atrophy in clinically isolated syndromes at presentation. J Neurol Neurosurg Psychiatry 2008; 79(11):1236–44.

47. Ceccarelli A, Rocca MA, Pagani E, et al. A voxel-based morphometry study of grey matter loss in

MS patients with different clinical phenotypes. Neuroimage 2008;42(1):315–22.

48. Chard DT, Griffin CM, Parker GJM, et al. Brain atrophy in clinically early relapsing-remitting multiple sclerosis. Brain 2002;125(Pt 2):327–37.

49. Morgen K, Sammer G, Courtney SM, et al. Evidence for a direct association between cortical atrophy and cognitive impairment in relapsing-remitting MS. Neuroimage 2006;30:891–8.

50. Calabrese M, Reynolds R, Magliozzi R, et al. Regional distribution and evolution of gray matter damage in different populations of multiple sclerosis patients. PLoS One 2015;10(8):e0135428.

51. Moffett JR, Ross B, Arun P, et al. N-Acetylaspartate in the CNS: from neurodiagnostics to neurobiology. Prog Neurobiol 2007;81(2):89–131.

52. Bitsch A, Bruhn H, Vougioukas V, et al. Inflammatory CNS demyelination: histopathologic correlation with in vivo quantitative proton MR spectroscopy. AJNR Am J Neuroradiol 1999;20(9):1619–27.

53. Mader I, Roser W, Kappos L, et al. Serial proton MR spectroscopy of contrast-enhancing multiple sclerosis plaques: absolute metabolic values over 2 years during a clinical pharmacological study. AJNR Am J Neuroradiol 2000;21(7):1220–7.

54. Wyss M, Kaddurah-Daouk R. Creatine and creatinine metabolism. Physiol Rev 2000;80(3):1107–213.

55. Rothman DL, Sibson NR, Hyder F, et al. In vivo nuclear magnetic resonance spectroscopy studies of the relationship between the glutamate-glutamine neurotransmitter cycle and functional neuroenergetics. Philos Trans R Soc Lond B Biol Sci 1999; 354(1387):1165–77.

56. Newcombe J, Uddin A, Dove R, et al. Glutamate receptor expression in multiple sclerosis lesions. Brain Pathol 2008;18(1):52–61.

57. Inglese M, Ge Y, Filippi M, et al. Indirect evidence for early widespread gray matter involvement in relapsing-remitting multiple sclerosis. Neuroimage 2004;21(4):1825–9.

58. Sharma R, Narayana PA, Wolinsky JS. Grey matter abnormalities in multiple sclerosis: proton magnetic resonance spectroscopic imaging. Mult Scler 2001;7(4):221–6.

59. Cifelli A, Arridge M, Jezzard P, et al. Thalamic neurodegeneration in multiple sclerosis. Ann Neurol 2002; 52(5):650–3.

60. Van Waesberghe JHTM, Kamphorst W, De Groot CJA, et al. Axonal loss in multiple sclerosis lesions: magnetic resonance imaging insights into substrates of disability. Ann Neurol 1999;46(5): 747–54.

61. Gass A, Barker GJ, Kidd D, et al. Correlation of magnetization transfer ratio with clinical disability in multiple sclerosis. Ann Neurol 1994;36(1):62–7.

62. Audoin B, Ranjeva JP, Van Au Duong M, et al. Voxel-based analysis of MTR images: a method to locate gray matter abnormalities in patients at the earliest stage of multiple sclerosis. J Magn Reson Imaging 2004;20(5):765–71.

63. Cercignani M, Bozzali M, Iannucci G, et al. Magnetisation transfer ratio and mean diffusivity of normal appearing white and grey matter from patients with multiple sclerosis. J Neurol Neurosurg Psychiatry 2001;70(3):311–7.

64. Derakhshan M, Caramanos Z, Narayanan S, et al. Surface-based analysis reveals regions of reduced cortical magnetization transfer ratio in patients with multiple sclerosis: a proposed method for imaging subpial demyelination. Hum Brain Mapp 2014; 35(7):3402–13.

65. Samson RS, Cardoso MJ, Muhlert N, et al. Investigation of outer cortical magnetisation transfer ratio abnormalities in multiple sclerosis clinical subgroups. Mult Scler 2014;20(10):1322–30.

66. Jonkman LE, Fleysher L, Steenwijk MD, et al. Ultrahigh field MTR and qR2* differentiates subpial cortical lesions from normal-appearing gray matter in multiple sclerosis. Mult Scler 2016;22(10):1306–14.

67. Mainero C, Louapre C, Govindarajan ST, et al. A gradient in cortical pathology in multiple sclerosis by in vivo quantitative 7 T imaging. Brain 2015; 138(Pt 4):932–45.

68. Agosta F, Rovaris M, Pagani E, et al. Magnetization transfer MRI metrics predict the accumulation of disability 8 years later in patients with multiple sclerosis. Brain 2006;129(Pt 10):2620–7.

69. Amann M, Papadopoulou A, Andelova M, et al. Magnetization transfer ratio in lesions rather than normal-appearing brain relates to disability in patients with multiple sclerosis. J Neurol 2015;262(8): 1909–17.

70. Le Bihan D. Molecular diffusion nuclear magnetic resonance imaging. Magn Reson Q 1991;7(1):1–30.

71. Basser PJ, Pierpaoli C. Microstructural and physiological features of tissues elucidated by quantitative-diffusion-tensor MRI. 1996. J Magn Reson 2011;213(2):560–70.

72. Calabrese M, Rinaldi F, Seppi D, et al. Cortical diffusion-tensor imaging abnormalities in multiple sclerosis: a 3-year longitudinal study. Radiology 2011;261(3):891–8.

73. Yaldizli Ö, Pardini M, Sethi V, et al. Characteristics of lesional and extra-lesional cortical grey matter in relapsing-remitting and secondary progressive multiple sclerosis: a magnetisation transfer and diffusion tensor imaging study. Mult Scler 2016;22(2):150–9.

74. Kaden E, Kelm ND, Carson RP, et al. Multi-compartment microscopic diffusion imaging. Neuroimage 2016;139:346–59.

75. Zhang H, Schneider T, Wheeler-Kingshott CA, et al. NODDI: practical in vivo neurite orientation dispersion and density imaging of the human brain. Neuroimage 2012;61(4):1000–16.

76. Calabrese M, Castellaro M, Bertoldo A, et al. Epilepsy in multiple sclerosis: the role of temporal lobe damage. Mult Scler 2016. http://dx.doi.org/10.1177/1352458516651502.

77. Ropele S, Kilsdonk ID, Wattjes MP, et al. Determinants of iron accumulation in deep grey matter of multiple sclerosis patients. Mult Scler 2014;20(13):1692–8.

78. Langkammer C, Liu T, Khalil M, et al. Quantitative susceptibility mapping in multiple sclerosis. Radiology 2013;267(2):551–9.

79. Bian W, Tranvinh E, Tourdias T, et al. In vivo 7T MR quantitative susceptibility mapping reveals opposite susceptibility contrast between cortical and white matter lesions in multiple sclerosis. AJNR Am J Neuroradiol 2016. http://dx.doi.org/10.3174/ajnr.A4830.

80. Langkammer C, Bredies K, Poser BA, et al. Fast quantitative susceptibility mapping using 3D EPI and total generalized variation. Neuroimage 2015;111:622–30.

81. Louapre C, Govindarajan ST, Giannì C, et al. Beyond focal cortical lesions in MS: an in vivo quantitative and spatial imaging study at 7T. Neurology 2015;85(19):1702–9.

82. D'haeseleer M, Hostenbach S, Peeters I, et al. Cerebral hypoperfusion: a new pathophysiologic concept in multiple sclerosis? J Cereb Blood Flow Metab 2015;35(9):1406–10.

83. Peruzzo D, Castellaro M, Calabrese M, et al. Heterogeneity of cortical lesions in multiple sclerosis: an MRI perfusion study. J Cereb Blood Flow Metab 2013;33(3):457–63.

84. D'haeseleer M, Cambron M, Vanopdenbosch L, et al. Vascular aspects of multiple sclerosis. Lancet Neurol 2011;10(7):657–66.

85. Debernard L, Melzer TR, Van Stockum S, et al. Reduced grey matter perfusion without volume loss in early relapsing-remitting multiple sclerosis. J Neurol Neurosurg Psychiatry 2014;85(5):544–51.

86. Marshall O, Lu H, Brisset J-C, et al. Impaired cerebrovascular reactivity in multiple sclerosis. JAMA Neurol 2014;71(10):1275–81.

87. Paling D, Thade Petersen E, Tozer DJ, et al. Cerebral arterial bolus arrival time is prolonged in multiple sclerosis and associated with disability. J Cereb Blood Flow Metab 2014;34(1):34–42.

88. Vercellino M, Masera S, Lorenzatti M, et al. Demyelination, inflammation, and neurodegeneration in multiple sclerosis deep gray matter. J Neuropathol Exp Neurol 2009;68(5):489–502.

89. Prinster A, Quarantelli M, Orefice G, et al. Grey matter loss in relapsing-remitting multiple sclerosis: a voxel-based morphometry study. Neuroimage 2006;29(3):859–67.

90. Bermel RA, Innus MD, Tjoa CW, et al. Selective caudate atrophy in multiple sclerosis: a 3D MRI parcellation study. Neuroreport 2003;14(3):335–9.

91. Geurts JJG, Reuling IEW, Vrenken H, et al. MR spectroscopic evidence for thalamic and hippocampal, but not cortical, damage in multiple sclerosis. Magn Reson Med 2006;55(3):478–83.

92. Mesaros S, Rocca MA, Absinta M, et al. Evidence of thalamic gray matter loss in pediatric multiple sclerosis. Neurology 2008;70(13 Pt 2):1107–12.

93. Quinn MP, Gati JS, Klassen ML, et al. Increased deep gray matter iron is present in clinically isolated syndromes. Mult Scler Relat Disord 2014;3(2):194–202.

94. Cavallari M, Ceccarelli A, Wang G-Y, et al. Microstructural changes in the striatum and their impact on motor and neuropsychological performance in patients with multiple sclerosis. PLoS One 2014;9(7):e101199.

Microstructural MR Imaging Techniques in Multiple Sclerosis

 CrossMark

Massimo Filippi, MD, FEAN*, Paolo Preziosa, MD,
Maria A. Rocca, MD

KEYWORDS

- Multiple sclerosis • Diffusion tensor • Magnetization transfer • MR imaging • White matter
- Gray matter • Spinal cord • Optic nerve

KEY POINTS

- Magnetization transfer (MT) and diffusion tensor (DT) MR imaging are validated techniques for the assessment of microstructural tissue abnormalities in multiple sclerosis (MS) patients.
- Using different methods of analysis, abnormalities of MT and DT MR imaging–derived indexes have been detected in different central nervous system (CNS) compartments in MS patients, including lesions, white matter (WM), gray matter (GM), the spinal cord, and the optic nerve.
- Such imaging abnormalities are more severe in patients with longer disease duration and with the progressive forms of the disease, they correlate with disease clinical manifestations (clinical disability, locomotor impairment, and cognitive impairment) and tend to worsen over time.
- The application of regional methods of analysis for the definition of the topographic distribution of damage holds promise for improving knowledge of the substrates determining the accumulation of irreversible disability and might provide new reliable markers to monitor disease progression and treatment efficacy.

INTRODUCTION

Due to its sensitivity in the detection of WM lesions, conventional MR imaging has become a paraclinical tool central to diagnosing MS and monitoring its evolution. Despite this, the correlation between patients' clinical manifestations and conventional MR imaging measures is often weak to moderate. The application of advanced MR imaging techniques with a higher specificity toward the heterogeneous pathologic substrates of the disease can contribute to improving knowledge of the substrates determining MS-related irreversible disability and identifying reliable

Disclosure Statement: M. Filippi is editor in chief of the *Journal of Neurology*; serves on a scientific advisory board for Teva Pharmaceutical Industries; has received compensation for consulting services and/or speaking activities from Biogen Idec, ExceMed, Novartis, and Teva Pharmaceutical Industries; and receives research support from Biogen Idec, Teva Pharmaceutical Industries, Novartis, Italian Ministry of Health, Fondazione Italiana Sclerosi Multipla, CurePSP, Alzheimer's Drug Discovery Foundation (ADDF), the Jacques and Gloria Gossweiler Foundation (Switzerland), and ARiSLA (Fondazione Italiana di Ricerca per la SLA). P. Preziosa received speaker honoraria from Biogen Idec, Novartis, and ExceMed. M.A. Rocca received speaker honoraria from Biogen Idec, Novartis, Teva Neurosciences, Genzyme, and ExceMed and receives research support from the Italian Ministry of Health and Fondazione Italiana Sclerosi Multipla.
Neuroimaging Research Unit, Institute of Experimental Neurology, Division of Neuroscience, San Raffaele Scientific Institute, Vita-Salute San Raffaele University, Via Olgettina, 60, Milan 20132, Italy
* Corresponding author. Neuroimaging Research Unit, Institute of Experimental Neurology, Division of Neuroscience, San Raffaele Scientific Institute, Vita-Salute San Raffaele University, Via Olgettina, 60, Milan 20132, Italy.
E-mail address: filippi.massimo@hsr.it

Neuroimag Clin N Am 27 (2017) 313–333
http://dx.doi.org/10.1016/j.nic.2016.12.004

neuroimaging.theclinics.com

markers to monitor disease progression and treatment efficacy.

MT MR imaging and DT MR imaging represent the 2 most relevant quantitative techniques applied to assess microstructural tissue abnormalities (ie, abnormalities beyond the resolution of conventional imaging) in patients suffering from this condition. Correlative MR imaging/pathologic studies have shown that the main pathologic correlates of MT and DT MR imaging alterations in MS are demyelination and axonal loss. This article provides an overview of the main results derived from the application of MT and DT MR imaging to study damage at the level of the brain, spinal cord, and optic nerve of patients with MS. The possibility of using these techniques to monitor treatment efficacy is also discussed.

METHODOLOGICAL CONSIDERATIONS

Several approaches can be used to analyze MS-related abnormalities on MT and DT MR imaging maps (Fig. 1):

1. Region-of-interest (ROI) analysis of specific tissues. This approach allows the study of individual MS lesions and discrete areas of the normal-appearing WM (NAWM) and GM.
2. Analysis of the average MT MR imaging/DT MR imaging values of T2 lesions. This approach allows investigators to obtain information about the severity of tissue damage of the overall lesion population.
3. Histogram analysis of large portions of brain and/or cord tissue. This strategy encompasses both microscopic and macroscopic lesion burdens of the examined tissues. It is possible, however, to mask lesions before the production of histograms, thus assessing only normal-appearing tissues. For each histogram, several parameters can be calculated, including the height and position of the histogram peak and the average value of a given parameter. Histograms can be obtained for the whole brain, WM, GM, or specific regions (eg, frontal lobe, cerebellum, and brainstem), which can be segmented according to standard neuroanatomic references.
4. Voxel-wise statistical analysis of MT MR imaging and DT MR imaging images. This approach, which is based on the use of standardized anatomic spaces and a voxel-by-voxel analysis, allows investigators to obtain an overall assessment of macroscopic and microscopic damages from the entire brain or specific brain tissues, such as the GM or the NAWM, without a priori knowledge about damage distribution.

Additional methods, applicable for the analysis of DT images, are discussed in the DT MR imaging section.

MAGNETIZATION TRANSFER MR IMAGING
Background

MT MR imaging is based on the interactions between protons in free fluid and protons bound to macromolecules.[1] When an off-resonance radiofrequency pulse is applied, the magnetization of bound protons becomes saturated. Magnetization is then transferred from these protons to more mobile protons, which reduces the signal intensity measured from the tissue.

MT MR imaging allows the calculation of an index, the MT ratio (MTR), which is a widely used measure of the amount of MT exchange taking place between the free (liquid) pool, in which protons are highly mobile, and a restricted (semisolid) pool consisting of protons bound to macromolecules, such as proteins or lipids, which are, therefore, relatively immobile.[1] The MTR reflects the efficiency of this exchange. It is obtained by calculating the difference in signal intensity between the images acquired before (nonsaturated [M_0]) and those acquired after (saturated [M_S]) the application of the radiofrequency pulse and then dividing this difference by the signal intensity before the pulse,[2] according to the following formula: ($M_0 - M_S$)/$M_0 \times 100$.

Therefore, a low MTR indicates that the signal reduction (due to the transfer of magnetization) is smaller than normal because of a reduced capacity of macromolecules in tissue to exchange magnetization with surrounding water molecules. As a consequence, this index provides an estimate of the extent of MS tissue disruption, and MTR is altered when myelin or other cellular structures (eg, neurons) are damaged. MTR is strongly affected by myelin, but it may also be influenced by water content, inflammation,[3] and axonal density.[4]

The most compelling evidence that the severity of MTR reduction reflects the severity of tissue injury comes from postmortem studies, which have shown a strong correlation between MTR and the degree of axonal and myelin damage.[4,5] A few studies also showed that remyelinated lesions have higher MTR values than demyelinated lesions,[4,6] suggesting the potential of MT MR imaging to monitor remyelination in MS.

Lesions

Several studies have reported variable and heterogeneous degrees an MTR reduction in focal WM MS lesions[7,8] (Fig. 2), with the most

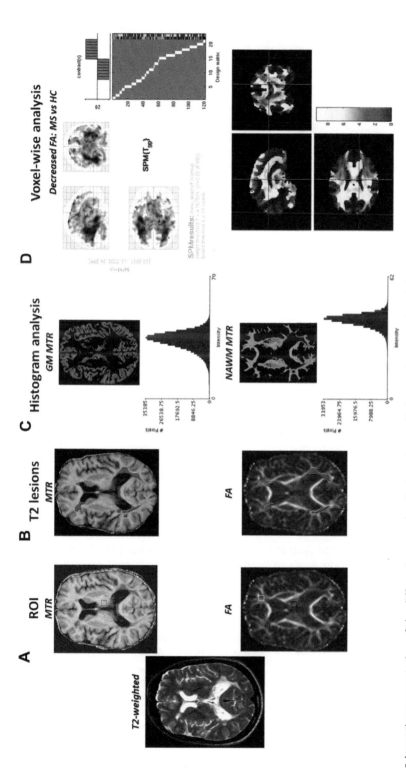

Fig. 1. Schematic representation of the different approaches that can be applied to analyze MS-related abnormalities on MT and DT MR imaging maps. (A) Analysis of ROIs with the selection of a WM lesion (*red*), a region of normal-appearing (NA) WM (*green*), and a region of GM (*blue*). (B) Analysis of the average MT MR imaging/DT MR imaging values of T2 lesions (*red*). (C) Histogram analysis of GM and NAWM. (D) Voxel-wise analysis. Comparison of FA values at a single voxel-level between MS patients (n = 61) and healthy controls (HC) (n = 23) using statistical parametric mapping (SPM) and a full factorial analysis of covariance, including age and gender as covariates in the design matrix (*top right*) (*P<.05 family-wise error corrected for multiple comparisons*). The graphic representation of the results is known as glass brain (*top left*), because the results of the analysis are reported on 3 views of the brain (sagittal, coronal, and axial) as if the brain were transparent. In the bottom part, regions with decreased FA (red-yellow coded) in MS patients versus HC are superimposed on a customized FA template.

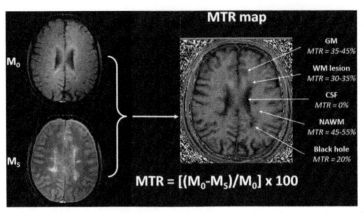

MTR map

GM
MTR = 35-45%

WM lesion
MTR = 30-35%

CSF
MTR = 0%

NAWM
MTR = 45-55%

Black hole
MTR = 20%

$$MTR = [(M_0-M_S)/M_0] \times 100$$

Fig. 2. Axial gradient-echo images of the brain, without (M_0) and with (M_S) the MT pulse applied, from a patient with RRMS. The corresponding MTR map obtained from the 2 previous coregistered images is also shown. MTR values of different brain regions are shown. MS lesions have highly variable MTR values.

prominent changes found in T1-hypointense lesions. Studies of newly formed lesions have shown that MTR drops substantially when a lesion forms (or starts to enhance) and then it generally recovers partially or completely during the subsequent 1 month to 6 months.[9–13] Such a finding is likely due to demyelination, possibly followed by different degrees of remyelination, where significantly higher values of MTR are observed.[4,6] MTR changes could also be due to edema and its subsequent resolution, because additional free extracellular water (edema) has a diluting effect on the measured MTR, although the magnitude of this diluting effect seems insufficient to fully explain the observed MTR changes.[14] Studies of individual enhancing lesions also suggest that the magnitude of the MTR changes is correlated with the severity of the associated tissue inflammation and the duration of the blood-brain barrier opening.[8,10,12,15]

Serial MR imaging studies have consistently demonstrated that MTR values drop in areas of NAWM several weeks before the formation of new gadolinium (Gd)-enhancing lesions.[10,11,16] These findings suggest the presence of focal biochemical changes preceding, the occurrence of MR imaging visible inflammatory activity. Different substrates might account for these abnormalities, including changes in the amount of unbound water caused by edema, astrocytic proliferation, early myelin injury, or axonal loss.[17–19]

Established chronic MS lesions also have a wide range of MTR values. T1-hypointense lesions (so-called black holes) have lower MTR than isointense lesions,[13,15] and MTR is inversely correlated with the degree of hypointensity.[15]

Recently, voxel-wise procedures have been applied to track longitudinal changes of MTR values in individual, newly formed MS lesions. Chen and colleagues[20] developed a method to monitor the evolution of MTR changes of individual lesion voxels and of mean normalized MTR over all lesion voxels during and after Gd enhancement and found significant changes of lesional MTR consistent with demyelination and remyelination that followed different temporal evolutions and which were still present in some lesions 3 years after their formation (**Fig. 3**). Brown and colleagues[21] demonstrated that focal demyelination may occur not only in NAWM before lesion formation but also in preexisting lesional tissue, suggesting that the heterogeneous patterns of focal lesions described by imaging and histopathologic studies might be the consequence of repeated episodes of demyelination associated with variable degree of remyelination and tissue recovery.

MS lesions are not limited to the WM but also involve, extensively, the GM. Using high and ultra-high field scanners, recent correlative MR imaging/pathologic studies reported a correlation between reduction of MTR values and the presence of focal cortical demyelination, supporting the notion that this technique is sensitive to demyelination/remyelination processes also in the cortex.[22–24] MTR reduction of the outer surface of the cortex has been detected in MS patients with the main disease phenotypes, with the lowest values seen in secondary progressive (SP) MS.[25,26] The spatial distributions of abnormal MTR preferentially involves cingulate cortex, insula, and the depths of sulci, in agreement with pathologic descriptions of subpial GM lesion distribution.[26] Moreover, the use of such a technique may contribute to the classification of different type of GM lesions.[27]

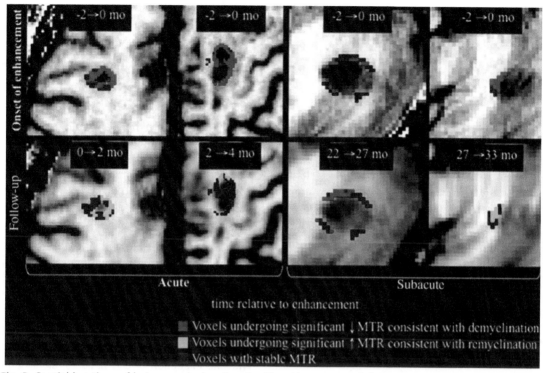

Fig. 3. Spatial locations of lesion voxels showing significant increases and decreases in MTR consistent with re-myelination and demyelination over time. MTR images from a single patient showing the heterogeneous evolution of initially enhancing lesion voxels (*top row*). Changes in MTR at the onset of enhancement in 4 lesions. Enhancement is associated with significant decreases in MTR consistent with demyelination over most voxels (*bottom row*). Changes in MTR at different time intervals after enhancement in the same lesion regions as shown in the top row. Most significant changes in MTR occur at the periphery of the initially enhancing lesion. In some cases, significant changes occur long after the time of enhancement. Red areas indicate voxels undergoing significant decreases in MTR consistent with demyelination; green areas indicate voxels undergoing significant increases in MTR consistent with remyelination; and blue areas indicate voxels with stable MTR. (*From* Chen JT, Collins DL, Atkins HL, et al. Magnetization transfer ratio evolution with demyelination and remyelination in multiple sclerosis lesions. Ann Neurol 2008;63(2):259; with permission.)

Normal-Appearing Brain Tissues, White Matter, and Gray Matter

The measurement of MTR in the whole normal-appearing brain tissue (NABT), after removal of focal WM lesions (defined as areas of abnormality seen on T2-weighted images), has been one of the first approaches used to investigate damage outside focal lesions in MS patients. Reduced NABT MTR has been found in asymptomatic relatives of MS patients,[28] in patients with clinically isolated syndrome (CIS),[29] and in patients with early relapsing-remitting (RR) MS with only mild clinical disability.[30,31] NABT MTR histograms are different[8,32,33] and evolve at a different pace in patients with the main MS clinical phenotypes.[8,32–34] Such NABT changes are only partially correlated with the extent of T2 visible lesions and the severity of intrinsic lesion damage,[33] suggesting that NABT MTR does not simply reflect wallerian degeneration of axons traversing the areas of focal pathology.

Decreased MTR values are also found in NAWM from MS patients, especially in areas adjacent to focal T2 lesions[35,36] and in the so-called dirty-appearing WM.[37]

Reduced MTR values have also been found in the cortical and deep GM of MS patients. GM abnormalities occur from the earliest phases of the disease,[38] become more severe in the progressive phenotypes,[39] and tend to worsen over time.[40–43]

Clinical Correlates

Average lesion MTR is lower in patients with RRMS than in those with CIS and benign (B) MS. A 3-year follow-up study[12] has also shown that newly formed lesions in SPMS patients have a more severe MTR deterioration than those in RRMS patients (**Fig. 4**). In addition, average lesion MTR percentage change after 12 months predicts the accumulation of clinical disability over the subsequent 8 years in patients with relapse-onset

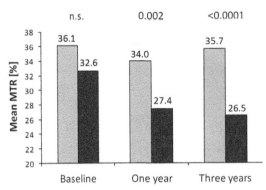

Fig. 4. MTR values of newly enhancing lesions from patients with RR (*light gray*) and SP (*dark gray*) MS at baseline and during 3 years of follow-up. Compared with RRMS, newly enhancing lesions in SPMS patients had lower MTR at the time of their appearance and presented a more severe and significant MTR reduction during the follow-up period. n.s., not significant. (*Adapted from* Rocca MA, Mastronardo G, Rodegher M, et al. Long-term changes of magnetization transfer-derived measures from patients with relapsing-remitting and secondary progressive multiple sclerosis. AJNR Am J Neuroradiol 1999;20(5):823; with permission.)

MS.[44] Brain MTR abnormalities are more severe in the more disabling stages of the disease[7,12,32,45] and correlate with the severity of clinical disability[45] and cognitive impairment.[46–49] A study in CIS patients has suggested that abnormal NABT MTR values at disease onset might have a predictive value for subsequent evolution to definite MS.[29] These results, however, have not been confirmed by subsequent studies.[50,51]

In patients with established MS, MTR reduction in the NAWM predicted the accumulation of clinical disability over the subsequent 5 years.[52,53] In relapse-onset MS patients, reduced GM MTR predicted worsening of disability after 8 years[44] and cognitive deterioration after 13 years.[54]

Regional analysis of brain MTR data may provide additional insights into the relationship between the location of brain tissue damage and its functional impact.[46–48] MTR decrease in specific cortical regions has been found to correlate with clinical disability and Paced Auditory Serial Addition Task performance in patients with primary progressive (PP) MS[48] and RRMS.[47]

Spinal Cord

MT MR imaging of the cervical cord and optic nerve presents technical difficulties, mainly because of the sizes of these 2 structures and their tendency to move during imaging. Nevertheless, several works have shown that it is possible to acquire good-quality MT MR images of the cervical cord (**Fig. 5**) and optic nerve.

With the exception of CIS patients, significant reduction of cervical cord MTR values have been found in MS patients with the main disease clinical phenotypes.[55–57] These MTR changes correlated with clinical disability,[56,58] whereas MTR abnormalities located in the dorsal and lateral columns of the spinal cord correlated with deficits of vibration sensation and strength, respectively.[59] In RRMS patients, reduced cervical cord GM MTR was correlated with the degree of disability.[60] A

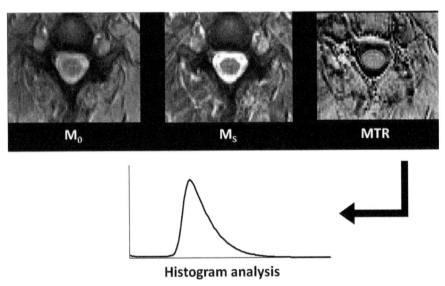

Fig. 5. Schematic representation of cervical cord spinal cord MT MR imaging analysis. Acquisition and coregistration of M_0 and M_s axial gradient-echo images of the cervical cord, creation of MTR maps, and histogram analysis, through the selection of regions of interest (*orange*).

recent study[61] showed that MTR abnormalities in the outer spinal cord region corresponding to the pia mater and subpial region occur already in patients with CIS and RRMS in the absence of atrophy and became more severe and associated with spinal cord atrophy in the progressive forms of the disease, thus suggesting that MTR abnormalities occur early in the course of MS and might represent useful predictors of subsequent accumulation of clinical disability, disease progression, and irreversible cord tissue loss.

Optic Nerve

Reduced MTR values of the optic nerve have been shown to correlate with several measures of optic nerve damage, including increased P100 latency at visual evoked potentials (VEP),[62,63] reduced retinal fiber layer thickness at optical coherence tomography (OCT),[63] and low visual acuity.[64] In a 1-year follow-up study of patients with acute optic neuritis, Hickman and colleagues[65] showed a progressive decline of average MTR of the affected optic nerve, which reached the nadir after approximately 8 months despite rapid initial visual recovery; such an MTR reduction was then followed by partial recovery. Another study evaluated patients with a first episode of acute optic neuritis using conventional and MT MR imaging at baseline and after 3 months and 12 months.[66] At the onset of acute optic neuritis, MTR values in the affected optic nerve were significantly higher than those of the healthy optic nerve, suggesting the presence of inflammatory cellular infiltrates due to the breakdown of the blood–optic nerve barrier. During follow-up, MTR values of affected optic nerve progressively decreased over time, without a subsequent increase, suggesting a progression of optic nerve damage despite the early visual recovery.[66]

Monitoring Multiple Sclerosis Treatment

Effort has been spent to set-up and standardize the acquisition of MT MR imaging sequences in multicenter studies.[51,67] Recovery of MTR in focal T2 lesions has been proposed as an outcome measure to assess the effect of remyelinating agents,[67,68] and sample size calculations have been performed for multicenter clinical trials using this metric.[67,68] A technique to quantify longitudinal MTR changes has been developed and applied to patients treated with autologous stem cell transplant.[68] A single-center MT MR imaging study showed that compared with interferon β-1a, natalizumab significantly promoted regional MTR recovery suggestive of remyelination and tissue recovery and prevented the further accumulation of microstructural tissue abnormalities both in the

NABT and in focal WM lesions.[69] Another single-center MT MR imaging study has suggested that alemtuzumab protects against GM and WM damage.[70] A combined MT and proton MR spectroscopy study[71] showed that compared with placebo, patients treated with laquinimod tend to accumulate less microscopic WM and GM damage. Another study showed that lamotrigine has no effect on the evolution of WM and GM damage measured using MTR in SPMS patients.[72] A recent post hoc analysis found that new brain lesions that developed during treatment with glatiramer acetate (GA) had evidence of greater MTR recovery than those formed during treatment with interferon β-1b.[73]

Future Perspectives

Using appropriate mathematical approaches to evaluate the MT effect in biological tissue models, it is possible to measure more fundamental quantitative MT parameters related to tissue structure, such as the restricted proton fraction, the T2 relaxation time of the restricted proton pool, the ratio of T1 to T2 for the free proton pool, and the forward exchange rate constant from the free to the restricted proton pool. These quantitative parameters are more robust and greatly influenced by the myelin content in the brain than MT MR imaging, because restricted protons are known to be attached to macromolecules, such as myelin, and have been demonstrated to be reliable and reproducible.[74,75] Giacomini and colleagues[76] studied 6 RRMS patients with acute Gd-enhancing lesions serially using quantitative MT imaging and demonstrated reductions in both MTR and the ratio of restricted to free protons in acute lesions, indicating a reduction in macromolecular content. Both parameters then recovered over a period of several months.

DIFFUSION MR IMAGING
Background

Diffusion-weighted MR imaging is a quantitative technique that exploits the diffusion of water molecules within biological tissues.[77] The diffusion coefficient measures the ease of this translational motion of water. In biological tissues like the brain, this coefficient is lower than that in free water because the various structures of the tissues (membranes, cell bodies, glia, inclusions, macromolecules, and so forth) influence the free movement of water molecules.[77] For this reason, when diffusion is evaluated in such biological systems, the measured diffusion coefficient is referred to as the apparent diffusion coefficient (ADC).[77] Pathologic processes that alter tissue integrity typically reduce the impediments to free water motion and, as a result, these processes tend to increase the measured ADC values.

A full characterization of diffusion can be provided in terms of a tensor,[78] which has a principal axis and 2 smaller axes that describe its width and depth. These 3 axes are perpendicular to each other and cross at the center point of the ellipsoid, and in this setting they are called eigenvectors and the measures of their length eigenvalues. The diffusivity along the principal axis is also called parallel or axial diffusivity (axD), whereas the diffusivities in the 2 minor axes are often averaged to produce a measure of radial diffusivity (radD). It is also possible to calculate the magnitude of diffusion, reflected by the mean diffusivity (MD) (Fig. 6), and the degree of anisotropy, which is a measure of tissue organization that can be expressed by several indexes, including a dimensionless one named fractional anisotropy (FA) (see Fig. 6).

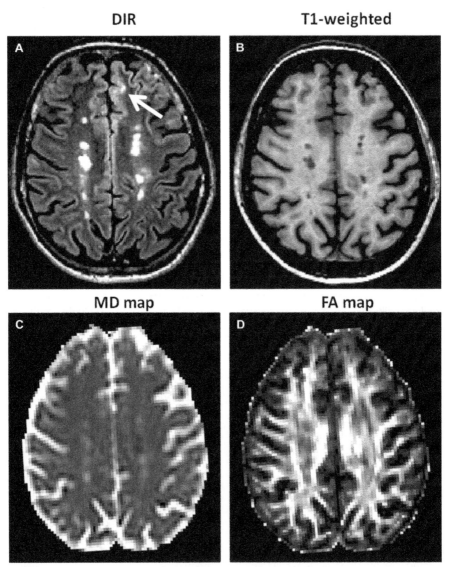

Fig. 6. Illustrative images from a patient with RRMS. (A) Double-inversion recovery (DIR) sequence, showing several WM hyperintense lesions and 1 GM lesion (arrow). (B) T1-weighted sequence showing several T1-hypointense lesions. (C) MD map. On this map, some of the lesions appear as hyperintense areas. The degree of hyperintensity is related to MD increase and indicates a loss of structural barriers to water molecular motion. (D) FA map. On this map, WM pixels are bright because of the directionality of the white matter fiber tracts. Dark areas corresponding to some of the macroscopic lesions indicate a loss of FA and suggest the presence of structural disorganization.

The pathologic elements of MS have the potential to alter the permeability or geometry of structural barriers to water diffusion in the CNS (Fig. 7). In particular, axonal damage has been shown to alter predominantly FA (which is typically decreased) and axD (which may result decreased or increased according to the stage of the insult and the direction and architecture of the underlying fibers),[78,79] whereas myelin breakdown has been associated with an increased radD,[78,79] even though pathologic studies have correlated myelin content also with FA and MD values.[80]

Lesions

DT MR imaging can contribute to grade the severity of damage within focal MS lesions, which typically show a heterogeneous pattern of diffusion abnormalities (ie, increased MD and decreased FA), which are always more pronounced than in the NAWM.[81,82] The more severe abnormalities are found in T1-hypointense lesions.[83,84] Conversely, conflicting results have been reported when comparing findings in Gd-enhancing versus nonenhancing lesions,[83–85] although most of the studies found lower FA values in enhancing lesions.[84,86] A longitudinal study of enhancing MS lesions followed-up for 1 to 3 months[85] showed that MD values were increased in all lesions but continued to increase during follow-up only in a subgroup of them. This finding highlights the notion that contrast enhancement does not allow profiling acute MS lesions, which might be characterized by varying degrees of tissue disruption. Importantly, despite a

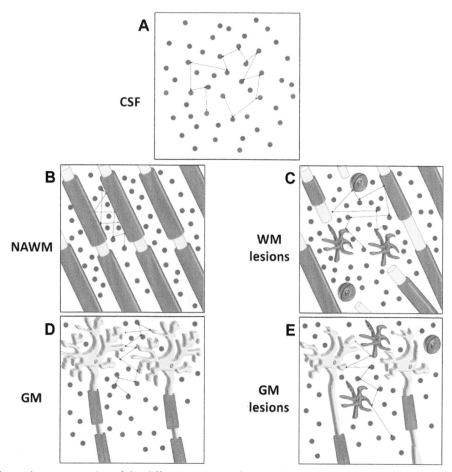

Fig. 7. Schematic representation of the different regimes of water diffusion in the different tissue compartments. (A) In the CSF, water molecule are constantly moving and colliding with other water molecules; (B) in the NAWM, diffusion is strongly dependent on the myelinated axonal direction; (C) in WM lesions, the movement of water molecules is increased, because it is influenced by edema, inflammation, demyelination, neuroaxonal damage, and gliosis (cells in green); (D) in the GM, diffusion of water molecule is also influenced by neuronal bodies and dendritic arborizations; and (E) in GM lesions, demyelination, neuroaxonal damage, reduction of dendritic arborization and gliosis might influence diffusion of water molecule, possibly increasing anisotropy.

majority of acute MS lesions presenting an increased diffusivity, a portion of demyelinating lesions might be characterized by an early restricted diffusivity, which might be or not in association with Gd-enhancement, possibly suggesting cytotoxic edema and increased cellularity combined with blood-brain barrier leakage.[87,88]

In line with MT MR imaging findings, DT MR imaging abnormalities are detectable in the NAWM several weeks before lesion formation.[89]

Several DT MR imaging studies have demonstrated that, compared with patients' normal appearing GM, intracortical MS lesions have increased FA values,[90–92] which might reflect an intralesional loss of dendrites, neuronal damage, and activation of microglial cells. One of these studies[92] also found that quantifying cortical lesions intrinsic damage using DT MR imaging can contribute distinguishing patients with SPMS from those with BMS (Fig. 8).

Normal-Appearing Brain Tissue, White Matter, and Gray Matter

DT MR imaging contributes to assess the presence, severity, and distribution of microstructural tissue abnormalities in the NABT, WM, and GM of MS patients.[81,82] Using different methods of analysis, increased MD and decreased FA have been consistently found in the NAWM of MS patients.[81,82] Such NAWM abnormalities tend to be more severe in perilesional areas[36,93] and at sites where MS lesions are typically located.[40,84]

DT MR imaging abnormalities have been demonstrated also in the GM of MS patients.[40,81,82,94,95] Higher MD values have been detected in deep GM nuclei of MS patients, especially in the thalamus.[96] These latter abnormalities were more pronounced in SPMS than in RRMS patients.[96]

NAWM and GM damage is only partially correlated with the extent of T2 lesions and the severity of intrinsic lesion damage, suggesting that diffusivity changes in NAWM and GM are not entirely dependent on retrograde degeneration of axons transected in focal lesions but rather they represent diffuse abnormalities beyond the resolution of conventional MR imaging. As support for this hypothesis, a study[97] correlated diffusivity with perfusion findings in the corpus callosum (CC) of RRMS patients. These results are more consistent with a primary ischemia than a secondary

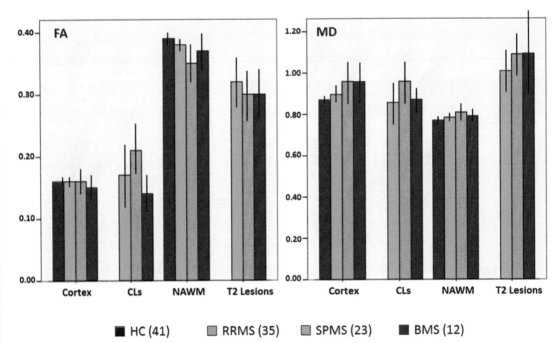

Fig. 8. DT imaging values from cortical lesions (CLs), cortex, NAWM, and T2 lesions in MS patients with different disease clinical phenotypes and a group of healthy controls (HC). Compared with RRMS patients, those with SPMS had a higher T2 lesion volume and a more severe damage to the cortex, NAWM, T2 lesions, and CLs. With the exception of CLs, damage to all these compartments was similar in SPMS and BMS patients. Conversely, compared with SPMS, BMS patients had lower FA and MD of CLs. No difference was detected between RRMS versus BMS patients. MD is expressed in units of mm²/s × 10⁻³; FA is dimensionless index. (*Adapted from* Filippi M, Preziosa P, Pagani E, et al. Microstructural MR imaging of cortical lesion in multiple sclerosis. Mult Scler 2013;19(4):418–26.)

hypoperfusion due to wallerian degeneration. These findings suggest a potentially reversible substrate of tissue damage, related to vascular impairment, whereas hypometabolism from axonal degeneration represents an advanced and irreversible condition.

Thanks to the ability of DT MR imaging to depict anisotropic tissues[98] and to detect their intrinsic structural abnormalities, several approaches have been developed to investigate damage to selected WM tracts, with the ultimate goal of improving the correlation with clinical measures. DT MR imaging tractography can be used to segment clinically eloquent WM pathways involved in different functions (**Fig. 9**), such as the corticospinal tract (CST),[99–101] CC,[102] optic

radiations (ORs)[103–105] and many others.[106–111] In line with studies performed using histogram or ROI analysis, these studies detected higher MD and lower FA of WM tracts in MS patients compared with healthy controls.

The application of tractography to the study of MS patients suffers from the drawback that the disease causes both focal and diffuse alterations of tissue organization, which result in a decreased anisotropy and consequent increase in uncertainty of the primary eigenvector of the DT. A possible approach to overcome this problem is the use of probability maps of tracts of interest obtained from healthy subjects to assess DT MR imaging metrics from the corresponding tracts of patients.[101]

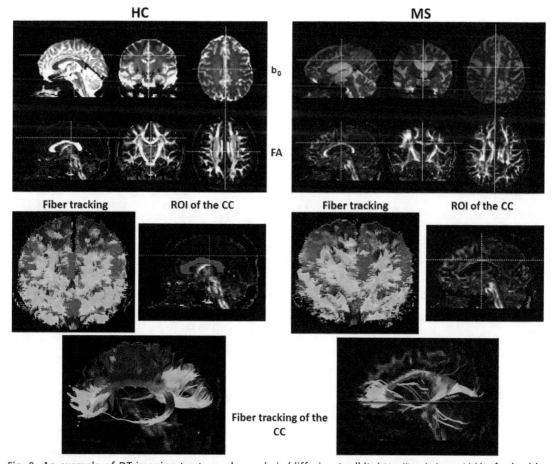

Fig. 9. An example of DT imaging tractography analysis (diffusion toolkit: http://trackvis.org/dtk) of a healthy control (HC) (*left*) and a patient with SPMS (*right*). The b_0 image FA map is shown in the top part of the figure. In the middle part, the global reconstruction of all fibers is shown. After the definition of an ROI for tracking the CC on the FA map, the reconstruction of the CC is shown at the bottom. In the MS patient, several periventricular lesions, causing a reduction of FA values, are visible on the b_0 image. Diffuse atrophy is also evident (enlargement of the ventricles and thinning of the CC on the midsagittal slice). The reconstruction of the CC shows the interruption of fiber propagation due to the presence of low FA values in lesions. Parameters used for tractography: FA threshold = 0.15; angle threshold = 35°; propagation algorithm: FACT with spline filter applied. b_0, image acquired without diffusion gradients applied.

Advances in DT MR imaging and tractography have promoted the development of brain neuroconnectivity techniques, which define and quantify anatomic links between remote brain regions by axonal fiber pathways.[112] The use of these approaches has revealed reduced network efficiency in the WM structural networks of MS patients,[113] including those with CIS.[114]

Voxel-wise approaches can also be used for the analysis of DT MR imaging data. A voxel-based study[115] showed that patients with RRMS and BMS differ in terms of topographic distribution of WM damage, whereas no between-group differences were found when the overall extent of WM diffusivity abnormalities was assessed. By combining tractography and voxel-based analysis, another study evaluated damage to several WM tracts, in terms of focal lesions and NAWM, from MS patients with the main disease clinical phenotypes.[106] Compared with healthy controls, diffusivity abnormalities were found in PPMS and CIS patients. The progressive MS forms showed

the most severe and distributed diffusivity abnormalities, whereas BMS patients had only a limited WM damage (Fig. 10). Using the same approach, 2 studies evaluated the correlations between impairment at visual[105] and cerebellar[110] functions with corresponding DT MR imaging abnormalities of the OR and cerebellar peduncles, demonstrating that such a strategy might contribute to explain clinical impairment in selective functional systems.

Tract-based spatial statistics is another technique that allows voxel-wise analysis of multisubject DT MR imaging data. Also, the use of such a technique has confirmed the presence of distributed WM tract FA and MD abnormalities in MS patients, which were related to deficits of specific cognitive domains.[116–119]

Clinical Correlates

Brain NAWM DT MR imaging abnormalities can be detected from the earliest stages of the disease in patients with CIS suggestive of MS,[106,120] and they

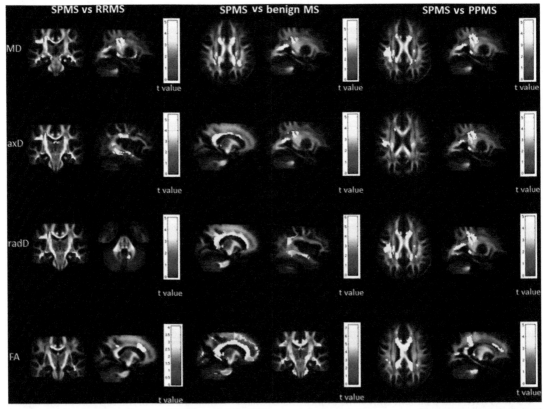

Fig. 10. Axial, sagittal, and coronal WM tract probability maps show statistical parametric mapping analysis (with color coding to show positive t values) of clusters with increased MD, axD, and radD, and decreased FA in different WM tracts of patients with SPMS versus RRMS, patients with SPMS versus BMS, and patients with SPMS versus PPMS (P<.001 for all comparisons). Images are presented in neurologic convention. axD, axial diffusivity; radD, radial diffusivity. (From Preziosa P, Rocca MA, Mesaros S, et al. Intrinsic damage to the major white matter tracts in patients with different clinical phenotypes of multiple sclerosis: a voxelwise diffusion-tensor MR study. Radiology 2011;260(2):547; with permission.)

become more pronounced with increasing disease duration and neurologic impairment.[40,81,82,106]

Using tractography, tract-derived DT MR imaging metrics correlate with several measures of locomotor disability and cognitive impairment.[99–104,107–111,121,122] For instance, MD and FA values of the CST correlated with clinical measures of motor (including locomotor) disability more than T2 lesion volume and the overall extent of diffusivity changes of the brain.[99,100,122] CIS patients with motor impairment had increased MD and T2 lesion volume in the CST compared with patients without pyramidal symptoms.[101] Increased MD of the CC has been associated with MS cognitive dysfunction.[100,102,123] Using DT MR imaging tractography of the ORs, 1 study showed that patients with optic neuritis had reduced connectivity values in both ORs compared with healthy controls, suggesting the occurrence of transsynaptic degeneration secondary to optic nerve damage.[103] In another study, OR DT MR imaging abnormalities correlated with retinal injury, assessed using OCT, and visual impairment.[104] By applying a random forest analysis to measures derived from DT MR imaging tractography, damage to critical WM tracts, such as the cingulum, was shown to contribute significantly to the cognitive impairment of MS patients.[121] The notion that cognitive impairment in MS patients is mainly due to a disconnection syndrome has also been demonstrated by a recent study that, using tractography-based parcellation of the thalamus and its WM connections, found that damage of specific cortico-thalamic tracts rather than thalamic damage itself, explained global cognitive dysfunction and impairment of selected cognitive domains.[124]

GM DT MR imaging changes tend to be more pronounced in patients with the progressive forms of the disease.[81,95,125] In patients with SPMS and PPMS,[126,127] as well as in those with RRMS[128] and CIS,[129] such DT MR imaging abnormalities worsen over time. The severity of GM damage has been correlated with the degree of cognitive impairment in mildly disabled RRMS patients[130] and has been found to predict accumulation of disability over a 5-year period in patients with PPMS.[127] In another study, average NAWM MD and FA thalamic change over 1 year follow-up were predictors of clinical deterioration after 5 years in PPMS patients.[131]

Spinal Cord

With the development of sophisticated MR imaging receiver coils and fast imaging techniques, it has been possible to obtain a more reliable imaging of the spinal cord, which also allows the acquisition of quantitative techniques, including DT MR imaging. Clark and colleagues[132] found higher MD values in spinal cord lesions of MS patients than in spinal cord from healthy controls. Abnormal DT MR imaging quantities from the cervical cord have been shown in patients with established MS[133,134] but not in those with CIS.[135] Cervical cord damage outside focal lesions is diffuse in SPMS, whereas it is more limited in BMS patients.[136] Several studies highlighted that brain and cord DT MR imaging metrics are independently associated with MS disability,[134,135,137] thus calling for an aggregate use of these measures to improve the understanding of disease progression.

Recent studies evaluated DT MR imaging abnormalities in the different cord compartments, including the main ascending and descending WM projections (eg, the CSTs and the posterior and lateral columns) and the central GM. Diffusivity abnormalities in the CST tracts and in the posterior columns[138] and at C2-C3 level[139] were associated with locomotor disability and sensory impairment, whereas spinal GM DT MR imaging abnormalities was associated with more severe clinical impairment and the presence of an SP phenotype.[140]

One longitudinal study, which obtained DT MR imaging from relapse-onset MS patients at baseline and after a mean period of 2.4 years, showed that baseline cord cross-sectional area and FA correlate with increased disability at follow-up.[60] In another study, lower radD at baseline and its improvement in the subsequent 6 months were associated with a better clinical outcome after a spinal cord relapse, suggesting that resolution of inflammation and remyelination might contribute to clinical recovery.[141]

Optic Nerve

Early DT MR imaging studies of the optic nerve measured diffusivity in a few directions.[142] With the introduction of high-resolution fat-suppressed and cerebral spinal fluid (CSF)-suppressed zonal oblique multisection echo-planar imaging sequences,[143–145] full DT MR imaging measurements from the optic nerve have been obtained.

In patients in the chronic phase after optic neuritis, MD of the diseased optic nerve is significantly higher than in either the fellow eye or those from healthy individuals.[143] DT MR imaging abnormalities correlated with abnormal VEP latencies,[143,146] loss of visual acuity,[143,147] and retinal nerve fiber layer thinning at OCT.[147] A multiparametric MR imaging study showed that 4 years after a unilateral optic neuritis, decreased optic nerve FA and volume are factors independently associated with visual dysfunction.[146] According to another study,[148] a significant lower axD during the acute optic neuritis was associated with a worse 6-month visual outcome and correlated with VEP and retinal nerve fiber layer measures of axon and myelin injury, whereas optic nerve radD after at least 6 months from an optic neuritis could differentiate normal, unaffected and affected optic nerve and categories of visual recovery.[149]

Monitoring Multiple Sclerosis Treatment

Only a few studies tried to set-up and standardize the acquisition of DT MR imaging sequences in multicenter studies.[119,124,150] Despite this, no clinical trial has yet been published with these metrics as outcome measures. A preliminary single-center study in 21 MS patients starting natalizumab showed that baseline Gd-enhancing lesions had increased FA after 1 year of treatment, which was mainly due to a decrease of radD. A significant decrease of FA was detected after 1 year in NABT, which was mainly driven by decreased axD. Globally, these results might reflect possible remyelination within acute lesions and chronic axonal degeneration in NABT, contributing to support the use of DT MR imaging as a measure of tissue integrity for studies of neuroprotective therapies.[151]

Future Perspectives

Several methods have been recently proposed to improve the evaluation, in vivo, of diffusivity abnormalities in biological tissues in course of disease. Diffusion kurtosis imaging (DKI) uses diffusion-sensitizing gradients similar to those used for DT MR imaging but acquires 3 or more diffusion-weighting b-values instead of 2.[152] Using such an approach, DKI can give information about restricted diffusion, which can be considered as those water molecules bound to cell membranes that are not studied using DT MR imaging. DKI measures include kurtosis anisotropy and mean, axial, and radial kurtosis. These measures can be considered indexes of tissue compartmentalization or complexity, with a lower mean kurtosis reflecting, for example, a decreased tissue complexity. Only a few studies have applied such a technique in MS, showing that DKI abnormalities occur in the NAWM,[153] GM,[154] and spinal cord[155] of these patients and are correlated with clinical disability.

Because the CNS is a complicated biological system characterized by many different tissue compartments, multicomponent relaxometry might allow to assess these different proton environments by exploiting their different relaxation characteristics. It has previously been shown that brain proton pools can be divided in 3 components based on their T2 relaxation times[156]: short (<35 ms), related to myelin water; intermediate (35–120 ms), associated with axonal and intra/extracellular water; and long (>120 ms), due to CSF. Unfortunately, the short T2 component pool is hardly detectable with standard MR imaging methods because the signal vanishes quickly and has a low intensity. This usually implies long acquisition times and the study of a single brain section. The ratio of the short T2 (myelin water) signal to the total water signal, termed the myelin water fraction,[156] has been shown to correlate with histologic measures of myelin content,[157,158] is independent of concomitant pathologic processes such as axonal degeneration and inflammation and has been explored in MS patients,[159] showing a reduction of myelin water fraction in PPMS, which was correlated with clinical disability.

Neurite orientation dispersion and density imaging (NODDI) is another promising new diffusion imaging technique that quantifies microstructural indexes of neurites in vivo.[160] NODDI is based on a 3-compartment tissue model fitted to high-angular resolution diffusion imaging acquired with 2 different diffusion weightings (ie, 1 shell with low and 1 shell with high b-value), optimized for clinical feasibility, and provides 2 key parameters, the neurite density (the intracellular volume fraction) and the orientation dispersion index, which characterizes the orientation dispersion of the axonal and/or dendritic projections. These parameters have been shown to disentangle the source of diffusion anisotropy, providing more specific measures of brain tissue microstructure than the standard parameters derived from the DT MR imaging eigenvalues.[160] A strong correlation of neurite density with the intensity of myelin stain under light microscopy has been demonstrated, indicating that neurite density may be an useful marker for demyelinating disorders.[161]

SUMMARY

Conventional MR imaging has limited specificity to the heterogeneous pathologic substrates of MS. MT MR imaging and DT MR imaging can quantify intrinsic tissue damage of focal lesions and can detect subtle abnormalities occurring in NAWM, GM, spinal cord, and optic nerves of MS patients (Table 1 for a summary). These techniques are contributing to improve the understanding of the mechanisms associated with the development of clinical disability and cognitive impairment in

Table 1
Summary of main magnetization transfer and diffusion tensor MR imaging findings in different brain regions in multiple sclerosis, their clinical correlates, and their possible role as predictors of subsequent clinical outcomes

	Measures	Magnetization Transfer Ratio	Mean Diffusivity	Fractional Anisotropy
Regions	WM lesions	↓↓↓	↑↑↑	↓↓↓
	GM lesions	↓	(=)	↓
	NABT	↓↓	↑↑	↓↓
	NAWM	↓↓	↑↑	↓↓
	GM	↓	↑	↓
	Spinal cord	↓	↑	↓
	Optic nerve	↓	↑	↓
Clinical correlates	Global disability (Expanded Disability Status Scale)	WM lesions, NAWM, GM, spinal cord	NAWM, GM, spinal cord	NAWM, GM, spinal cord
	Locomotor disability	WM lesions, NAWM, GM, spinal cord	NAWM, spinal cord	NAWM, spinal cord
	Cognitive functions	WM lesions, NAWM, GM	WM lesions, NAWM, GM	WM lesions, NAWM
	Visual functions	Optic nerve	Optic nerve, OR	Optic nerve, OR
	Progressive MS forms	WM lesions, NABT, NAWM, GM	NAWM, GM	NAWM, GM lesions, spinal cord
Predictors	Clinical disability	WM lesions, NAWM, GM, spinal cord	NAWM	GM, spinal cord
	Cognitive impairment	GM	GM	—

Abbreviations: ↑, decreased; ↓, increased; (=), unchanged.

these patients. In addition, they allow a better characterization of the main disease clinical phenotypes.

Several approaches have been applied to analyze MT and DT MR imaging data. Each of them has the potential to provide useful pieces of information to improve understanding of MS pathophysiology. The best acquisition and postprocessing strategies, however, especially in the context of multicenter studies remain a matter of debate and further validation studies need to be performed. The role of these techniques as markers of treatments efficacy and as predictors of subsequent disease progression deserves further and more extensive investigations.

REFERENCES

1. Wolff SD, Balaban RS. Magnetization transfer imaging: practical aspects and clinical applications. Radiology 1994;192(3):593–9.
2. van Buchem MA, McGowan JC, Kolson DL, et al. Quantitative volumetric magnetization transfer analysis in multiple sclerosis: estimation of macroscopic and microscopic disease burden. Magn Reson Med 1996;36(4):632–6.
3. Vavasour IM, Laule C, Li DK, et al. Is the magnetization transfer ratio a marker for myelin in multiple sclerosis? J Magn Reson Imaging 2011;33(3):713–8.
4. Schmierer K, Scaravilli F, Altmann DR, et al. Magnetization transfer ratio and myelin in postmortem multiple sclerosis brain. Ann Neurol 2004; 56(3):407–15.
5. van Waesberghe JH, Kamphorst W, De Groot CJ, et al. Axonal loss in multiple sclerosis lesions: magnetic resonance imaging insights into substrates of disability. Ann Neurol 1999;46(5):747–54.
6. Barkhof F, Bruck W, De Groot CJ, et al. Remyelinated lesions in multiple sclerosis: magnetic resonance image appearance. Arch Neurol 2003; 60(8):1073–81.
7. Filippi M. Magnetization transfer imaging to monitor the evolution of individual multiple sclerosis lesions. Neurology 1999;53(5 Suppl 3):S18–22.
8. Filippi M, Rocca MA, Sormani MP, et al. Short-term evolution of individual enhancing MS lesions studied with magnetization transfer imaging. Magn Reson Imaging 1999;17(7):979–84.
9. Dousset V, Gayou A, Brochet B, et al. Early structural changes in acute MS lesions assessed by serial magnetization transfer studies. Neurology 1998;51(4):1150–5.

10. Filippi M, Rocca MA, Martino G, et al. Magnetization transfer changes in the normal appearing white matter precede the appearance of enhancing lesions in patients with multiple sclerosis. Ann Neurol 1998;43(6):809–14.

11. Goodkin DE, Rooney WD, Sloan R, et al. A serial study of new MS lesions and the white matter from which they arise. Neurology 1998;51(6):1689–97.

12. Rocca MA, Mastronardo G, Rodegher M, et al. Long-term changes of magnetization transfer-derived measures from patients with relapsing-remitting and secondary progressive multiple sclerosis. AJNR Am J Neuroradiol 1999;20(5):821–7.

13. van Waesberghe JH, van Walderveen MA, Castelijns JA, et al. Patterns of lesion development in multiple sclerosis: longitudinal observations with T1-weighted spin-echo and magnetization transfer MR. AJNR Am J Neuroradiol 1998;19(4):675–83.

14. Dousset V, Grossman RI, Ramer KN, et al. Experimental allergic encephalomyelitis and multiple sclerosis: lesion characterization with magnetization transfer imaging. Radiology 1992;182(2):483–91.

15. Hiehle JF Jr, Grossman RI, Ramer KN, et al. Magnetization transfer effects in MR-detected multiple sclerosis lesions: comparison with gadolinium-enhanced spin-echo images and non-enhanced T1-weighted images. AJNR Am J Neuroradiol 1995;16(1):69–77.

16. Fazekas F, Ropele S, Enzinger C, et al. Quantitative magnetization transfer imaging of pre-lesional white-matter changes in multiple sclerosis. Mult Scler 2002;8(6):479–84.

17. Arstila AU, Riekkinen P, Rinne UK, et al. Studies on the pathogenesis of multiple sclerosis. Participation of lysosomes on demyelination in the central nervous system white matter outside plaques. Eur Neurol 1973;9(1):1–20.

18. Allen IV, McKeown SR. A histological, histochemical and biochemical study of the macroscopically normal white matter in multiple sclerosis. J Neurol Sci 1979;41(1):81–91.

19. Evangelou N, Konz D, Esiri MM, et al. Regional axonal loss in the corpus callosum correlates with cerebral white matter lesion volume and distribution in multiple sclerosis. Brain 2000;123(Pt 9):1845–9.

20. Chen JT, Collins DL, Atkins HL, et al. Magnetization transfer ratio evolution with demyelination and remyelination in multiple sclerosis lesions. Ann Neurol 2008;63(2):254–62.

21. Brown RA, Narayanan S, Arnold DL. Imaging of repeated episodes of demyelination and remyelination in multiple sclerosis. Neuroimage Clin 2014;6:20–5.

22. Schmierer K, Parkes HG, So PW, et al. High field (9.4 Tesla) magnetic resonance imaging of cortical grey matter lesions in multiple sclerosis. Brain 2010;133(Pt 3):858–67.

23. Tardif CL, Bedell BJ, Eskildsen SF, et al. Quantitative magnetic resonance imaging of cortical multiple sclerosis pathology. Mult Scler Int 2012;2012:742018.

24. Chen JT, Easley K, Schneider C, et al. Clinically feasible MTR is sensitive to cortical demyelination in MS. Neurology 2013;80(3):246–52.

25. Samson RS, Cardoso MJ, Muhlert N, et al. Investigation of outer cortical magnetisation transfer ratio abnormalities in multiple sclerosis clinical subgroups. Mult Scler 2014;20(10):1322–30.

26. Derakhshan M, Caramanos Z, Narayanan S, et al. Surface-based analysis reveals regions of reduced cortical magnetization transfer ratio in patients with multiple sclerosis: a proposed method for imaging subpial demyelination. Hum Brain Mapp 2014;35(7):3402–13.

27. Jonkman LE, Fleysher L, Steenwijk MD, et al. Ultra-high field MTR and qR2* differentiates subpial cortical lesions from normal-appearing gray matter in multiple sclerosis. Mult Scler 2016;22(10):1306–14.

28. Siger-Zajdel M, Filippi M, Selmaj K. MTR discloses subtle changes in the normal-appearing tissue from relatives of patients with MS. Neurology 2002;58(2):317–20.

29. Iannucci G, Tortorella C, Rovaris M, et al. Prognostic value of MR and magnetization transfer imaging findings in patients with clinically isolated syndromes suggestive of multiple sclerosis at presentation. AJNR Am J Neuroradiol 2000;21(6):1034–8.

30. De Stefano N, Narayanan S, Francis SJ, et al. Diffuse axonal and tissue injury in patients with multiple sclerosis with low cerebral lesion load and no disability. Arch Neurol 2002;59(10):1565–71.

31. Rocca MA, Falini A, Colombo B, et al. Adaptive functional changes in the cerebral cortex of patients with nondisabling multiple sclerosis correlate with the extent of brain structural damage. Ann Neurol 2002;51(3):330–9.

32. Kalkers NF, Hintzen RQ, van Waesberghe JH, et al. Magnetization transfer histogram parameters reflect all dimensions of MS pathology, including atrophy. J Neurol Sci 2001;184(2):155–62.

33. Tortorella C, Viti B, Bozzali M, et al. A magnetization transfer histogram study of normal-appearing brain tissue in MS. Neurology 2000;54(1):186–93.

34. Filippi M, Inglese M, Rovaris M, et al. Magnetization transfer imaging to monitor the evolution of MS: a 1-year follow-up study. Neurology 2000;55(7):940–6.

35. Filippi M, Campi A, Dousset V, et al. A magnetization transfer imaging study of normal-

appearing white matter in multiple sclerosis. Neurology 1995;45(3 Pt 1):478–82.

36. Guo AC, Jewells VL, Provenzale JM. Analysis of normal-appearing white matter in multiple sclerosis: comparison of diffusion tensor MR imaging and magnetization transfer imaging. AJNR Am J Neuroradiol 2001;22(10):1893–900.

37. Ge Y, Grossman RI, Babb JS, et al. Dirty-appearing white matter in multiple sclerosis: volumetric MR imaging and magnetization transfer ratio histogram analysis. AJNR Am J Neuroradiol 2003;24(10):1935–40.

38. Davies GR, Altmann DR, Rashid W, et al. Emergence of thalamic magnetization transfer ratio abnormality in early relapsing-remitting multiple sclerosis. Mult Scler 2005;11(3):276–81.

39. Rocca MA, Mesaros S, Pagani E, et al. Thalamic damage and long-term progression of disability in multiple sclerosis. Radiology 2010;257(2):463–9.

40. Cercignani M, Bozzali M, Iannucci G, et al. Magnetisation transfer ratio and mean diffusivity of normal appearing white and grey matter from patients with multiple sclerosis. J Neurol Neurosurg Psychiatry 2001;70(3):311–7.

41. Dehmeshki J, Chard DT, Leary SM, et al. The normal appearing grey matter in primary progressive multiple sclerosis: a magnetisation transfer imaging study. J Neurol 2003;250(1):67–74.

42. Davies GR, Altmann DR, Hadjiprocopis A, et al. Increasing normal-appearing grey and white matter magnetisation transfer ratio abnormality in early relapsing-remitting multiple sclerosis. J Neurol 2005;252(9):1037–44.

43. Fernando KT, Tozer DJ, Miszkiel KA, et al. Magnetization transfer histograms in clinically isolated syndromes suggestive of multiple sclerosis. Brain 2005;128(Pt 12):2911–25.

44. Agosta F, Rovaris M, Pagani E, et al. Magnetization transfer MRI metrics predict the accumulation of disability 8 years later in patients with multiple sclerosis. Brain 2006;129(Pt 10):2620–7.

45. Ramio-Torrenta L, Sastre-Garriga J, Ingle GT, et al. Abnormalities in normal appearing tissues in early primary progressive multiple sclerosis and their relation to disability: a tissue specific magnetisation transfer study. J Neurol Neurosurg Psychiatry 2006;77(1):40–5.

46. Audoin B, Ranjeva JP, Au Duong MV, et al. Voxel-based analysis of MTR images: a method to locate gray matter abnormalities in patients at the earliest stage of multiple sclerosis. J Magn Reson Imaging 2004;20(5):765–71.

47. Ranjeva JP, Audoin B, Au Duong MV, et al. Local tissue damage assessed with statistical mapping analysis of brain magnetization transfer ratio: relationship with functional status of patients in the earliest stage of multiple sclerosis. AJNR Am J Neuroradiol 2005;26(1):119–27.

48. Khaleeli Z, Sastre-Garriga J, Ciccarelli O, et al. Magnetisation transfer ratio in the normal appearing white matter predicts progression of disability over 1 year in early primary progressive multiple sclerosis. J Neurol Neurosurg Psychiatry 2007;78(10):1076–82.

49. Amato MP, Portaccio E, Stromillo ML, et al. Cognitive assessment and quantitative magnetic resonance metrics can help to identify benign multiple sclerosis. Neurology 2008;71(9):632–8.

50. Brex PA, Leary SM, Plant GT, et al. Magnetization transfer imaging in patients with clinically isolated syndromes suggestive of multiple sclerosis. AJNR Am J Neuroradiol 2001;22(5):947–51.

51. Rocca MA, Agosta F, Sormani MP, et al. A three-year, multi-parametric MRI study in patients at presentation with CIS. J Neurol 2008;255(5):683–91.

52. Santos AC, Narayanan S, de Stefano N, et al. Magnetization transfer can predict clinical evolution in patients with multiple sclerosis. J Neurol 2002;249(6):662–8.

53. Rovaris M, Agosta F, Sormani MP, et al. Conventional and magnetization transfer MRI predictors of clinical multiple sclerosis evolution: a medium-term follow-up study. Brain 2003;126(Pt 10):2323–32.

54. Filippi M, Preziosa P, Copetti M, et al. Gray matter damage predicts the accumulation of disability 13 years later in MS. Neurology 2013;81(20):1759–67.

55. Bozzali M, Rocca MA, Iannucci G, et al. Magnetization-transfer histogram analysis of the cervical cord in patients with multiple sclerosis. AJNR Am J Neuroradiol 1999;20(10):1803–8.

56. Rovaris M, Gallo A, Riva R, et al. An MT MRI study of the cervical cord in clinically isolated syndromes suggestive of MS. Neurology 2004;63(3):584–5.

57. Filippi M, Bozzali M, Horsfield MA, et al. A conventional and magnetization transfer MRI study of the cervical cord in patients with MS. Neurology 2000;54(1):207–13.

58. Charil A, Caputo D, Cavarretta R, et al. Cervical cord magnetization transfer ratio and clinical changes over 18 months in patients with relapsing-remitting multiple sclerosis: a preliminary study. Mult Scler 2006;12(5):662–5.

59. Zackowski KM, Smith SA, Reich DS, et al. Sensorimotor dysfunction in multiple sclerosis and column-specific magnetization transfer-imaging abnormalities in the spinal cord. Brain 2009;132(Pt 5):1200–9.

60. Agosta F, Absinta M, Sormani MP, et al. In vivo assessment of cervical cord damage in MS patients: a longitudinal diffusion tensor MRI study. Brain 2007;130(Pt 8):2211–9.

61. Kearney H, Yiannakas MC, Samson RS, et al. Investigation of magnetization transfer ratio-derived pial and subpial abnormalities in the multiple sclerosis spinal cord. Brain 2014;137(Pt 9): 2456–68.

62. Thorpe JW, Barker GJ, Jones SJ, et al. Magnetisation transfer ratios and transverse magnetisation decay curves in optic neuritis: correlation with clinical findings and electrophysiology. J Neurol Neurosurg Psychiatry 1995;59(5):487–92.

63. Trip SA, Schlottmann PG, Jones SJ, et al. Optic nerve magnetization transfer imaging and measures of axonal loss and demyelination in optic neuritis. Mult Scler 2007;13(7):875–9.

64. Inglese M, Ghezzi A, Bianchi S, et al. Irreversible disability and tissue loss in multiple sclerosis: a conventional and magnetization transfer magnetic resonance imaging study of the optic nerves. Arch Neurol 2002;59(2):250–5.

65. Hickman SJ, Toosy AT, Jones SJ, et al. Serial magnetization transfer imaging in acute optic neuritis. Brain 2004;127(Pt 3):692–700.

66. Melzi L, Rocca MA, Marzoli SB, et al. A longitudinal conventional and magnetization transfer magnetic resonance imaging study of optic neuritis. Mult Scler 2007;13(2):265–8.

67. van den Elskamp IJ, Knol DL, Vrenken H, et al. Lesional magnetization transfer ratio: a feasible outcome for remyelinating treatment trials in multiple sclerosis. Mult Scler 2010;16(6):660–9.

68. Brown RA, Narayanan S, Arnold DL. Segmentation of magnetization transfer ratio lesions for longitudinal analysis of demyelination and remyelination in multiple sclerosis. Neuroimage 2013;66:103–9.

69. Zivadinov R, Dwyer MG, Hussein S, et al. Voxelwise magnetization transfer imaging study of effects of natalizumab and IFNbeta-1a in multiple sclerosis. Mult Scler 2012;18(8):1125–34.

70. Button T, Altmann D, Tozer D, et al. Magnetization transfer imaging in multiple sclerosis treated with alemtuzumab. Mult Scler 2013;19(2):241–4.

71. Filippi M, Rocca MA, Pagani E, et al. Placebo-controlled trial of oral laquinimod in multiple sclerosis: MRI evidence of an effect on brain tissue damage. J Neurol Neurosurg Psychiatry 2014; 85(8):851–8.

72. Hayton T, Furby J, Smith KJ, et al. Longitudinal changes in magnetisation transfer ratio in secondary progressive multiple sclerosis: data from a randomised placebo controlled trial of lamotrigine. J Neurol 2012;259(3):505–14.

73. Brown RA, Narayanan S, Stikov N, et al. MTR recovery in brain lesions in the BECOME study of glatiramer acetate vs interferon beta-1b. Neurology 2016;87(9):905–11.

74. Schmierer K, Wheeler-Kingshott CA, Tozer DJ, et al. Quantitative magnetic resonance of postmortem multiple sclerosis brain before and after fixation. Magn Reson Med 2008;59(2): 268–77.

75. Levesque IR, Sled JG, Narayanan S, et al. Reproducibility of quantitative magnetization-transfer imaging parameters from repeated measurements. Magn Reson Med 2010;64(2): 391–400.

76. Giacomini PS, Levesque IR, Ribeiro L, et al. Measuring demyelination and remyelination in acute multiple sclerosis lesion voxels. Arch Neurol 2009;66(3):375–81.

77. Le Bihan D, Mangin JF, Poupon C, et al. Diffusion tensor imaging: concepts and applications. J Magn Reson Imaging 2001;13(4):534–46.

78. Pierpaoli C, Barnett A, Pajevic S, et al. Water diffusion changes in Wallerian degeneration and their dependence on white matter architecture. Neuroimage 2001;13(6 Pt 1):1174–85.

79. Wheeler-Kingshott CA, Cercignani M. About "axial" and "radial" diffusivities. Magn Reson Med 2009; 61(5):1255–60.

80. Schmierer K, Wheeler-Kingshott CA, Boulby PA, et al. Diffusion tensor imaging of post mortem multiple sclerosis brain. Neuroimage 2007;35(2): 467–77.

81. Rovaris M, Agosta F, Pagani E, et al. Diffusion tensor MR imaging. Neuroimaging Clin N Am 2009;19(1):37–43.

82. Rovaris M, Gass A, Bammer R, et al. Diffusion MRI in multiple sclerosis. Neurology 2005;65(10): 1526–32.

83. Filippi M, Iannucci G, Cercignani M, et al. A quantitative study of water diffusion in multiple sclerosis lesions and normal-appearing white matter using echo-planar imaging. Arch Neurol 2000; 57(7):1017–21.

84. Filippi M, Cercignani M, Inglese M, et al. Diffusion tensor magnetic resonance imaging in multiple sclerosis. Neurology 2001;56(3):304–11.

85. Castriota-Scanderbeg A, Sabatini U, Fasano F, et al. Diffusion of water in large demyelinating lesions: a follow-up study. Neuroradiology 2002; 44(9):764–7.

86. Werring DJ, Clark CA, Barker GJ, et al. Diffusion tensor imaging of lesions and normal-appearing white matter in multiple sclerosis. Neurology 1999;52(8):1626–32.

87. Preziosa P, Martinelli V, Moiola L, et al. Dynamic pattern of clinical and MRI findings in a tumefactive demyelinating lesion: a case report. J Neurol Sci 2016;361:184–6.

88. Rovira A, Pericot I, Alonso J, et al. Serial diffusion-weighted MR imaging and proton MR spectroscopy of acute large demyelinating brain lesions: case report. AJNR Am J Neuroradiol 2002;23(6): 989–94.

89. Rocca MA, Cercignani M, Iannucci G, et al. Weekly diffusion-weighted imaging of normal-appearing white matter in MS. Neurology 2000;55(6):882–4.

90. Poonawalla AH, Hasan KM, Gupta RK, et al. Diffusion-tensor MR imaging of cortical lesions in multiple sclerosis: initial findings. Radiology 2008; 246(3):880–6.

91. Calabrese M, Rinaldi F, Seppi D, et al. Cortical diffusion-tensor imaging abnormalities in multiple sclerosis: a 3-year longitudinal study. Radiology 2011;261(3):891–8.

92. Filippi M, Preziosa P, Pagani E, et al. Microstructural MR imaging of cortical lesion in multiple sclerosis. Mult Scler 2013;19(4):418–26.

93. Hasan KM, Gupta RK, Santos RM, et al. Diffusion tensor fractional anisotropy of the normal-appearing seven segments of the corpus callosum in healthy adults and relapsing-remitting multiple sclerosis patients. J Magn Reson Imaging 2005; 21(6):735–43.

94. Bozzali M, Cercignani M, Sormani MP, et al. Quantification of brain gray matter damage in different MS phenotypes by use of diffusion tensor MR imaging. AJNR Am J Neuroradiol 2002;23(6):985–8.

95. Rovaris M, Bozzali M, Iannucci G, et al. Assessment of normal-appearing white and gray matter in patients with primary progressive multiple sclerosis: a diffusion-tensor magnetic resonance imaging study. Arch Neurol 2002;59(9):1406–12.

96. Fabiano AJ, Sharma J, Weinstock-Guttman B, et al. Thalamic involvement in multiple sclerosis: a diffusion-weighted magnetic resonance imaging study. J Neuroimaging 2003;13(4):307–14.

97. Saindane AM, Law M, Ge Y, et al. Correlation of diffusion tensor and dynamic perfusion MR imaging metrics in normal-appearing corpus callosum: support for primary hypoperfusion in multiple sclerosis. AJNR Am J Neuroradiol 2007;28(4):767–72.

98. Mori S, van Zijl PC. Fiber tracking: principles and strategies - a technical review. NMR Biomed 2002;15(7–8):468–80.

99. Wilson M, Tench CR, Morgan PS, et al. Pyramidal tract mapping by diffusion tensor magnetic resonance imaging in multiple sclerosis: improving correlations with disability. J Neurol Neurosurg Psychiatry 2003;74(2):203–7.

100. Lin X, Tench CR, Morgan PS, et al. 'Importance sampling' in MS: use of diffusion tensor tractography to quantify pathology related to specific impairment. J Neurol Sci 2005;237(1–2):13–9.

101. Pagani E, Filippi M, Rocca MA, et al. A method for obtaining tract-specific diffusion tensor MRI measurements in the presence of disease: application to patients with clinically isolated syndromes suggestive of multiple sclerosis. Neuroimage 2005; 26(1):258–65.

102. Mesaros S, Rocca MA, Riccitelli G, et al. Corpus callosum damage and cognitive dysfunction in benign MS. Hum Brain Mapp 2009;30(8):2656–66.

103. Ciccarelli O, Toosy AT, Hickman SJ, et al. Optic radiation changes after optic neuritis detected by tractography-based group mapping. Hum Brain Mapp 2005;25(3):308–16.

104. Reich DS, Smith SA, Gordon-Lipkin EM, et al. Damage to the optic radiation in multiple sclerosis is associated with retinal injury and visual disability. Arch Neurol 2009;66(8):998–1006.

105. Rocca MA, Mesaros S, Preziosa P, et al. Wallerian and trans-synaptic degeneration contribute to optic radiation damage in multiple sclerosis: a diffusion tensor MRI study. Mult Scler 2013;19(12): 1610–7.

106. Preziosa P, Rocca MA, Mesaros S, et al. Intrinsic damage to the major white matter tracts in patients with different clinical phenotypes of multiple sclerosis: a voxelwise diffusion-tensor MR study. Radiology 2011;260(2):541–50.

107. Audoin B, Guye M, Reuter F, et al. Structure of WM bundles constituting the working memory system in early multiple sclerosis: a quantitative DTI tractography study. Neuroimage 2007;36(4):1324–30.

108. Rocca MA, Pagani E, Absinta M, et al. Altered functional and structural connectivities in patients with MS: a 3-T study. Neurology 2007;69(23):2136–45.

109. Rocca MA, Valsasina P, Ceccarelli A, et al. Structural and functional MRI correlates of Stroop control in benign MS. Hum Brain Mapp 2009;30(1):276–90.

110. Preziosa P, Rocca MA, Mesaros S, et al. Relationship between damage to the cerebellar peduncles and clinical disability in multiple sclerosis. Radiology 2014;271(3):822–30.

111. Kacar K, Rocca MA, Copetti M, et al. Overcoming the clinical-MR imaging paradox of multiple sclerosis: MR imaging data assessed with a random forest approach. AJNR Am J Neuroradiol 2011; 32(11):2098–102.

112. Guye M, Bettus G, Bartolomei F, et al. Graph theoretical analysis of structural and functional connectivity MRI in normal and pathological brain networks. MAGMA 2010;23(5–6):409–21.

113. Shu N, Liu Y, Li K, et al. Diffusion tensor tractography reveals disrupted topological efficiency in white matter structural networks in multiple sclerosis. Cereb Cortex 2011;21:2565–77.

114. Li Y, Jewells V, Kim M, et al. Diffusion tensor imaging based network analysis detects alterations of neuroconnectivity in patients with clinically early relapsing-remitting multiple sclerosis. Hum Brain Mapp 2013;34(12):3376–91.

115. Ceccarelli A, Rocca MA, Pagani E, et al. The topographical distribution of tissue injury in benign MS: a 3T multiparametric MRI study. Neuroimage 2008; 39(4):1499–509.

116. Dineen RA, Vilisaar J, Hlinka J, et al. Disconnection as a mechanism for cognitive dysfunction in multiple sclerosis. Brain 2009;132(Pt 1):239–49.

117. Roosendaal SD, Geurts JJ, Vrenken H, et al. Regional DTI differences in multiple sclerosis patients. Neuroimage 2009;44(4):1397–403.

118. Hulst HE, Steenwijk MD, Versteeg A, et al. Cognitive impairment in MS: impact of white matter integrity, gray matter volume, and lesions. Neurology 2013;80(11):1025–32.

119. Preziosa P, Rocca MA, Pagani E, et al. Structural MRI correlates of cognitive impairment in patients with multiple sclerosis: a multicenter study. Hum Brain Mapp 2016;37(4):1627–44.

120. Gallo A, Rovaris M, Riva R, et al. Diffusion-tensor magnetic resonance imaging detects normal-appearing white matter damage unrelated to short-term disease activity in patients at the earliest clinical stage of multiple sclerosis. Arch Neurol 2005;62(5):803–8.

121. Mesaros S, Rocca MA, Kacar K, et al. Diffusion tensor MRI tractography and cognitive impairment in multiple sclerosis. Neurology 2012; 78(13):969–75.

122. Lin F, Yu C, Jiang T, et al. Diffusion tensor tractography-based group mapping of the pyramidal tract in relapsing-remitting multiple sclerosis patients. AJNR Am J Neuroradiol 2007; 28(2):278–82.

123. Lin X, Tench CR, Morgan PS, et al. Use of combined conventional and quantitative MRI to quantify pathology related to cognitive impairment in multiple sclerosis. J Neurol Neurosurg Psychiatry 2008;79(4):437–41.

124. Bisecco A, Rocca MA, Pagani E, et al. Connectivity-based parcellation of the thalamus in multiple sclerosis and its implications for cognitive impairment: a multicenter study. Hum Brain Mapp 2015; 36(7):2809–25.

125. Pulizzi A, Rovaris M, Judica E, et al. Determinants of disability in multiple sclerosis at various disease stages: a multiparametric magnetic resonance study. Arch Neurol 2007;64(8):1163–8.

126. Rovaris M, Gallo A, Valsasina P, et al. Short-term accrual of gray matter pathology in patients with progressive multiple sclerosis: an in vivo study using diffusion tensor MRI. Neuroimage 2005;24(4): 1139–46.

127. Rovaris M, Judica E, Gallo A, et al. Grey matter damage predicts the evolution of primary progressive multiple sclerosis at 5 years. Brain 2006;129(Pt 10):2628–34.

128. Oreja-Guevara C, Rovaris M, Iannucci G, et al. Progressive gray matter damage in patients with relapsing-remitting multiple sclerosis: a longitudinal diffusion tensor magnetic resonance imaging study. Arch Neurol 2005;62(4):578–84.

129. Rovaris M, Judica E, Ceccarelli A, et al. A 3-year diffusion tensor MRI study of grey matter damage progression during the earliest clinical stage of MS. J Neurol 2008;255(8):1209–14.

130. Rovaris M, Iannucci G, Falautano M, et al. Cognitive dysfunction in patients with mildly disabling relapsing-remitting multiple sclerosis: an exploratory study with diffusion tensor MR imaging. J Neurol Sci 2002;195(2):103–9.

131. Mesaros S, Rocca MA, Pagani E, et al. Thalamic damage predicts the evolution of primary-progressive multiple sclerosis at 5 years. AJNR Am J Neuroradiol 2011;32(6):1016–20.

132. Clark CA, Werring DJ, Miller DH. Diffusion imaging of the spinal cord in vivo: estimation of the principal diffusivities and application to multiple sclerosis. Magn Reson Med 2000;43(1):133–8.

133. Agosta F, Benedetti B, Rocca MA, et al. Quantification of cervical cord pathology in primary progressive MS using diffusion tensor MRI. Neurology 2005;64(4):631–5.

134. Valsasina P, Rocca MA, Agosta F, et al. Mean diffusivity and fractional anisotropy histogram analysis of the cervical cord in MS patients. Neuroimage 2005;26(3):822–8.

135. Agosta F, Filippi M. MRI of spinal cord in multiple sclerosis. J Neuroimaging 2007;17(Suppl 1): 46S–9S.

136. Benedetti B, Rocca MA, Rovaris M, et al. A diffusion tensor MRI study of cervical cord damage in benign and secondary progressive MS patients. J Neurol Neurosurg Psychiatry 2009;81(1):26–30.

137. Benedetti B, Valsasina P, Judica E, et al. Grading cervical cord damage in neuromyelitis optica and MS by diffusion tensor MRI. Neurology 2006; 67(1):161–3.

138. Naismith RT, Xu J, Klawiter EC, et al. Spinal cord tract diffusion tensor imaging reveals disability substrate in demyelinating disease. Neurology 2013;80(24):2201–9.

139. Toosy AT, Kou N, Altmann D, et al. Voxel-based cervical spinal cord mapping of diffusion abnormalities in MS-related myelitis. Neurology 2014; 83(15):1321–5.

140. Kearney H, Schneider T, Yiannakas MC, et al. Spinal cord grey matter abnormalities are associated with secondary progression and physical disability in multiple sclerosis. J Neurol Neurosurg Psychiatry 2015;86(6):608–14.

141. Freund P, Wheeler-Kingshott C, Jackson J, et al. Recovery after spinal cord relapse in multiple sclerosis is predicted by radial diffusivity. Mult Scler 2010;16(10):1193–202.

142. Iwasawa T, Matoba H, Ogi A, et al. Diffusion-weighted imaging of the human optic nerve: a new approach to evaluate optic neuritis in multiple sclerosis. Magn Reson Med 1997;38(3):484–91.

143. Hickman SJ, Wheeler-Kingshott CA, Jones SJ, et al. Optic nerve diffusion measurement from diffusion-weighted imaging in optic neuritis. AJNR Am J Neuroradiol 2005;26(4):951–6.

144. Trip SA, Wheeler-Kingshott C, Jones SJ, et al. Optic nerve diffusion tensor imaging in optic neuritis. Neuroimage 2006;30(2):498–505.

145. Wheeler-Kingshott CA, Parker GJ, Symms MR, et al. ADC mapping of the human optic nerve: increased resolution, coverage, and reliability with CSF-suppressed ZOOM-EPI. Magn Reson Med 2002;47(1):24–31.

146. Kolbe S, Chapman C, Nguyen T, et al. Optic nerve diffusion changes and atrophy jointly predict visual dysfunction after optic neuritis. Neuroimage 2009; 45(3):679–86.

147. Smith SA, Williams ZR, Ratchford JN, et al. Diffusion tensor imaging of the optic nerve in multiple sclerosis: association with retinal damage and visual disability. AJNR Am J Neuroradiol 2011;32(9):1662–8.

148. Naismith RT, Xu J, Tutlam NT, et al. Diffusion tensor imaging in acute optic neuropathies: predictor of clinical outcomes. Arch Neurol 2012;69(1):65–71.

149. Naismith RT, Xu J, Tutlam NT, et al. Radial diffusivity in remote optic neuritis discriminates visual outcomes. Neurology 2010;74(21):1702–10.

150. Pagani E, Hirsch JG, Pouwels PJ, et al. Intercenter differences in diffusion tensor MRI acquisition. J Magn Reson Imaging 2010;31(6):1458–68.

151. Fox RJ, Cronin T, Lin J, et al. Measuring myelin repair and axonal loss with diffusion tensor imaging. AJNR Am J Neuroradiol 2011;32(1):85–91.

152. Jensen JH, Helpern JA. MRI quantification of non-Gaussian water diffusion by kurtosis analysis. NMR Biomed 2010;23(7):698–710.

153. de Kouchkovsky I, Fieremans E, Fleysher L, et al. Quantification of normal-appearing white matter tract integrity in multiple sclerosis: a diffusion kurtosis imaging study. J Neurol 2016; 263(6):1146–55.

154. Bester M, Jensen JH, Babb JS, et al. Non-Gaussian diffusion MRI of gray matter is associated with cognitive impairment in multiple sclerosis. Mult Scler 2015;21(7):935–44.

155. Raz E, Bester M, Sigmund EE, et al. A better characterization of spinal cord damage in multiple sclerosis: a diffusional kurtosis imaging study. AJNR Am J Neuroradiol 2013;34(9):1846–52.

156. MacKay A, Whittall K, Adler J, et al. In vivo visualization of myelin water in brain by magnetic resonance. Magn Reson Med 1994;31(6):673–7.

157. Laule C, Kozlowski P, Leung E, et al. Myelin water imaging of multiple sclerosis at 7 T: correlations with histopathology. Neuroimage 2008;40(4): 1575–80.

158. Laule C, Leung E, Lis DK, et al. Myelin water imaging in multiple sclerosis: quantitative correlations with histopathology. Mult Scler 2006;12(6):747–53.

159. Kolind S, Matthews L, Johansen-Berg H, et al. Myelin water imaging reflects clinical variability in multiple sclerosis. Neuroimage 2012;60(1):263–70.

160. Zhang H, Schneider T, Wheeler-Kingshott CA, et al. NODDI: practical in vivo neurite orientation dispersion and density imaging of the human brain. Neuroimage 2012;61(4):1000–16.

161. Jespersen SN, Bjarkam CR, Nyengaard JR, et al. Neurite density from magnetic resonance diffusion measurements at ultrahigh field: comparison with light microscopy and electron microscopy. NeuroImage 2010;49(1):205–16.

Iron Mapping in Multiple Sclerosis

Stefan Ropele, PhD*, Christian Enzinger, MD, Franz Fazekas, MD

KEYWORDS

- Iron • Ferritin • Multiple sclerosis • MR imaging • Magnetic susceptibility • Neurodegeneration
- Biomarker

KEY POINTS

- Most nonheme brain iron is stored in the globular storage protein ferritin, which can be assessed by MR imaging through relaxation enhancement and susceptibility effects.
- R_2^* mapping and quantitative susceptibility mapping represent the currently most relevant approaches for assessing iron levels in vivo.
- Cerebral iron levels are highest in deep gray matter and are associated with age, and disease duration and disability in multiple sclerosis.
- Iron mapping in multiple sclerosis lesions and white matter remains an unmet need.

INTRODUCTION

Owing to the existence of the blood–brain barrier, the iron content of the brain is largely decoupled from the iron stores of the remaining body. This inaccessibility makes brain iron more difficult to study and also explains why less is known about iron metabolism in the brain compared with other organs.

Consequently, extrapolation of iron levels in the brain from those measured in serum or other organs is misleading. So far, MR imaging thus represents the only noninvasive tool on hand for this purpose, because it can use several mechanisms affected by the presence of iron, including relaxation enhancement and susceptibility effects.

Improvements in MR imaging methodology over recent years have already allowed gaining important insights into multiple sclerosis (MS)-related alterations of brain iron metabolism. This review, therefore, gives an overview on current MR imaging techniques for brain iron mapping and their application to MS. In addition, possible limitations and future directions that promise advances in this field are discussed briefly.

IRON DISTRIBUTION AND METABOLISM IN THE NORMAL BRAIN

The normal adult brain contains approximately 60 mg of nonheme iron, which corresponds with 1% of the total iron content of the human body.[1] Iron in the brain is needed for oxygen transport, myelination, electron transport, storage and activation, and many other relevant metabolic processes.[2]

Most of the iron is tightly complexed in proteins, but iron may also be present in a soluble 'pool' of low-molecular-weight complexes such as Fe(III) ATP and ferric citrate. The concentration of free iron is very low and is estimated to be less than 10^{-18} M Fe^{3+} and 10^{-8} M Fe^{2+}.[3] Most of the nonheme iron is stored in ferritin that keeps iron in a soluble and nontoxic state. Ferritin consists of a spherical protein shell, 12 nm in diameter, that encapsulates up to 4500 iron ions as hydrated iron oxide (Fe^{3+}) nanocrystal with a diameter of up to 8 nm.[4] Ferritin is composed of 24 subunits of varying composition, a heavy (H) polypeptide chain and a light (L) polypeptide. These peptides have different physiologic roles, including the uptake and oxidation of ferrous iron, growth of the

Disclosures: Nothing to disclose.
Department of Neurology, Medical University of Graz, Graz, Austria
* Corresponding author. Department of Neurology, Medical University of Graz, Auenbruggerplatz 22, Graz 8036, Austria.
E-mail address: stefan.ropele@medunigraz.at

neuroimaging.theclinics.com

iron oxide nanocrystal, and reduction and release. The H-subunit has a specific ferroxidase activity for rapid iron uptake, whereas the L-subunit facilitates mineralization.[4,5] The relative abundance of H- and L-ferritin varies between cell types[6] and between brain regions.[7] Although oligodendrocytes express similar amounts of L- and H-subunits, neurons express mostly H-ferritin. Ferritin is not distributed uniformly across the brain, but most of the iron is intracellular and in lysosomes and mitochondria. The highest ferritin concentrations are found in oligodendrocytes and their processes, in motor neurons, and in myelinated axons close to the inner shell of the myelin sheet.[8–10] Ferritin found at the surface of myelin is associated with the ferritin in the processes of the oligodendrocytes.[10]

It is commonly accepted that iron accumulates in the brain as a function of age, with almost no iron present at birth.[1] The accumulation can be best described by an exponential saturation function, reaching a ceiling effect after the fourth decade of life.[11,12] In the adult brain, iron concentration varies greatly across different brain regions. Concentrations of up to 200 mg/kg wet weight can be found in the globus pallidus whereas cerebral white matter usually has iron levels around 40 mg/kg.[1,13] Interestingly, the reason for this iron accumulation is still unclear because, in the adult brain, only a few percent of all stored iron is really needed for iron-dependent processes. A possible explanation for this implies that iron transport to the brain mostly represents a 1-way traffic.

As indicated, transferrin or other iron transporters cannot simply cross the blood–brain barrier, which is also why brain iron levels are independent from serum iron levels.[14] Iron transport into the brain over the blood–brain barrier is an active process that is regulated through transferrin receptors on capillary endothelial cells in the parenchyma and the choroid plexus.[15] In contrast, iron leaves the brain with the bulk outflow of cerebrospinal fluid (CSF) through the arachnoid villi and other channels.[16]

Brain maturation and other developmental processes can cause a delay or shift between inflow and outflow. A recent study has elucidated an unbalanced import and outflow of brain iron using a staggered design, where rats were fed with 3 stable iron isotope tracers.[17] The turnover rate of iron entering the brain resulted in a half-life of approximately 9 months. The observed tracer accumulation in brain iron over the study period was extrapolated to an increase of brain iron in the rat brain by approximately 30% from early adulthood to the end of life, which corresponds well with observations in the human brain.[1]

ALTERED IRON HOMEOSTASIS IN THE BRAIN WITH MULTIPLE SCLEROSIS

Perturbation of iron homeostasis in MS seems to occur at several metabolic levels and, because an excess of iron may induce oxidative stress, it has been speculated that iron may be involved in the pathophysiology and pathogenesis of MS.[18]

So far, histology has detected iron within microglia at the edge of MS lesions,[19,20] corresponding with the dark rings observed on susceptibility weighted MR imaging in vivo.[21] The iron in the microglia has been assumed to originate from extracellular space, where it had presumably been released by myelin and oligodendrocytes upon their destruction. It was speculated consequently that iron in microglia cells might propagate chronic, low-grade inflammation unlinked to demyelination per se, that might in turn promote neurodegeneration and disease progression.[20]

In contrast, the center of most MS lesions is characterized by a loss of iron while only very few chronic active lesions demonstrate increased iron levels. In normal-appearing white matter (NAWM), a loss of iron has been found to be paralleled by a loss of myelin and oligodendrocytes with disease progression, and these processes in turn could be related to chronic inflammation.[20]

MS-related iron accumulation in deep gray matter (GM), its relation to iron levels in and around MS lesions, and the cellular distribution have not been studied by histology so far. In CSF, transferrin and ferritin levels in MS patients are within normal ranges. Elevated ferritin levels in CSF have been reported only in progressive MS so far.[22]

MAGNETIC PROPERTIES OF IRON COMPOUNDS

MR imaging can assess most iron compounds in the brain owing to their distinct magnetic properties. The magnetic susceptibility, that is, the response of a material or atom to an external magnetic field, is determined largely by unpaired electrons in unfilled shells. Because of its 4 unpaired electrons in the d-shell, iron has great potential for a high paramagnetism (ie, positive magnetic susceptibility, which allows a material to become magnetized), but the effective susceptibility largely depends on the binding and spin state. The 4 iron atoms in an oxygenated hemoglobin molecule, for instance, have a spin number of zero and are therefore diamagnetic, that is, they cannot be magnetized.[23] In contrast, Fe^{3+} in some sulfur proteins can reach a maximum spin of 5/2,[24] which corresponds with a magnetic moment of 5.92 Bohr magnetons.[25]

The magnetic behavior of iron in the most relevant iron compounds is summarized in **Table 1**.

Iron in ferritin, the most relevant nonheme iron compound in the brain, has a spin number of 3/2 and therefore lies in the middle of the paramagnetic spectrum of iron atoms. Although ferritin is among the most studied biocrystals, the magnetic phases of the crystal are still unclear, which makes an accurate assessment by MR imaging challenging. Although the outer crystal core is considered paramagnetic, electron nanodiffraction and high-resolution transmission electron microscopy studies have reported phases such as hematite (Fe_2O_3), magnetite (Fe_3O_4), and maghemite (γ-Fe_2O_3) for the inner core.[26,27] These phases would give rise for ferrimagnetic behavior, that is, most of the magnetic moments compensate each other with only little remaining net magnetization, which clearly reduces the detectability by MR imaging.

Hemosiderin is another large iron compound that contains conglomerates of denatured proteins, denatured ferritin particles, and lipids. The iron within hemosiderin is insoluble, but is in equilibrium with the soluble ferritin pool. The magnetic properties of hemosiderin are not clear yet because it has no fixed composition and no maximum size owing to the absence of a size-limiting protein shell.[28]

The magnetic susceptibility of other iron compounds such as iron sulfur proteins or transferrin is negligible. Although transferrin is the most relevant iron transporter, its 2 Fe^{3+} ions with a spin of 1/2 cannot produce a significant susceptibility shift in the tissue at physiologic concentrations. In this context, it should be noted that the paramagnetism of all iron compounds is opposed by the diamagnetism (ie, negative magnetic susceptibility) of the tissue matrix. Water as the predominant component of brain tissue has a susceptibility of approximately -9 ppm and, therefore, is diamagnetic.[23] Even though iron compounds can evoke a paramagnetic shift of the susceptibility by a few ppm (toward positive susceptibility) the tissue remains weakly diamagnetic. However, iron is not equally distributed across the brain and therefore may cause local susceptibility shifts that are well above the detection limit of MR imaging.

Iron-induced susceptibility changes can also be confounded by the presence of other paramagnetic metal ions. The 2 most relevant candidates are copper and manganese. Copper has a low effective magnetic moment and is much less abundant in the brain than iron. Because of 5 unpaired electrons, manganese shows a high mass susceptibility, but the concentration of iron compared with manganese is approximately 200 times higher in deep GM and 300 times higher in white matter.[13]

IRON MAPPING IN THE HUMAN BRAIN WITH MR IMAGING

Most MR imaging approaches for iron mapping are based on 1 of 2 essential biophysical phenomena (**Table 2**). Iron-induced variations of the

---

Table 1
Iron compounds in the brain and their detectability by MR imaging

Fe Compound	Valence/Binding of Fe	Effective Magnetic Moment μ_{eff} of Fe [Bohr Magnetons]	Estimated Total Nonheme Iron in the Adult Brain (%)	Magnetic Susceptibility
Ferritin	Fe^{3+} (covalent/ionic)	3.87	>90	+520 ppm/molecule
Hemosiderin	Fe^{3+} (covalent/ionic)	3.87	Not found in healthy brain	Similar to ferritin but depends on size
Oxyhemoglobin	Fe^{2+} (covalent)	0	—	−9.9 ppm/molecule, −8.5 ppm/red blood cell
Deoxyhemoglobin	Fe^{2+} (ionic)	4.9	—	+0.2 ppm/molecule, −6.5 ppm/red blood cell
Transferrin	Fe^{3+} (covalent)	1.73	<1	+0.03 ppm/molecule
Other	Fe^{2+}, Fe^{3+}	0–5.92	<2	—

The detectability is given by the relative concentration and the intrinsic susceptibility. The effective moment is directly proportional to the spin number. Estimated susceptibility values were taken from reference.[23] Note that the paramagnetism of the iron compounds is counteracted by the diamagnetism of other tissue components including tissue water (−9.05 ppm).

Table 2
MR imaging techniques for iron mapping

Technique	Effect	Sequence	Sensitivity[a]	Effort, Complexity
$R_2{}^a$ mapping	Microscopic susceptibility variations	Dual or multi-echo FLASH	$R^2 = 0.90$[29]	Simple
R_2 mapping	Microscopic susceptibility variations and diffusion	Dual or multi-echo spin echo	$R^2 = 0.67$[29]	Simple
Field-dependent relaxometry	Microscopic susceptibility variations and field dependency of transversal relaxation	Dual echo or multiecho spin echo	$R^2 = 0.96$[62]	Two scanners with different field strength are needed
Quantitative susceptibility mapping	Macroscopic susceptibility changes	Dual echo or multiecho spoiled gradient echo sequence (magnitude and phase data)	$R^2 = 0.76$[36,63]	Complex. Outcome needs a reference and may vary across proposed methods

[a] For a better comparison, references from validation studies at 3 T are provided that included gray and white matter in the regression analysis. Field-dependent relaxometry was done at 0.5 T and 1.5 T.

magnetic susceptibility on a microscopic level represent the first mechanism. Protons of surrounding tissue water are exposed to these gradients and experience a phase shift that scales with the iron concentration. Considering a larger ensemble of water protons at a macroscopic level (ie, in 1 voxel), these individual phase shifts cause dephasing and consequently accelerated signal loss because the phase shift is slightly different for each water proton. An iron-induced increase of the transversal relaxation rate $R_2{}^*$ is, therefore, considered as a sensitive measure for iron.[29] $R_2{}^*$ can be assessed with a spoiled gradient echo sequence (FLASH) in a 2-dimensional or 3-dimensaionl acquisition mode and shows a high reproducibility, even on different scanners.[11] Iron also affects the transversal relaxation rate R_2, obtained from a spin echo sequence, which is normally insensitive for magnetic field gradients or inhomogeneities. However, molecular diffusion through these gradient fields hinders that the refocusing radio frequency pulse unwinds the iron-induced phase shifts. Consequently, R_2 also shows a high sensitivity for iron,[29] but FLASH imaging seems to be more practicable, in particular at higher resolutions and at higher field strengths, because of the inherently low specific absorption rate. R_2 and $R_2{}^*$ can be obtained from the ratio of 2 echoes or alternatively from a single exponential fit to multiecho data. Because the iron-induced gradient fields scale with field strengths, field-dependent relaxometry has been proposed as another

method for iron mapping.[30] However, this approach needs R_2 mapping at 2 different field strengths (eg, 1.5 T and 3 T) and, therefore, is not feasible in a clinical setting.

The second effect that can be used for iron mapping is the local frequency shift. The bulk susceptibility of a voxel can be considered as the sum of the susceptibilities of all tissue components. The local Larmor frequency is related directly to the bulk susceptibility and can be assessed with phase images from a spoiled FLASH sequence. However, owing to the dipole effect (convolution with a dipole kernel), the local phase and frequency also contain nonlocals contributions and therefore cannot be used as a reliable measure for iron concentration.[31]

For the same reason, susceptibility weighted imaging, which essentially combines phase and magnitude images from a spoiled FLASH sequence,[32] cannot be used to quantify iron concentration, although susceptibility weighted imaging has turned out to be otherwise helpful to enhance tissue contrast for iron-containing structures.[21] Quantitative susceptibility mapping (QSM) is the latest development in this field, aiming at assessment of the frequency shift caused by local iron concentration, that is, at the voxel level. QSM has become feasible by new approaches for dipole inversion or deconvolution[33–35] and provides a linear and sensitive measure for iron concentration in brain tissue.[36] When combined with echo 3-dimensional planar imaging, high-resolution iron mapping of the brain can be done in a few minutes.[37] However, through phase filtering and removal of the background phase, it is not possible to obtain absolute susceptibility values. Therefore, usually CSF or regions in NAWM are used as a reference, whereupon the latter can introduce bias in MS affected brains.

Comparing results from QSM and R_2^* mapping, it becomes evident that, although based on the same FLASH sequence, both techniques are differently affected by the diamagnetic components of the tissue (**Fig. 1**). With QSM, the diamagnetism of tissue water and various myelin components counteracts the paramagnetism of iron, and it contributes to R_2^* additively.[38,39] In other words, demyelination reduces R_2^* and it increases the susceptibility as assessed by QSM. Additionally, myelinated axons can be considered as diamagnetic hollow cylinders giving rise to an orientational dependency of the susceptibility effect with respect to the main magnetic field.[40,41] Both conditions render iron mapping in white matter less reliable.[29,36] So far, the only way to eliminate the diamagnetic background is to assess the Curie effect and to map R_2^* at different temperatures,[42] but this has not yet proven possible in vivo.[43]

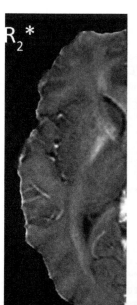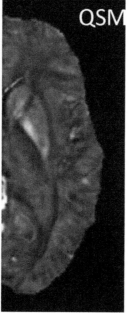

Fig. 1. Comparison of R_2^* (*left*) and quantitative susceptibility mapping (QSM; *right*) maps. Note that both maps were calculated from the same raw data from a single normal subject. Myelin-rich structures seem to be brighter in the R_2^* map because they provide an additional source of microscopic field gradients and therefore enhance transversal relaxation.

Also other techniques have been proposed for iron mapping, including magnetic field correlation imaging, direct saturation imaging, and mapping of the longitudinal relaxation rate, with the latter showing only a limited sensitivity for iron.[44] Magnetic field correlation assesses microscopic field gradients by a series of asymmetric spin echoes, which provide information about R_2 and R_2^*.[45,46] Asymmetric spin echo sequences are usually not available on clinical scanners. Direct saturation imaging is an indirect measure of R_2 because the absorption spectrum of water protons scales with R_2.[47] So far, direct saturation imaging and mapping of the longitudinal relaxation time have not been applied in MS.

IRON MAPPING USING MR IMAGING OF THE BRAIN IN MULTIPLE SCLEROSIS: INSIGHTS, LIMITATIONS, AND PROSPECTS

The first indirect evidence for the iron metabolism to be distorted in MS dates back to the early days of clinical MR imaging. Drayer and colleagues[48] noticed in 1986 that the basal ganglia seem to be dark on T2-weighted spin echo scans even in normal aging subjects. In a postmortem correlation study applying Perls staining, they indeed demonstrated that this T2 shortening to be owing to iron. Consequently, they proposed a visual score to rate the signal intensity in the globus pallidus, using the putamen and thalamus as references. Consequently, it was found that patients with more severe MS show a more pronounced reduction of these signal intensities.[49]

In subsequent studies, similar observations were made in larger MS cohorts and with quantitative MR imaging approaches, including R_2 mapping,[50] local frequency shift imaging,[51] magnetic field correlation imaging,[46] and R_2^* mapping.[52] So far, the greatest sensitivity for disease-related changes in deep GM has been achieved using QSM.[53] A possible explanation for the slight advantage over R_2^* mapping is that susceptibility further increases with demyelination (ie, less diamagnetic contribution), a condition that is already seen in the deep GM of patients with early MS.[54]

Current studies suggest that iron accumulation in deep GM in MS may represent an epiphenomenon of the disease. Considering both the limited iron outflow rate of the brain and the fact that deep GM acts as storage place for brain iron, an increased iron concentration may be indicative of more deliberated iron from demyelination, a reduced demand for metabolic relevant iron, or both.

Increased iron levels in the deep GM have been associated independently with disease duration and disability in MS, and a role for cerebral atrophy has also been suggested.[55,56] On the contrary, the absence of increased iron levels in patients with a clinically isolated syndrome (CIS) indicates that iron accumulation is unlikely to precede the development of MS.[56] It should be noted, however, that age-related iron accumulation exceeds MS disease related effects, in particular in the first 4 decades of life. Correction for age is, therefore, mandatory for iron mapping studies in MS.[11,55]

Importantly, the dynamics of iron accumulation in deep GM and their relation to disease progression remain unclear. Walsh and colleagues[57] investigated R_2^* changes in 17 patients with remitting–relapsing MS over a follow-up period of 2 years. On a group level, a significant R_2^* increase was found in several deep GM structure with the globus pallidus showing a 6.7% increase. Longitudinal R2* changes much better correlated with the Expanded Disability Status Scale as a measure of disability than with R_2^* levels at baseline. In contrast, a larger longitudinal study with a mean follow-up period of 3 years could neither replicate the strong R_2^* increase in patients with remitting–relapsing MS nor a correlation with the Expanded Disability Status Scale.[58] However, in this study, iron accumulation was more pronounced in patients with a CIS suggestive of MS, indicating that iron accumulation may be more relevant in earlier phases of the disease.

A limited number of QSM studies have also aimed at assessing iron levels in MS lesions and NAWM. Early to intermediately aged nonenhancing lesions present with a much higher magnetic susceptibility than enhancing lesions or chronic nonenhancing lesions and with a slow rate of change until the susceptibility of NAWM is reached in a chronic stage.[59] This pattern can be explained by both an increased iron content and demyelination.[60] This is most likely also the reason why a post mortem study found that reliable assessment of iron content in MS lesions is not possible with current MR imaging methods.[61] Future concepts also considering water and myelin content as well as fiber orientation from diffusion tensor imaging are expected to allow a more specific interpretation of susceptibility changes in lesions and NAWM.

SUMMARY

Among the many approaches available for iron mapping, R_2^* mapping and in particular QSM have been established in recent years as state-of-the-art methods. These methods are readily available, provide low variability, can be performed even at ultrahigh field strengths, and are highly correlated with true iron concentration. Although the application of these methods in MS has already provided new insights into region-specific iron accumulation and its relation to clinical status and morphologic changes of the brain, further technical developments are needed to improve the reliability for iron mapping in white matter.

REFERENCES

1. Hallgren B, Sourander P. The effect of age on the non-haemin iron in the human brain. J Neurochem 1958;3(1):41–51.
2. Crichton R. Inorganic biochemistry of iron metabolism: from molecular mechanisms to clinical consequences. In: Crichton RR, editor. Brain iron homeostasis and its perturbation in various neurodegenerative diseases. Third edition. West Sussex (England): John Wiley & Sons, Ltd; 2001. p. 371–2398.
3. Williams RJP. Free manganese(II) and iron cations can act as intracellular cell controls. FEBS Lett 1982;140(1):3–10.
4. Chasteen ND, Harrison PM. Mineralization in ferritin: an efficient means of iron storage. J Struct Biol 1999; 126(3):182–94.
5. Harrison PM, Arosio P. The ferritins: molecular properties, iron storage function and cellular regulation. Biochim Biophys Acta 1996;1275(3):161–203.
6. Connor JR, Boeshore KL, Benkovic SA, et al. Isoforms of ferritin have a specific cellular distribution in the brain. J Neurosci Res 1994;37(4):461–5.
7. Galazka-Friedman J, Friedman A, Bauminger ER. Iron in the brain. In: Kuzmann E, Lazar K, editors. Proceedings of the international symposium on the industrial applications of the Mössbauer effect (ISIAME 2008). Dordrecht (Netherlands): Springer; 2008. p. 31–8.
8. Connor JR, Menzies SL, St Martin SM, et al. Cellular distribution of transferrin, ferritin, and iron in normal and aged human brains. J Neurosci Res 1990; 27(4):595–611.
9. Meguro R, Asano Y, Odagiri S, et al. Cellular and subcellular localizations of nonheme ferric and ferrous iron in the rat brain: a light and electron microscopic study by the perfusion-Perls and -Turnbull methods. Arch Histol Cytol 2008;71(4):205–22.
10. Quintana C, Bellefqih S, Laval JY, et al. Study of the localization of iron, ferritin, and hemosiderin in Alzheimer's disease hippocampus by analytical microscopy at the subcellular level. J Struct Biol 2006; 153(1):42–54.
11. Ropele S, Wattjes MP, Langkammer C, et al. Multicenter R2* mapping in the healthy brain. Magn Reson Med 2014;71:1103–7.
12. Li W, Wu B, Batrachenko A, et al. Differential developmental trajectories of magnetic susceptibility in human brain gray and white matter over the lifespan. Hum Brain Mapp 2014;35(6):2698–713.

13. Krebs N, Langkammer C, Goessle W, et al. Assessment of trace elements in human brain using inductively coupled plasma mass spectrometry. J Trace Elem Med Biol 2014;28(1):1–7.

14. Pirpamer L, Hofer E, Gesierich B, et al. Determinants of iron accumulation in the normal aging brain. Neurobiol Aging 2016;43:149–55.

15. Burdo JR, Connor JR. Brain iron uptake and homeostatic mechanisms: an overview. Biometals 2003; 16(1):63–75.

16. Bradbury MW. Transport of iron in the blood-brain-cerebrospinal fluid system. J Neurochem 1997; 69(2):443–54.

17. Chen J-H, Singh N, Tay H, et al. Imbalance of iron influx and efflux causes brain iron accumulation over time in the healthy adult rat. Metallomics 2014;6(8):1417–26.

18. LeVine SM. Iron deposits in multiple sclerosis and Alzheimer's disease brains. Brain Res 1997;760(1–2):298–303.

19. Bagnato F, Hametner S, Yao B, et al. Tracking iron in multiple sclerosis: a combined imaging and histopathological study at 7 Tesla. Brain 2011;134(Pt 12):3602–15.

20. Hametner S, Wimmer I, Haider L, et al. Iron and neurodegeneration in the multiple sclerosis brain. Ann Neurol 2013;74(6):848–61.

21. Haacke EM, Makki M, Ge Y, et al. Characterizing iron deposition in multiple sclerosis lesions using susceptibility weighted imaging. J Magn Reson Imaging 2009;29(3):537–44.

22. LeVine SM, Lynch SG, Ou C-N, et al. Ferritin, transferrin and iron concentrations in the cerebrospinal fluid of multiple sclerosis patients. Brain Res 1999; 821(2):511–5.

23. Schenck JF. The role of magnetic susceptibility in magnetic resonance imaging: MR imaging magnetic compatibility of the first and second kinds. Med Phys 1996;23(6):815–50.

24. Beinert H. Iron-sulfur proteins: ancient structures, still full of surprises. J Biol Inorg Chem 2000;5(1):2–15.

25. Ropele S, Langkammer C. Iron quantification with susceptibility. NMR Biomed 2016. http://dx.doi.org/10.1002/nbm.3534.

26. Quintana C, Cowley JM, Marhic C. Electron nanodiffraction and high-resolution electron microscopy studies of the structure and composition of physiological and pathological ferritin. J Struct Biol 2004; 147(2):166–78.

27. Resnick D. Modeling of the magnetic behavior of γ-Fe[sub 2]O[sub 3] nanoparticles mineralized in ferritin. J Appl Phys 2004;95(11):7127.

28. Chua-anusorn W, St Pierre T. Pathological biomineralization of iron. In: Königsberger E, Königsberger L, editors. Biomineralization - medical aspects of solubility. Chapter 5. Chichester (UK): John Wiley and Sons, Ltd; 2006. p. 219–67.

29. Langkammer C, Krebs N, Goessler W, et al. Quantitative MRI of brain iron: a postmortem validation study. Radiology 2010;257(2):455–62.

30. Bartzokis G, Aravagiri M, Oldendorf WH, et al. Field dependent transverse relaxation rate increase may be a specific measure of tissue iron stores. Magn Reson Med 1993;29(4):459–64.

31. Yao B, Li T, Gelderen P, et al. Susceptibility contrast in high field MRI of human brain as a function of tissue iron content. Neuroimage 2009;44(4):1259–66.

32. Haacke EM, Mittal S, Wu Z, et al. Susceptibility-weighted imaging: technical aspects and clinical applications, part 1. AJNR Am J Neuroradiol 2009; 30:19–30.

33. Reichenbach JR, Schweser F, Serres B, et al. Quantitative susceptibility mapping: concepts and applications. Clin Neuroradiol 2015;25(Suppl 2):225–30.

34. Wang Y, Liu T. Quantitative susceptibility mapping (QSM): decoding MRI data for a tissue magnetic biomarker. Magn Reson Med 2015;73(1):82–101.

35. Liu C, Li W, Tong KA, et al. Susceptibility-weighted imaging and quantitative susceptibility mapping in the brain. J Magn Reson Imaging 2015;42(1):23–41.

36. Langkammer C, Schweser F, Krebs N, et al. Quantitative susceptibility mapping (QSM) as a means to measure brain iron? A post mortem validation study. Neuroimage 2012;62(3):1593–9.

37. Langkammer C, Bredies K, Poser BA, et al. Fast quantitative susceptibility mapping using 3D EPI and total generalized variation. Neuroimage 2015; 111:622–30.

38. Schweser F, Deistung A, Lehr BW, et al. Quantitative imaging of intrinsic magnetic tissue properties using MRI signal phase: an approach to in vivo brain iron metabolism? Neuroimage 2011;54(4):2789–807.

39. Liu C, Li W, Johnson GA, et al. High-field (9.4 T) MRI of brain dysmyelination by quantitative mapping of magnetic susceptibility. Neuroimage 2011;56(3):930–8.

40. Bender B, Klose U. The in vivo influence of white matter fiber orientation towards B(0) on T2* in the human brain. NMR Biomed 2010;23(9):1071–6.

41. Liu C. Susceptibility tensor imaging. Magn Reson Med 2010;63(6):1471–7.

42. Birkl C, Langkammer C, Krenn H, et al. Iron mapping using the temperature dependency of the magnetic susceptibility. Magn Reson Med 2015; 73(3):1282–8.

43. Birkl C, Carassiti D, Langkammer C, et al. Assessment of ferritin in the multiple sclerosis brain using temperature induced R2* changes. In: Proceedings of the ISMRM, 24th Annual Meeting. Singapore, May 7–13, 2016.

44. Gelman N, Ewing JR, Gorell JM, et al. Interregional variation of longitudinal relaxation rates in human brain at 3.0 T: relation to estimated iron and water contents. Magn Reson Med 2001;45(1):71–9.

45. Raz E, Jensen JH, Ge Y, et al. Brain iron quantification in mild traumatic brain injury: a magnetic field correlation study. AJNR Am J Neuroradiol 2011; 32(10):1851–6.

46. Ge Y, Jensen JH, Lu H, et al. Quantitative assessment of iron accumulation in the deep gray matter of multiple sclerosis by magnetic field correlation imaging. AJNR Am J Neuroradiol 2007;28(9):1639–44.

47. Smith S, Bulte J, Van Zijl P. Direct saturation MRI: theory and application to imaging brain iron. Magn Reson Med 2009;62(2):384–93.

48. Drayer B, Burger P, Darwin R, et al. MRI of brain iron. AJR Am J Roentgenol 1986;147(1):103–10.

49. Drayer B, Burger P, Hurwitz B, et al. Reduced signal intensity on MR images of thalamus and putamen in multiple sclerosis: increased iron content? AJR Am J Roentgenol 1987;149(2):357–63.

50. Burgetova A, Seidl Z, Krasensky J, et al. Multiple sclerosis and the accumulation of iron in the Basal Ganglia: quantitative assessment of brain iron using MRI t(2) relaxometry. Eur Neurol 2010;63(3):136–43.

51. Hammond KE, Lupo JM, Xu D, et al. Development of a robust method for generating 7.0 T multichannel phase images of the brain with application to normal volunteers and patients with neurological diseases. Neuroimage 2008;39(4):1682–92.

52. Khalil M, Enzinger C, Langkammer C, et al. Quantitative assessment of brain iron by R(2)* relaxometry in patients with clinically isolated syndrome and relapsing-remitting multiple sclerosis. Mult Scler 2009;15(9):1048–54.

53. Langkammer C, Liu T, Khalil M, et al. Quantitative susceptibility mapping in multiple sclerosis. Radiology 2013;267(2):551–9.

54. Haider L, Simeonidou C, Steinberger G, et al. Multiple sclerosis deep grey matter: the relation between demyelination, neurodegeneration, inflammation and iron. J Neurol Neurosurg Psychiatry 2014; 85(12):1386–95.

55. Ropele S, Kilsdonk ID, Wattjes MP, et al. Determinants of iron accumulation in deep grey matter of multiple sclerosis patients. Mult Scler 2014;20(13): 1692–8.

56. Khalil M, Langkammer C, Ropele S, et al. Determinants of brain iron in multiple sclerosis: a quantitative 3T MRI study. Neurology 2011;77(18):1691–7.

57. Walsh AJ, Blevins G, Lebel RM, et al. Longitudinal MR imaging of iron in multiple sclerosis: an imaging marker of disease. Radiology 2014;270(1):186–96.

58. Khalil M, Langkammer C, Pichler A, et al. Dynamics of brain iron levels in multiple sclerosis: a longitudinal 3T MRI study. Neurology 2015;84:2396–402.

59. Chen W, Gauthier SA, Gupta A, et al. Quantitative susceptibility mapping of multiple sclerosis lesions at various ages. Radiology 2014;271(1):183–92.

60. Wisnieff C, Ramanan S, Olesik J, et al. Quantitative susceptibility mapping (QSM) of white matter multiple sclerosis lesions: interpreting positive susceptibility and the presence of iron. Magn Reson Med 2015;74(2):564–70.

61. Walsh AJ, Lebel RM, Eissa A, et al. Multiple sclerosis: validation of MR imaging for quantification and detection of iron. Radiology 2013;267(2): 531–42.

62. Bartzokis G, Beckson M, Hance D, et al. MR evaluation of age-related increase of brain iron in young adult and older normal males. Magn Reson Imaging 1997;15(1):29–35.

63. Zheng W, Nichol H, Liu S, et al. Measuring iron in the brain using quantitative susceptibility mapping and X-ray fluorescence imaging. Neuroimage 2013;78: 68–74.

Molecular and Metabolic Imaging in Multiple Sclerosis

Marcello Moccia, MD[a,b], Olga Ciccarelli, PhD, FRCP[a,c],*

KEYWORDS

- Multiple sclerosis • MR imaging • Spectroscopy • PET • Molecular • Metabolic

KEY POINTS

- Molecular and metabolic imaging techniques assess dynamically and in vivo the pathogenetic mechanisms that lead to MS pathology and reflect the heterogeneity of pathologic abnormalities occurring in MS.
- [1]H-MR spectroscopy estimates brain levels of several metabolites, which reflect important biologic processes, such as mitochondrial function and/or neuronal integrity (N-acetyl-aspartate), and glial cell activation and proliferation (myo-inositol).
- [23]Na MR imaging estimates the total concentration of sodium within regions-of-interest in the brain. Increased total sodium concentration is thought to reflect axonal impaired energy metabolism and neurodegeneration.
- PET permits the characterization of the biologic processes occurring at the cellular and molecular levels. The following radioligands are often used: ^{18}F-fluoro-2'-deoxyglucose to investigate inflammation, translocator protein tracers to study microglia activation, amyloid tracers to study demyelination, and ^{11}C-flumazenil to investigate neuronal damage.
- Although technically challenging and expensive, the translation of these techniques to clinical trials and the clinical setting may allow stratification of patients for treatments.

INTRODUCTION

Recent advances in conventional MR imaging have remarkably improved the diagnosis of multiple sclerosis (MS), which can now be achieved earlier and with greater precision. T2 lesions and brain atrophy estimated with MR imaging are currently used in clinical trials as outcome measures. However, conventional neuroimaging techniques lack of specificity with regard to different pathophysiologic substrates of MS, and are not able to explain the heterogeneous and long-term clinical evolution of this disease.[1–4]

MS usually starts with a relapsing–remitting course (RRMS), characterized by the subacute occurrence of neurologic symptoms (namely relapses) that may be followed up by a clinical improvement. In view of this, the presence of focal areas of inflammatory demyelination in the white

Funding Sources: None.
Conflict of Interest: Professor O. Ciccarelli is a consultant for Biogen Idec, Genzyme, Novartis, Roche, Teva, and General Electric. She is an associate editor of Neurology. Dr M. Moccia: None.
[a] NMR Research Unit, Queen Square MS Centre, University College London, Institute of Neurology, 10-12 Russell Square, London WC1B 5EH, UK; [b] MS Clinical Care and Research Centre, Department of Neuroscience, Federico II University, Via Sergio Pansini 5, Naples 80131, Italy; [c] NIHR University College London Hospitals, Biomedical Research Centre, Maple House Suite A 1st floor, 149 Tottenham Court Road, London W1T 7DN, UK
* Corresponding author. NMR Research Unit, Queen Square MS Centre, University College London, Institute of Neurology, 10-12 Russell Square, London WC1B 5EH, UK.
E-mail address: o.ciccarelli@ucl.ac.uk

Neuroimag Clin N Am 27 (2017) 343–356
http://dx.doi.org/10.1016/j.nic.2016.12.005

matter (WM), known as plaques and responsible for relapses, has been considered the main pathologic feature of MS. After 15 to 25 years from disease onset, the clinical course of MS typically shifts into a progressive course, which is termed secondary progressive MS (SPMS). However, a small group of patients (10%–15%) develop a progressive course of the disease since onset, and this type of MS is called primary progressive MS (PPMS).

The main pathologic mechanism underling the progressive course of MS is thought to be neurodegeneration. The occurrence of neurodegenerative features is considered to be a consequence of the inflammatory activity,[1,5,6] and a primary neurodegenerative component.[7] Neurodegeneration occurs diffusely in the brain and spinal cord of patients with MS, and is reflected by changes in structural imaging parameters that are measured within and outside lesions, namely in the normal appearing WM (NAWM) and gray matter (GM).[8]

The pathogenesis of MS is not fully understood, and it is thought that there is a series of pathobiologic events, starting with focal lymphocytic infiltration and microglia activation, and ending with demyelination and neuroaxonal degeneration (Fig. 1). In particular, a primary stimulus (either endogenous or exogenous) may be responsible for an inflammatory, demyelinating response, which induces a compensatory response within neurons. This response, which includes the redistribution of sodium channels along the demyelinated axolemma and increased mitochondrial metabolism, might have a transient functional benefit, but may be deleterious in the long-term. Specifically, oxidative stress, mitochondrial injury, and ion channel dysfunction have been suggested as possible "maladaptive" changes, leading to neuroaxonal damage (see Fig. 1).[1,9] Molecular and metabolic imaging have the unique ability to reflect in vivo some of the molecular and metabolic pathways involved in the development and progression of neurodegeneration in MS.[2,10]

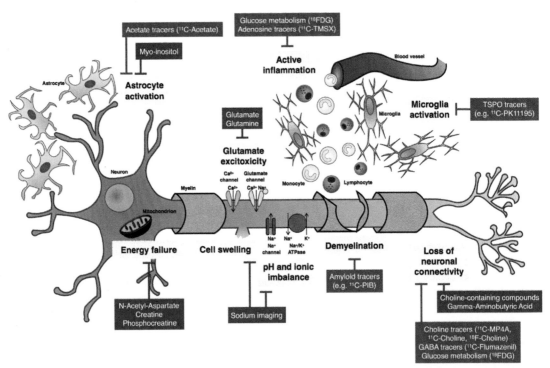

Fig. 1. Mechanisms of neurodegeneration and the molecular and metabolic imaging targets studied in MS. Inflammatory cells (eg, lymphocytes, monocytes, microglia) produce reactive oxygen species and reactive nitrogen species, which contribute to mitochondrial injury. This leads to metabolic stress, energy deficiency, and progressive loss of neuroaxonal function. Activation and proliferation of astrocytes occur to restore neuroaxonal function, although reactive astroglial cells also have harmful consequences on axonal survival. After acute demyelination, there is a redistribution of ion channels (eg, Na^+ channels) that, along with accumulation of glutamate (the main excitatory neurotransmitter of the central nervous system), promotes ionic imbalance, with increased intracellular concentration of calcium and consequent neuronal apoptosis. The metabolites most commonly studied in MS are highlighted in the red boxes, and the targets of PET radioligands are shown in the blue boxes. TSPO, translocator protein.

This article describes and discusses clinical studies that used molecular and metabolic imaging techniques to investigate the role of specific molecular, cellular, subcellular, and metabolic processes in causing neurodegeneration in MS. The most successful techniques are [1]H-magnetic resonance spectroscopy (MRS), sodium imaging, and PET. These techniques have been often used to provide insights into the pathogenesis of MS in vivo and explain the clinical heterogeneity of patients with MS. Translation of these techniques to clinical trials and the clinical setting may facilitate the development of effective treatments in MS and help to stratify patients for treatments.

MAGNETIC RESONANCE SPECTROSCOPY

MRS is used to study metabolites in the brain, as long as they are available in relatively high concentrations and present one or more MR visible nuclei (for more details on MRS see Ref.[11]). The most common nucleus that is used is [1]H (proton). In MS, ^{1}H-MRS is used to provide in vivo quantification of brain levels of several metabolites. Each metabolite appears at a specific part per million, and each one reflects specific cellular and biochemical processes; therefore, their concentrations may change in association with pathologic abnormalities. The most commonly estimated metabolites are total N-acetyl-aspartate (NAA), which includes NAA and N-acetylaspartylglutamate; glutamate (Glu); γ-aminobutyric acid (GABA); creatinine (Cr); choline-containing compounds (Cho); and myo-inositol (**Fig. 2, Table 1**). These metabolites can be estimated within lesions or in the normal-appearing brain.

Next we review the most recent clinical studies that detected abnormal levels of metabolites in patients with MS when compared with healthy control subjects, by going through the metabolites from the right of the spectrum to the left, and discuss the findings of abnormal levels of metabolites in the brain (lesions, NAWM, and GM) and spinal cord.

N-Acetyl-Aspartate

NAA is synthesized by neural mitochondria and is almost exclusively located within neural cells in the mature brain.[2,10,12–14] Although its biochemical functions are not completely understood, NAA might reflect neuronal mitochondrial metabolism and/or neuronal integrity (see **Fig. 1**).[10] Because metabolic (mitochondrial) dysfunction is considered to play a role in neurodegeneration, the in vivo estimation of NAA levels may provide insight into the mechanisms of damage and recovery in MS.

NAA levels can either be calculated as absolute concentrations or as values normalized to intravoxel Cr (NAA/Cr); advantages and disadvantages of both methods have been previously discussed.[15] In their meta-analytic review including 30 studies evaluating NAA in MS, Caramanos and colleagues[12] found that the directions of change in mean NAA values and mean NAA/Cr ratios were concordant in most studies, suggesting the use of these measures as a practical compromise to the acquisition of a surrogate measure of "cerebral tissue integrity."[16]

In acute lesions there is a reduction of NAA levels when compared with the surrounding NAWM,[17] and with the WM of healthy control subjects,[18] suggesting neuronal loss and/or metabolic dysfunction; the reduction of NAA may be, at least in part, caused by the local edema, which is associated with acute inflammation. Similarly, in

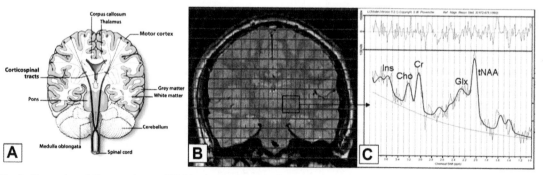

Fig. 2. Examples of the spectra on MRS in the corticospinal tract. Anatomy of the corticospinal tract (A), with the corresponding chemical shift imaging grid on a single image (B); spectrum from the voxel located above the left cerebral peduncle in a healthy control subject (C). Cho, choline; Cr, creatinine; Glx, glutamate and glutamine; Ins, inosine; tNAA, N- acetylaspartate and N-acetylaspartylglutamate. (*From* Tur C, Wheeler-Kingshott CAM, Altmann DR, et al. Spatial variability and changes of metabolite concentrations in the cortico-spinal tract in multiple sclerosis using coronal CSI. Hum Brain Mapp 2014;35(3):993–1003.)

Table 1
Metabolites measured with ¹H-MRS

Metabolites	Pathophysiologic Mechanisms if Abnormal Concentration	Imaging Finding in MS Versus Healthy Control Subjects	Clinical Correlations
N-Acetyl-aspartate	Impaired energy metabolism and/or neural integrity	Acute WM lesions: ↑ Chronic WM lesions: ↓ NAWM: ↓ GM: ↓ Spinal cord: ↓	Motor disability and in general, neurologic disability
Glutamate and glutamine	Inflammation, if increased; reduction of synapses and neuroaxonal degeneration, if reduced	Acute WM lesions: ↑ NAWM: ↑ GM: ↓ Spinal cord: ↓	Physical disability and cognitive dysfunction, especially for GM
γ-Aminobutyric acid	If reduced, impaired compensatory mechanisms and neuroaxonal damage	GM: ↓	Motor disability
Creatine and phosphocreatine	Impaired energy metabolism	Lesions: ↑ NAWM: ↑ Corticospinal tract: ↑	Motor disability
Choline-containing compounds	Elevate cell turnover and inflammation	Acute WM lesions: ↑ NAWM: ↑	Motor disability
Myo-inositol	Astrocytic activation and proliferation	Acute WM lesions: ↑ NAWM: ↑ Corticospinal tract: ↑ GM: ↑ Spinal cord: ↑	Motor disability

Different metabolites with a specific pathogenetic relevance in MS are evaluated with ¹H-MRS. Imaging findings and clinical correlations are reported.

chronic WM lesions (hypointense on T1-weighted images), there is an overall mean decrease in NAA levels of about 20%.[12]

When the temporal behavior of NAA is examined over time, MRS studies in the brain and spinal cord have found that reduced NAA levels in acute lesion partially recover over time, although it does not return to normal.[17,19,20] Because at the same time progressive atrophy occurred, it is possible that increased NAA levels indicate the enhanced mitochondrial activity that is necessary to restore and maintain axonal conduction after acute inflammatory demyelination. The resolution of edema or a change in the relative partial volume of neuronal processes may also play a role in increasing NAA levels after an acute damage.

In MS NAWM, there is an overall mean decrease of NAA of about 7% when compared with healthy WM[12]; greater reductions in NAA were found in the progressive forms of MS. Patients with clinically isolated syndrome (CIS) showed reduced[21,22] or normal NAA levels in the NAWM when compared with control subjects.[23,24] In a previous study in CIS patients, WM NAA/Cr was significantly lower in patients who developed new T2 lesions on MR imaging and/or relapses during the follow-up than in stable patients,[25] suggesting that neuroaxonal damage may be already well established in patients at such an early disease stage and thus indicates a more aggressive disease course. Similarly, a relationship between lower NAA levels in several WM regions and higher clinical disability, as assessed by the MS Functional Composite (MSFC), has been described in patients with RRMS.[26] Interestingly, 18 recently diagnosed, mildly disabled, patients with RRMS, all on immunomodulatory medication, showed a 6% lower WM NAA than control subjects at study entry, but an increase in NAA over 3 years, at a rate of 0.1 mM per year[27]; this increase of NAA levels may indicate a neuronal dysfunction, which may improve with treatment.

In the GM, NAA levels were found to be consistently reduced in the thalamus and inconsistently reduced in the cortex of patients with MS when compared with healthy control subjects,[12,28–30] suggesting neuroaxonal damage and loss. Two different studies conducted in patients with PPMS, RRMS, and SPMS showed that GM NAA alterations involve the thalamus and the lymbic system,[26,29] although they might be more diffuse and involve also the prefrontal and motor areas. Lower NAA in the bilateral caudate nucleus was found to correlate with higher clinical disability.[26]

Lower NAA levels were found in the spinal cord of 21 patients with early PPMS when compared with healthy control subjects, and were associated with higher motor disability, as measured by the Expanded Disability Scale Score (EDSS),[31] suggesting that neurodegeneration may occur in the spinal cord in the early phase of progressive MS, even in the absence of significant spinal cord atrophy.

Overall, all these studies have supported the use of NAA as marker of axonal loss and/or metabolic dysfunction, and a few clinical trials have used it as a secondary outcome measure to assess the efficacy of experimental treatments in MS.[32,33] Recommendations and advice on how to introduce the measurement of NAA levels in clinical trials have been previously provided by the MAGNIMS group.[15]

Glutamate and Glutamine

In ^{1}H-MRS, Glu is generally quantified together with glutamine (Gln), which is both its precursor and catabolite, although Glu makes up most of the Glx signal (Glx = Glu + Gln). Glu is an important excitatory neurotransmitter, and its in vivo quantification is obtained by using specific techniques, allowing unobstructed Glu signal detection.

Increased extracellular Glu concentration in MS is determined by enhanced production by inflammatory cells (macrophages and microglial cells), reduced uptake in oligodendrocytes and in astrocytes, and increased receptor expression. Increased Glu levels may contribute to neuroaxonal degeneration, through the mechanism of "excitotoxicity" (see **Fig. 1**).[10,34] An elevation of Glu levels has been found in active WM lesions.[35]

Glu and Gln levels have been found to be increased in the NAWM in different disease subtypes (PPMS, RRMS, and SPMS) when compared with healthy control subjects.[34,36] Over the course of MS, there is evidence of a progressive reduction in their concentrations within the NAWM, compared with other markers, such as NAA, which, on the opposite, remains substantially stable. Therefore, Glu might increase at an early stage (with suggested toxic effects), and then progressively decline, reflecting progressive neurodegeneration.[36] A longitudinal study on 343 patients with MS (mainly RRMS) showed that higher Glu concentration in the NAWM was associated with higher rate of NAA decline after 2 years,

higher rate of brain volume loss after 3 years, and greater disability progression after 4 years, measured with the MS functional composite score.[34] Therefore, the authors suggested that the Glu/NAA ratio might be a more biologically relevant predictor than either metabolite alone, because when using this ratio the Glu concentrations are adjusted for the amount of the neuronal dysfunction (as measured by NAA).[34]

Glu and Glx concentration have been found to be reduced in the parietal and cingulate GM regions in patients with RRMS when compared with control subjects.[26,37] In addition, impairment of the visuospatial memory was significantly associated with lower hippocampal, cingulate, and thalamic Glu levels, independently from other measures of GM damage.[37] Similarly, a previous study found reduced Glx in the cortical GM in the brains of patients with early PPMS when compared with control subjects.[38] Because Glu is more abundant inside cells and in the synaptic terminals than in the extracellular space, a possible interpretation of its reduced concentration is a reduction in the number of synapses and neuroaxonal degeneration, which have been described in postmortem studies of MS brains.[39]

Reduced Glx levels were also found in the spinal cord of 21 patients with early PPMS when compared with 24 control subjects,[31] suggesting that reduced glutamatergic metabolism occurs in the early phase of the disease. It is more challenging to perform MRS and, in particular, to estimate the levels of Glx, in the spinal cord than in the brain.

Blocking Glu receptors seems a promising therapeutic approach to slow down disease progression and, for instance, memantine has been used in different clinical trials to improve cognitive function in MS.[40] In future, the efficacy of medications targeting the glutamatergic metabolism could be monitored by using MRS.

γ-Aminobutyric Acid

GABA is the major inhibitory neurotransmitter in the brain, and is evaluated with ^{1}H-MRS by using spectral editing method that allows its discrimination from more abundant metabolites. Measurements of GABA in brain lesions and NAWM have not been reported so far.

With regard to the GM, GABA levels have been found to be reduced in the hippocampus and sensorimotor cortex in 30 patients with SPMS when compared with 17 healthy control subjects.[41] The reduction of GABA in the sensorimotor cortex was associated with a more impaired motor function of the contralateral limbs.[41] Previous postmortem studies have detected a loss of GABAergic inhibitory interneurons in the temporal cortex of MS patients with seizures,[42] and a decrease in presynaptic and postsynaptic components of GABAergic neurotransmission and in the density of inhibitory interneuron processes in MS cortex.[43] Therefore, GABA has been suggested to be a marker of neurodegeneration. Additionally, it is thought that reduced cerebral levels of GABA reflect impaired compensatory mechanisms occurring in the damaged areas of the brain in progressive MS.[2,41]

Agonists of the GABA receptor may be used to manage symptoms associated with MS; for example, baclofen is commonly used to ameliorate spasticity and topiramate is used by some patients with established MS who also have epilepsy or migraines. It has been demonstrated that increasing GABAergic activity may be beneficial for animals with experimental autoimmune encephalomyelitis (animal model of MS) and that this effect occurred, at least in part, through a direct effect of the GABAergic agents on the immune system,[44] suggesting that further studies are needed to establish whether GABAergic agents may have an effect on underlying MS disease activity and whether MRS can be used to monitor it.

Creatine

Cr reflects energy metabolism. A meta-analysis has reported no significant overall change in the Cr in MS lesions and GM when compared with WM and GM of healthy control subjects, and a medium-effect-sized overall increase in the Cr of NAWM relative to WM. In a recent study, Cr has been found to be increased within the corticospinal tract, which is characterized by a high metabolic rate, of patients with RRMS and PPMS when compared with control subjects.[45] Lower Cr levels within the corticospinal tract were associated with higher motor disability in 13 PPMS and 14 patients with RRMS, suggesting that an impaired energy metabolism is responsible for clinical features of MS.[18,45]

Choline-Containing Compounds

Cho is a marker of cell membrane, and its increase reflects elevated cellular turnover. It is often reported to be raised in the NAWM of patients with MS when compared with control subjects.[27] Narayana and colleagues[17] described the elevation of Cho before the appearance of a gadolinium-enhancing lesion, suggesting that Cho might be a marker of inflammation preceding demonstrable blood-brain barrier breakdown.

When Cho was measured along the whole corticospinal tract, it was higher in 13 RRMS when compared with 16 healthy control subjects, but similar between patients with RRMS and PPMS. In addition, in the PPMS group, lower Cho levels were associated with worse walking abilities and greater disability, as measured by the EDSS, suggesting that abnormal membrane turnover from demyelination and remyelination, which is reflected by lower Cho levels, might be responsible for disability accrual.[45] However, these correlations were not confirmed by the study of Kirov and colleagues[27] carried out in 18 patients with RRMS with short disease duration and minimal disease activity; additionally, this work did not detect significant changes in Cho levels in the GM between patients and control subjects, suggesting that the injury may be focal, subtle, or heterogeneous between cortex and deep GM. Similarly, Donadieu and colleagues[26] did not find any difference in GM Cho levels between 19 patients with RRMS and 19 healthy control subjects, possibly because of their voxelwise between-group analysis, which might have made it difficult to detect the random distribution of Cho.

Myo-Inositol

Myo-inositol is a glial cell marker, and its increase reflects glial cell (or astrocytic) activation and proliferation (see Fig. 1).[10,35,46]

Different disease subtypes (eg, PPMS and RRMS) show increased myo-inositol levels in the acute and chronic WM lesions of the brain and the spinal cord when compared with healthy control subjects.[18,26,31,35,47] In a study carried out in 14 patients with RRMS, higher myo-inositol levels within acute lesions of the spinal cord were associated with greater disability, as measured by the EDSS.[18]

Myo-inositol levels were found to be higher in the NAWM of 19 RRMS when compared with 19 healthy control subjects, especially in the periventricular regions within bilateral temporal and frontal lobes, in the left thalamus, and superior temporal gyrus.[26] A significantly higher myo-inositol concentration was found in the corticospinal tract of 13 patients with RRMS when compared with 16 healthy control subjects, and higher myo-inositol levels were associated with greater walking difficulties. However, in the same study, no difference was found between PPMS and healthy control subjects, suggesting a more widespread glial activation in the corticospinal tract of patients with RRMS.[45] A study carried out in patients with CIS has reported elevated myo-inositol levels in the NAWM when compared with control subjects,[23] which did not correlate with T2 lesion load, suggesting that *myo*-inositol may reflect a process of pathogenic importance, independently of WM lesions. However, other studies in CIS patients did not confirm increased *myo*-inositol in NAWM when compared with control subjects.[21,24]

Higher *myo*-inositol levels were found in the cortical GM and in the thalamus of 19 patients with RRMS when compared with control subjects,[26] suggesting that astrocytic activation and proliferation involve cortical and deep GM regions in MS.

Finally, *myo*-inositol levels have been found to be increased in the lesional upper cervical cord of MS patients, when compared with control subjects and with patients with neuromyelitis optica,[47] with potentially important diagnostic implications. Reduced *myo*-inositol values might reflect the extent of the damage of astrocytes, which are highly damaged in neuromyelitis optica, but not in MS, where they are typically activated and increased in number (ie, gliosis).

Limitations

From a technical point of view, there are several limitations of MRS imaging,[11] which may hamper its use in the clinical setting and in clinical trials.[15] These include (1) long acquisition times, more significantly for chemical-shift imaging than for single-voxel MRS; (2) lower spatial resolution compared with MR imaging,[46] with minimal spatial information provided by single-voxel MRS acquisition; (3) difficulties in differentiating between the intracellular and the extracellular pool of different metabolites and between GM and WM compartments within volumes of interest; (4) use of different scanners and acquisition protocols, which can be responsible for incomplete agreement on metabolite concentrations; and (5) spectra are influenced by variations in B0 and B1 magnetic fields, and there are pathology-related changes in the T1 and T2 relaxation times of the spectral metabolites that need to be considered when investigating patients. Furthermore, spinal cord MRS presents additional technical limitations, such as the small size of the cord; the susceptibility artifacts because of tissue-bone interfaces; and the motion artifacts arising from respiratory, arterial, and cardiac activities, and systolic-related cerebrospinal fluid and spinal cord pulsations.

SODIUM IMAGING

In the central nervous system, sodium concentration is maintained at a markedly lower concentration (12 mM/L) in the larger intracellular compartment (tissue fraction of 80%), when compared with the higher concentration (140 mM/L) in the smaller extracellular compartment (tissue fraction of 20%), as a result of complex energy-dependent mechanisms (eg, Na/K pump) (see **Fig. 1**).[1] Increased concentration of intracellular sodium is caused by impaired mitochondrial metabolism and is considered to play a role in the cascade of event that leads to neuronal death. Additionally, in acute inflammatory demyelinated lesions, there is extracellular edema, with increased fluid in the interstitial compartments. Increased extracellular sodium in MS may also occur because of the expansion of the extracellular space secondary to neuroaxonal loss.

Previous sodium MR imaging studies have estimated the total sodium concentration in the brain, without distinguishing between its intracellular and extracellular component.[48,49] These studies have reported higher total sodium concentrations in lesions, NAWM, and cortical GM in patients with MS when compared with control subjects, with especially high concentrations detected in patients with higher clinical disability and progressive MS.[49] These findings suggest that raised total sodium concentration may reflect neuroaxonal damage, which is responsible for progression and increased disability. However, also patients with early RRMS show abnormally high total sodium concentrations, although limited to a certain number of brain regions (brainstem, bilateral cerebellum, left temporal pole) and the GM.[50]

More recently, the use of ultra-high field MR imaging has allowed the discrimination of intracellular and extracellular sodium concentrations. Petracca and colleagues[48] have performed a triple-quantum filtered ^{23}Na MR imaging with an MR pulse sequence and applied a single-quantum and triple-quantum filtered imaging at 7 T to quantify intracellular sodium concentration and intracellular sodium volume fraction, an indirect measure of the extracellular sodium. Both total and intracellular sodium concentrations were increased in the NAWM and in the GM of 19 RRMS, compared with 17 control subjects, whereas extracellular sodium concentrations were reduced; furthermore, reduced levels of extracellular sodium were associated with disability, as measured by the EDSS.[48] These findings suggest that sodium accumulation is not only a consequence of demyelination and neuroaxonal loss, but also a marker of metabolic dysfunction. Therefore, measuring the intracellular component might provide the unique opportunity to identify metabolically dysfunctional brain areas, which might be targeted by new drugs restoring their function and, so, preventing irreversible structural alterations.

PET

PET is a quantitative imaging technique that investigates cellular and molecular processes in vivo. It requires the reconstruction of an image of the tissue of interest after the distribution of an exogenously administered positron-emitting molecule, ideally binding a selective target.[46,51]

Because MS is a complex and multifactorial disease, there are different possible radioligands, which can be used in PET imaging with high selectivity. Examples of the targets of the PET radioligands used in MS are shown in **Fig. 1**.

We next discuss the results of the studies using PET tracers by grouping them according to the underlying pathologic processes that they reflect: inflammation, demyelination, neuronal damage, and astrocyte activation (**Table 2**).

Inflammatory Markers

The acute, inflammatory activity in MS is characterized by breakdown of the blood–brain barrier, inflammatory cell infiltrates, microglial activation, and production of immune soluble mediators and harmful inflammatory enzymes. In the short-term, inflammation is responsible for the development of acute demyelinating lesions, with consequent clinical relapses.[9,10] In the long-term, demyelinated axons undergo neurodegeneration. Additionally, microglial cell activation is thought to have a short-term positive effect on tissue repair, but a long-term contribution to neuronal cell death.[13,46,52] These inflammatory processes may be associated with increased PET signal detected in patients with MS when compared with healthy control subjects.

Translocator protein PET

The translocator protein (TSPO, formerly known as the peripheral benzodiazepine receptor [PBR]) is an 18-kDa macromolecular complex that is expressed at low levels in the outer mitochondrial membrane and is strongly up-regulated in activated microglial cells. Hence, TSPO ligands can reflect in vivo the presence of activated microglial cells.[13,46,52,53]

TSPO studies using ^{11}C-PK11195 (a 3-isoquinolinecarboxamide antagonist with nanomolar affinity for TSPO) have reported increased uptake of this radiotracer in active MS lesions and in the NAWM than healthy control subjects,[54,55] suggesting that this radiotracer might detect the widespread microglial cell activation in the active inflammatory rim of chronically active plaques and in the NAWM. Increased ^{11}C-PK11195 uptake has been found also in the cortical GM of 10 RRMS and eight patients with SPMS when compared with eight healthy control subjects.[54] Higher TSPO binding levels were associated with disability scores, particularly if located in clinically meaningful anatomic regions.[55]

A few PET studies were carried out in small groups of patients with MS using the second generation of TSPO tracers, such as ^{11}C-vinpocetine, ^{11}C-PBR28, ^{18}F-FEDAA1106, ^{18}F-PBR111, and ^{18}F-DPA714. An example of a PET scan showing the ^{11}C-PBR28 uptake in MS is given in **Fig. 3**. These novel radioligands are expected to overcome the low brain uptake and nonspecific

Table 2
Cellular and molecular processes measured with PET

Pathophysiologic Mechanisms	Tracers	Imaging Finding in MS Versus Healthy Control Subjects	Clinical Correlations
Inflammation	^{11}C-PK11195 and other TSPO tracers	Chronic WM lesions: ↑ NAWM: ↑ GM: ↑ Hippocampus: ↑	Motor disability Low mood
	^{18}F-FDG	Acute WM lesions: ↑	
	^{11}C-TMSX	NAWM: ↑	Motor disability
Demyelination	^{11}C-PIB, ^{18}F-florbetaben and other β-amyloid tracers	Acute WM lesions: ↓ Chronic WM lesions: ↓	Motor disability
Neuronal damage	^{11}C-flumazenil	GM: ↓	Cognitive disability
Astrocyte activation	^{11}C-acetate	NAWM: ↑ GM: ↑	

PET tracers reflect different pathologic processes with a specific pathogenetic relevance in MS (inflammation, demyelination, neuronal damage, and astrocyte activation). Imaging findings and clinical correlations are reported.

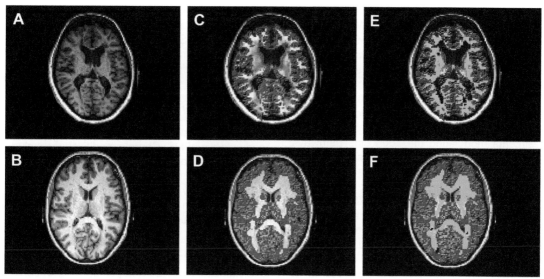

Fig. 3. Example of TSPO PET scans in MS. T1 axial section from a 45-year-old woman with aggressive disease course (disease duration of 14 years) (A), and a 42-year-old woman with benign disease course with EDSS of 1.0 (B). The corresponding T1 overlaid with voxel-wise TSPO PET image of ^{11}C-PBR28 distribution volume ratio (DVR) for patient A (C) and patient B (D). Bright yellow indicates high DVR and red is lower DVR. Overlaid on the images from C and D in E and F, respectively, are the normal-appearing white matter (green) and T2 white matter lesion (blue) mask. (Courtesy of Dr Gourab Datta and Professor Paul Matthews, OBE, MD, DPhil, FRCP, FMedSci, Imperial College London, United Kingdom.)

binding of ^{11}C-PK1119 with subsequent higher signal-to-noise ratios.[10,46,51,53,56] However, the TSPO polymorphisms, which explains differences in binding affinity of the PET radioligand between subjects, need to be considered when using the second-generation TSPO ligands.[13,57] Increased uptake of ^{18}F-PBR111 was detected in WM lesions and NAWM of 11 patients with MS, when compared with 11 healthy control subjects.[56] Reduced uptake of ^{18}F-PBR111 in the hippocampus of 13 patients with RRMS, when compared with 22 healthy control subjects, was associated with higher scores at the Beck Depression Inventory, suggesting the involvement of this area in mood symptoms of MS.[58] In an exploratory analysis comparing four patients with RRMS with four healthy control subjects, ^{11}C-PBR28 presented a good test-retest reproducibility (less than 9%), and so might be suitable for future longitudinal assessments.[59]

^{18}F-FDG PET
Brain 2'-[^{18}F] fluoro-2'-deoxyglucose (^{18}F-FDG) PET measures the cerebral metabolic rate of glucose utilization and, hence, has been used as a marker of inflammation. Higher metabolic rates are found in regions with ongoing inflammation because of an avid uptake from activated inflammatory cells.[13,51] Specifically, ^{18}F-FDG PET has been used in MS to classify WM lesions as either acute (hypermetabolism) or chronic (hypometabolism) based on local glucose metabolism.[60]

However, ^{18}F-FDG uptake is not specific for inflammatory cells and is limited by the high background glucose uptake within the brain, which reduces its ability to detect small active lesions.[13,51] It has been suggested that ^{18}F-FDG uptake reflects glucose transport and metabolism by neurons and astrocytes, and, so, their integrity and functional state.[10,60] In agreement with this hypothesis, a pilot ^{18}F-FDG PET study of the spinal cord in eight patients with MS reported a lower uptake of this radioligand when compared with eight healthy control subjects. Furthermore, a decreased ^{18}F-FDG binding was associated with worse autonomic and walking symptoms,[61] suggesting that an impaired metabolic activity in the spinal cord may be responsible for neurologic disability.

Purine PET
Adenosine is a ubiquitous purine that binds to a group of G-protein-coupled receptors (A1R, A2AR, A2BR, and A3R). A2A receptors are upregulated at sites of inflammation and tissue damage, thereby attenuating inflammation.[51,62] ^{11}C-TMSX radioligand binds to adenosine A2A receptors. Rissanen and colleagues[62] have carried out a PET study using this tracer in 10 patients with SPMS and 10 age- and sex-matched healthy

control subjects. They found increased distribution volumes of ^{11}C-TMSX in the NAWM of SPMS when compared with control subjects. Furthermore, the increased A2AR binding was associated with increased tissue loss and reduced fiber integrity, as measured by diffusion tensor imaging, and higher disability, as measured by the EDSS.[62]

It is worth noting that this technique might be particularly valuable in measuring the impact of treatments modulating the adenosine pathways, such as caffeine-related compounds.[51,63–65]

Purinergic pathways can be studied also by targeting the P2X7 receptor. Different tracers have been developed (eg, ^{11}C-JNJ-54173717, ^{11}C-A-740003, ^{11}C-GSK-1482160),[57,66,67] and some of them have been tested on animal models of MS.[57,66] These tracers might measure the activation of microglia and the associated release of inflammatory cytokines, and are expected to be tested soon in vivo.[68]

Myelin Markers

Demyelination is a hallmark of MS and can occur in GM and WM. The inflammatory process causes the development of acute demyelinating lesions, which is associated with axonal transection.[69] Demyelination can be followed by remyelination, or, in the long-term, neurodegeneration.[9]

Amyloid PET

PET images with amyloid tracers, such as a carbon-labelled version of the Pittsburgh compound B (^{11}C-PIB) and ^{18}F-florbetaben, show normal uptake in healthy WM, thereby making the amyloid tracers potentially useful for studying MS.[51,70,71]

In acute WM lesions, ^{11}C-PIB and ^{18}F-florbetaben uptake was decreased when compared with NAWM, and a decreasing gradient in binding levels was found when going from the NAWM to the lesions,[72,73] reflecting a more extensive myelin loss in acute lesions than in the NAWM. Both positive and negative variations in the binding of these PET ligands were observed in the chronic phase of the WM lesions, reflecting the net result of dynamic processes of myelin loss and remyelination. Additionally, in patients with RRMS, a higher ^{11}C-PIB uptake within the WM lesions was associated with a more benign clinical evolution.[72] Progressive forms of MS showed a more pronounced reduction of the uptake in the damaged WM, in comparison with the RRMS type.[73] These studies suggest that in future amyloid-PET may be used to monitor MS progression and may be used to provide outcome measures in clinical trials designed to measure the effects of remyelinating agents.[46,71]

^{11}C-BMB (^{11}C-1,4-bis(p-aminostyryl)-2-methoxybenzene) and its derivatives (ie, ^{11}C-CIC, along with ^{11}C-MeDAS), which have shown promising results in animal models of MS, with concentration-dependent binding to WM tracts, will be investigated in humans.[13,52]

Neuronal Markers

Neurodegenerative alterations occur even in the early stages of MS. Chronic modifications include activation of glial cells; infiltration of macrophages; and, ultimately, neuronal functional alterations and death.[1] In view of this, a variety of PET radioligands has been used to measure different components of these chronic neurodegenerative changes.

^{11}C-flumazenil PET

^{11}C-flumazenil is an antagonist of the central benzodiazepine receptor, a component of the ubiquitous GABA-A receptor complex present in the neuronal synapses in the GM. Thus, ^{11}C-flumazenil PET is a specific marker of neuronal integrity.[2,13,74]

In a pilot study, Freeman and colleagues[74] found a reduced ^{11}C-flumazenil cortical binding in nine patients with RRMS and nine patients with SPMS, compared with eight healthy control subjects. Interestingly, this difference was already seen in patients with RRMS, who did not show a significant degree of GM atrophy. In addition, reduced GABA-A receptor binding was associated with impairment of information processing speed,[74] further suggesting the clinical relevance of this quantitative measure. These findings suggest that synaptic/dendritic damage may occur before a quantifiable GM volume loss, and contribute to clinical impairment. In future, neuroprotective and reparative treatment trials that aim to stop or slow down the progression of MS may consider developing the ^{11}C-flumazenil cortical binding as outcome measure for clinical trials or to select the patients who show early neurodegenerative changes in GM.

Markers of Astrocyte Activation

Glial (or astrocytic) cell activation and proliferation is known to occur since the early stage of MS, as discussed previously in the *myo*-inositol section. Astrocytes are thought to play an important role in the pathogenesis of MS.[75]

^{11}C-acetate PET

In MS lesions, activated glial cells overexpress metabolic enzymes, such as the monocarboxylate transporter,[76] which absorbs acetate into astrocytes. The acetate is then converted into fatty acids. Takata and colleagues[77] carried out an ^{11}C-acetate PET study in six patients with RRMS and six healthy control subjects. An increased uptake of this radioligand was observed in both the WM and the GM of patients with MS when compared with control subjects, but was more pronounced in the WM, particularly in the regions of axonal damage, as detected by diffusion-tensor MR imaging. Therefore, the detection of acetate has been suggested as a marker of astrocytic-associated damage in MS, although a development of a clinically feasible protocol for acetate PET and future investigations are warranted.

Choline PET

A preliminary study by Virta and colleagues[78] did not find any difference in the cortical uptake of the PET tracer ^{11}C-MP4A, which reflects the acetylcholinesterase activity, between 10 patients with SPMS and 10 healthy control subjects. Nevertheless, ^{11}C-choline and ^{18}F-choline PET can evaluate the cholinergic metabolic profile of specific areas, such as large demyelinated lesions.[79,80]

Limitations

Possible limitations of PET imaging include (1) the injection of radioactive tracers, although generally at low dosages; (2) PET costs, which are still high for its application in clinical practice; (3) lack of standardized procedures (there is a need for data modeling techniques based on methods not dependent on reference plasma input or manual delineation of reference tissue region)[54]; (4) relatively low resolution of PET with subsequent difficulties in evaluating small plaques[77]; and (5) static image acquisition in most protocols with subsequent difficulties in tracking the tracer over time.

SUMMARY

Despite the high costs of PET and the technical challenges of PET and MRS studies, these techniques have provided insights into the pathogenesis of MS and helped to understand the clinical heterogeneity of patients with MS. The next step is to translate these techniques from the research laboratories to clinical trials and the clinical setting, to identify groups of patients who are more likely to respond to a medication and to monitor the treatment response. For example, reparative clinical trials testing the efficacy of remyelinating agents may in future benefit from inclusion of myelin PET into their trial design, perhaps to select patients who have the greatest remyelination potential.

REFERENCES

1. Friese MA, Schattling B, Fugger L. Mechanisms of neurodegeneration and axonal dysfunction in multiple sclerosis. Nat Rev Neurol 2014;10(4):225–38.
2. Bodini B, Louapre C, Stankoff B. Advanced imaging tools to investigate multiple sclerosis pathology. Presse Med 2015;44(4):e159–67.
3. Sormani MP, Arnold DL, De Stefano N. Treatment effect on brain atrophy correlates with treatment effect on disability in multiple sclerosis. Ann Neurol 2014; 75(1):43–9.
4. Popescu V, Agosta F, Hulst HE, et al. Brain atrophy and lesion load predict long-term disability in multiple sclerosis. J Neurol Neurosurg Psychiatry 2013; 84(10):1082–91.
5. Inglese M, Oesingmann N, Casaccia P, et al. Progressive multiple sclerosis and gray matter pathology: an MRI perspective. Mt Sinai J Med 2011; 78(2):258–67.
6. Scalfari A, Neuhaus A, Daumer M, et al. Early relapses, onset of progression, and late outcome in multiple sclerosis. JAMA Neurol 2013;70(2):214–22.
7. Stys P, Zamponi G, van Minnen J, et al. Will the real multiple sclerosis please stand up? Nat Rev Neurosci 2012;13(7):507–14.
8. Koini M, Filippi M, Rocca M, et al. Correlates of executive functions in multiple sclerosis based on structural and functional MR imaging: insights from a multicenter study. Radiology 2016;280(3):869–79.
9. Dendrou C, Fugger L, Friese M. Immunopathology of multiple sclerosis. Nat Rev Immunol 2015;15(9): 545–58.
10. Ciccarelli O, Barkhof F, Bodini B, et al. Pathogenesis of multiple sclerosis: insights from molecular and metabolic imaging. Lancet Neurol 2014;13(8):807–22.
11. Gülin Ö. Magnetic resonance spectroscopy of degenerative brain diseases. Contemporary. Switzerland: Springer; 2016.
12. Caramanos Z, Narayanan S, Arnold DL. 1H-MRS quantification of tNA and tCr in patients with multiple sclerosis: a meta-analytic review. Brain 2005; 128(11):2483–506.
13. Matthews PM, Comley R. Advances in the molecular imaging of multiple sclerosis. Expert Rev Clin Immunol 2009;5(6):765–77.
14. van Horssen J, Witte M, Ciccarelli O. The role of mitochondria in axonal degeneration and tissue repair in MS. Mult Scler J 2012;18(8):1058–67.
15. De Stefano N, Filippi M, Miller D, et al. Guidelines for using proton MR spectroscopy in multicenter clinical MS studies. Neurology 2007;69(20):1942–52.
16. Roosendaal SD, Barkhof F. Imaging phenotypes in multiple sclerosis. Neuroimaging Clin N Am 2015; 25(1):83–96.
17. Narayana PA, Doyle TJ, Lai D, et al. Serial proton magnetic resonance spectroscopic imaging,

contrast-enhanced magnetic resonance imaging, and quantitative lesion volumetry in multiple sclerosis. Ann Neurol 1998;43(1):56–71.

18. Ciccarelli O, Wheeler-Kingshott CA, McLean MA, et al. Spinal cord spectroscopy and diffusion-based tractography to assess acute disability in multiple sclerosis. Brain 2007;130(8):2220–31.

19. Ciccarelli O, Altmann DR, McLean MA, et al. Spinal cord repair in MS: does mitochondrial metabolism play a role? Neurology 2010;74(9):721–7.

20. De Stefano N, Matthews P, Antel J, et al. Chemical pathology of acute demyelinating lesions and its correlation with disability. Ann Neurol 1995;38(6):901–9.

21. Wattjes MP, Harzheim M, Lutterbey GG, et al. High field MR imaging and 1H-MR spectroscopy in clinically isolated syndromes suggestive of multiple sclerosis: correlation between metabolic alterations and diagnostic MR imaging criteria. J Neurol 2008; 255(1):56–63.

22. Rocca MA, Mezzapesa DM, Falini A, et al. Evidence for axonal pathology and adaptive cortical reorganization in patients at presentation with clinically isolated syndromes suggestive of multiple sclerosis. Neuroimage 2003;18(4):847–55.

23. Fernando KTM, McLean MA, Chard DT, et al. Elevated white matter myo-inositol in clinically isolated syndromes suggestive of multiple sclerosis. Brain 2004;127(6):1361–9.

24. Brex PA, Gomez-Anson B, Parker GJM, et al. Proton MR spectroscopy in clinically isolated syndromes suggestive of multiple sclerosis. J Neurol Sci 1999; 166(1):16–22.

25. Sbardella E, Tomassini V, Stromillo M, et al. Pronounced focal and diffuse brain damage predicts short-term disease evolution in patients with clinically isolated syndrome suggestive of multiple sclerosis. Mult Scler J 2011;17(12):1432–40.

26. Donadieu M, Le Fur Y, Lecocq A, et al. Metabolic voxel-based analysis of the complete human brain using fast 3D-MRSI: proof of concept in multiple sclerosis. J Magn Reson Imaging 2016;44(2):411–9.

27. Kirov II, Tal A, Babb JS, et al. Serial proton MR spectroscopy of gray and white matter in relapsing-remitting MS. Neurology 2013;80(1):39–46.

28. Chard DT, Griffin CM, McLean MA, et al. Brain metabolite changes in cortical grey and normal-appearing white matter in clinically early relapsing-remitting multiple sclerosis. Brain 2002;125(Pt 10): 2342–52.

29. Geurts JJG, Reuling IEW, Vrenken H, et al. MR spectroscopic evidence for thalamic and hippocampal, but not cortical, damage in multiple sclerosis. Magn Reson Med 2006;55(3):478–83.

30. Tiberio M, Chard DT, Altmann DR, et al. Metabolite changes in early relapsing-remitting multiple sclerosis: a two year follow-up study. J Neurol 2006; 253(2):224–30.

31. Abdel-Aziz K, Schneider T, Solanky BS, et al. Evidence for early neurodegeneration in the cervical cord of patients with primary progressive multiple sclerosis. Brain 2015;138(Pt 6):1568–82.

32. Filippi M, Rocca MA, Pagani E, et al. Placebo-controlled trial of oral laquinimod in multiple sclerosis: MRI evidence of an effect on brain tissue damage. J Neurol Neurosurg Psychiatry 2014; 85(8):852–9.

33. Sajja BR, Narayana PA, Wolinsky JS, et al. Longitudinal magnetic resonance spectroscopic imaging of primary progressive multiple sclerosis patients treated with glatiramer acetate: multicenter study. Mult Scler 2008;14(1):73–80.

34. Azevedo CJ, Kornak J, Chu P, et al. In vivo evidence of glutamate toxicity in multiple sclerosis. Ann Neurol 2014;76(2):269–78.

35. Srinivasan R, Sailasuta N, Hurd R, et al. Evidence of elevated glutamate in multiple sclerosis using magnetic resonance spectroscopy at 3 T. Brain 2005; 128(5):1016–25.

36. MacMillan EL, Tam R, Zhao Y, et al. Progressive multiple sclerosis exhibits decreasing glutamate and glutamine over two years. Mult Scler J 2016;22(1): 112–6.

37. Muhlert N, Atzori M, De Vita E, et al. Memory in multiple sclerosis is linked to glutamate concentration in grey matter regions. J Neurol Neurosurg Psychiatry 2014;85:834–40.

38. Sastre-Garriga J, Ingle GT, Chard DT, et al. Metabolite changes in normal-appearing gray and white matter are linked with disability in early primary progressive multiple sclerosis. Arch Neurol 2005;62(4): 569–73.

39. Wegner C, Esiri MM, Chance SA, et al. Neocortical neuronal, synaptic, and glial loss in multiple sclerosis. Neurology 2006;67(6):960–7.

40. Lovera J, Ramos A, Devier D, et al. Polyphenon E, non-futile at neuroprotection in multiple sclerosis but unpredictably hepatotoxic: phase I single group and phase II randomized placebo-controlled studies. J Neurol Sci 2015;358(1–2):46–52.

41. Cawley N, Solanky BS, Muhlert N, et al. Reduced gamma-aminobutyric acid concentration is associated with physical disability in progressive multiple sclerosis. Brain 2015;138(9):2584–95.

42. Nicholas R, Magliozzi R, Campbell G, et al. Temporal lobe cortical pathology and inhibitory GABA interneuron cell loss are associated with seizures in multiple sclerosis. Mult Scler 2016;22(1):25–35.

43. Dutta R, McDonough J, Yin X, et al. Mitochondrial dysfunction as a cause of axonal degeneration in multiple sclerosis patients. Ann Neurol 2006;59(3): 478–89.

44. Bhat R, Axtell R, Mitra A, et al. Inhibitory role for GABA in autoimmune inflammation. Proc Natl Acad Sci U S A 2010;107(6):2580–5.

45. Tur C, Wheeler-Kingshott CAM, Altmann DR, et al. Spatial variability and changes of metabolite concentrations in the cortico-spinal tract in multiple sclerosis using coronal CSI. Hum Brain Mapp 2014; 35(3):993–1003.

46. Matthews PM, Datta G. Positron-emission tomography molecular imaging of glia and myelin in drug discovery for multiple sclerosis. Expert Opin Drug Discov 2015;10(5):557–70.

47. Ciccarelli O, Thomas DL, De Vita E, et al. Low *myo*-inositol indicating astrocytic damage in a case series of neuromyelitis optica. Ann Neurol 2013;74(2): 301–5.

48. Petracca M, Vancea RO, Fleysher L, et al. Brain intra- and extracellular sodium concentration in multiple sclerosis: a 7 T MRI study. Brain 2016;139(3): 795–806.

49. Paling D, Solanky BS, Riemer F, et al. Sodium accumulation is associated with disability and a progressive course in multiple sclerosis. Brain 2013;136: 2305–17.

50. Zaaraoui W, Konstandin S, Bertrand A, et al. Distribution of brain sodium accumulation correlates with disability in multiple sclerosis: a cross-sectional 23Na MR imaging study. Radiology 2012; 264(3):859–67.

51. De Paula Faria D, Copray S, Buchpiguel C, et al. PET imaging in multiple sclerosis. J Neuroimmune Pharmacol 2014;9(4):468–82.

52. Niccolini F, Su P, Politis M. PET in multiple sclerosis. Clin Nucl Med 2015;40(1):e46–52.

53. Janssen B, Vugts DJ, Funke U, et al. Imaging of neuroinflammation in Alzheimer's disease, multiple sclerosis and stroke: recent developments in positron emission tomography. Biochim Biophys Acta 2015; 1862(3):425–41.

54. Rissanen E, Tuisku J, Rokka J, et al. In vivo detection of diffuse inflammation in secondary progressive multiple sclerosis using PET imaging and the radioligand C-11-PK11195. J Nucl Med 2014; 55(6):939–44.

55. Politis M, Giannetti P, Su P, et al. Increased PK11195 PET binding in the cortex of patients with MS correlates with disability. Neurology 2012;79(6):523–30.

56. Colasanti A, Guo Q, Muhlert N, et al. In vivo assessment of brain white matter inflammation in multiple sclerosis with (18)F-PBR111 PET. J Nucl Med 2014;55(7):1112–8.

57. Janssen B, Vugts DJ, Funke U, et al. Synthesis and initial preclinical evaluation of the P2X7 receptor antagonist [11C]A-740003 as a novel tracer of neuroinflammation. J Labelled Comp Radiopharm 2014; 57(8):509–16.

58. Colasanti A, Guo Q, Giannetti P, et al. Hippocampal neuroinflammation, functional connectivity, and depressive symptoms in multiple sclerosis. Biol Psychiatry 2015;80(1):62–72.

59. Park E, Gallezot JD, Delgadillo A, et al. 11C-PBR28 imaging in multiple sclerosis patients and healthy controls: test-retest reproducibility and focal visualization of active white matter areas. Eur J Nucl Med Mol Imaging 2015;42(7):1081–92.

60. Schiepers C, Van Hecke P, Vandenberghe R, et al. Positron emission tomography, magnetic resonance imaging and proton NMR spectroscopy of white matter in multiple sclerosis. Mult Scler 1997;3(1): 8–17.

61. Kindred JH, Koo PJ, Rudroff T. Glucose uptake of the spinal cord in patients with multiple sclerosis detected by (1)(8)F-fluorodeoxyglucose PET/CT after walking. Spinal Cord 2014;52(Suppl 3):S11–3.

62. Rissanen E, Virta JR, Paavilainen T, et al. Adenosine A2A receptors in secondary progressive multiple sclerosis: a [(11)C]TMSX brain PET study. J Cereb Blood Flow Metab 2013;33(9):1394–401.

63. Hedström AK, Mowry EM, Gianfrancesco MA, et al. High consumption of coffee is associated with decreased multiple sclerosis risk; results from two independent studies. J Neurol Neurosurg Psychiatry 2016;87(5):454–60.

64. Liu Y, Zou H, Zhao P, et al. Activation of the adenosine A2A receptor attenuates experimental autoimmune encephalomyelitis and is associated with increased intracellular calcium levels. Neuroscience 2016;330:150–61.

65. Wang T, Xi NN, Chen Y, et al. Chronic caffeine treatment protects against experimental autoimmune encephalomyelitis in mice: therapeutic window and receptor subtype mechanism. Neuropharmacology 2014;86:203–11.

66. Ory D, Celen S, Gijsbers R, et al. Preclinical evaluation of a P2X7 receptor selective radiotracer: PET studies in a rat model with local overexpression of the human P2X7 receptor and in non-human primates. J Nucl Med 2016;57(9):1436–41.

67. Gao M, Wang M, Green MA, et al. Synthesis of [11C]GSK1482160 as a new PET agent for targeting P2X7 receptor. Bioorg Med Chem Lett 2015;25(9): 1965–70.

68. Hagens M, van Berckel B, Barkhof F. Novel MRI and PET markers of neuroinflammation in multiple sclerosis. Curr Opin Neurol 2016;29:229–36.

69. Trapp B, Peterson J, Ransohoff R, et al. Axonal transection in the lesions of multiple sclerosis. N Engl J Med 1998;338(5):278–85.

70. Stankoff B, Freeman L, Aigrot MS, et al. Imaging central nervous system myelin by positron emission tomography in multiple sclerosis using [methyl-11C]-2-(4-methylaminophenyl)- 6-hydroxybenzothiazole. Ann Neurol 2011;69(4):673–80.

71. Mallik S, Samson RS, Wheeler-Kingshott CAM, et al. Imaging outcomes for trials of remyelination in multiple sclerosis. J Neurol Neurosurg Psychiatry 2014; 85(12):1396–404.

72. Bodini B, Veronese M, García-Lorenzo D, et al. Dynamic imaging of individual remyelination profiles in multiple sclerosis. Ann Neurol 2016. [Epub ahead of print].

73. Matías-Guiu JA, Cabrera-Martín MN, Matías-Guiu J, et al. Amyloid PET imaging in multiple sclerosis: an 18F-florbetaben study. BMC Neurol 2015;15(1):243.

74. Freeman L, Garcia-Lorenzo D, Bottin L, et al. The neuronal component of gray matter damage in multiple sclerosis: a [(11) C]flumazenil positron emission tomography study. Ann Neurol 2015;78(4): 554–67.

75. Ludwin SK, Rao VT, Moore CS, et al. Astrocytes in multiple sclerosis. Mult Scler J 2016;22(9):1114–24.

76. Nijland PG, Michailidou I, Witte ME, et al. Cellular distribution of glucose and monocarboxylate transporters in human brain white matter and multiple sclerosis lesions. Glia 2014;62(7):1125–41.

77. Takata K, Kato H, Shimosegawa E, et al. 11C-acetate PET imaging in patients with multiple sclerosis. PLoS One 2014;9(11):e111598.

78. Virta JR, Laatu S, Parkkola R, et al. Cerebral acetylcholinesterase activity is not decreased in MS patients with cognitive impairment. Mult Scler 2011; 17(8):931–8.

79. Padma MV, Adineh M, Pugar K, et al. Functional imaging of a large demyelinating lesion. J Clin Neurosci 2005;12(2):176–8.

80. Bolcaen J, Acou M, Mertens K, et al. Structural and metabolic features of two different variants of multiple sclerosis: a PET/MRI study. J Neuroimaging 2013;23(3):431–6.

Insights from Ultrahigh Field Imaging in Multiple Sclerosis

Matthew K. Schindler, MD, PhD, Pascal Sati, PhD, Daniel S. Reich, MD, PhD*

KEYWORDS

• Multiple sclerosis • Ultrahigh field imaging • MR imaging

KEY POINTS

- Ultrahigh-field (UHF) MR imaging enables superior detection of MS abnormalities in the white matter and gray matter.
- The detection of the "central vein sign" within multiple sclerosis (MS) lesions is improved with UHF MR imaging.
- UHF MR imaging provides new insights about the mechanisms of lesion development.
- Susceptibility-based MR imaging at UHF may provide new information about the outcome of MS lesions.

INTRODUCTION

The application of magnetic resonance (MR) imaging to multiple sclerosis (MS) occurred soon after human scanners were developed. Today, MR imaging is paramount for the MS clinician and researcher and is used for diagnosis, disease monitoring, clinical trial outcomes, and studying disease pathophysiology. As MR imaging technologies have advanced from the first studies of MS patients at 0.25 T,[1] the term "ultrahigh field" (UHF) imaging itself has evolved as ever more powerful magnets have been adopted into routine clinical practice.

Currently, 1.5-T magnets are available in most clinical centers, and 3-T magnets are found in many major academic centers. UHF imaging now applies to 7-T and higher MR imaging, and imaging at these magnetic field strengths has become increasingly common in the last 5 years. Although these advances have generally started in academic medical centers, many have ultimately made their way into routine clinical care.

The 2 main advantages that come with increasing magnetic field strength are (1) the increase in the signal-to-noise ratio (SNR) that approximately scales with the field; and (2) the increased contrast-to-noise ratio caused by substantial changes in T1, T2, and T2* relaxation times. These advantages can be used to improve spatial resolution and detection of anatomic features; for an in-depth review of the technical improvements inherent with 7T MR imaging, see Ref.[2] At 7 T, resolutions can be pushed to less than 0.5 mm with isotropic voxels yielding volumes

Disclosures: The authors have no financial or commercial disclosures. Funding for the study from the intramural research program of National Institute of Neurologic Disorders and Stroke, National Institutes of Health (Z01NS003119), and the National Multiple Sclerosis Society.
Translational Neuroradiology Section, National Institute of Neurological Disorders and Stroke, National Institutes of Health, Medical Center Boulevard, 10 Center Drive, MSC 1400, Bethesda, MD 20892, USA
* Corresponding author. Translational Neuroradiology Section, National Institute of Neurological Disorders and Stroke, National Institutes of Health, 10 Center Drive, MSC 1400, Building 10 Room 5C103, Bethesda, MD 20892.
E-mail address: reichds@ninds.nih.gov

Neuroimag Clin N Am 27 (2017) 357–366
http://dx.doi.org/10.1016/j.nic.2016.12.006
1052-5149/17/Published by Elsevier Inc.

of 125 nL or less, thus providing exquisite levels of detail.[3] As a result, MS abnormality that could previously only be appreciated under the microscopic can now be seen with MR imaging. This review describes the advances and applications of UHF strength imaging (7 T and greater) as it applies to MS. The authors focus on advances in the understanding of the biology of MS, current limitations, and future directions of UHF imaging.

LESION DETECTION AND CHARACTERIZATION
White Matter

Studies of MS brains show a panoply of inflammatory demyelinating lesions of various sizes, including very small white matter (WM) and cortical gray matter (GM) lesions. The ability of MR imaging to detect these lesions is constrained by the physical properties of limits on spatial resolution. Clinically, this may be most important at the time of first presentation, because missing existing lesions and new lesions could delay diagnosis due to reduced ability to meet current MR imaging diagnostic criteria, resulting in delayed initiation of disease-modifying therapy. In addition, detecting new lesions, especially early in their development, could in principle allow clinicians to intervene to limit the extent of damage. The finer spatial resolution of UHF MR imaging has improved the ability to detect ever smaller lesions, in both WM and GM, and to improve their localization of such lesions. It is important to note that the limits on improved spatial resolution from UHF are not known.[2] In addition, finer spatial resolution does not necessarily mean improved imaging, as artifacts related to B0 and B1 field inhomogeneities, exquisite sensitivity to patient motion, and safety concerns from implants and objects not tested at 7 T can limit both the target population and the interpretability of the acquired images. Even with these limitations, imaging at 7 T has proven safe, and advances in pulse sequences continue to improve upon these limitations.

The first in vivo studies at 7 T in MS showed ~25% improvement in the number of WM lesions detected at 7 T compared with 1.5 T.[4] The fact that this improvement was only modest indicates how well sequences have been tuned on conventional scanners to detect focal WM lesions. In addition, early studies used T2-weighted sequences, which are the preferred imaging sequence for WM lesion detection at 3 T, but have proven difficult to implement at 7 T due to the high specific absorption rate (SAR) of radiofrequency energy caused by the refocusing pulses. On the other hand, T1-weighted sequences, which typically have lower SAR, show more sensitivity to detecting MS lesions at 7 T. Indeed, T1-weighted imaging at 7 T showed nearly 50% more MS lesions than T1-weighted imaging at 1.5 T.[5] In a direct comparison of 7 T T1-weighted imaging to 3-T T2-weighted fluid-attenuated inversion recovery (FLAIR) imaging—the gold standard in WM lesion detection—in 14 people with MS, 1075 lesions were detected on 7-T MPRAGE (magnetization-prepared rapid gradient echo) compared with 812 lesions on 3-T FLAIR.[6] Importantly, many of the lesions only detected on 7 T were within what would have been interpreted as normal-appearing WM at 3 T. This improved lesion detection was tempered by the presence of 3-T FLAIR lesions not seen on 7 T, mostly in the infratentorium, where signal dropout was noticed at 7 T. However, this issue might be resolved through the use of the advanced magnetization-prepared 2 rapid acquisition gradient echoes (MP2RAGE) technique, which corrects the image intensity variations due to large spatial B1 field inhomogeneities and thus can provide homogeneous T1 contrast across the entire brain at 7 T.[7] Fig. 1 shows representative images from a person with MS imaged both at 1.5 T, with a conventional T1-weighted sequence, and at 7 T, using MP2RAGE. The improvement in contrast between GM and WM structures, and in the conspicuity of MS lesions, is easily appreciable.

Gray Matter

In addition to detecting WM lesions, the increased spatial resolution and improved tissue contrast of UHF imaging have been instrumental for detecting GM lesions, both in the cortex and in the deep GM nuclei. Demyelination in deep GM structures has been described in the context of MS, and these lesions share characteristics with WM inflammatory demyelinating lesions.[8] However, few radiological studies have assessed for focal lesions in these structures. Instead, studies have primarily focused on iron deposition (see later discussion) and changes in metabolites. Harrison and colleagues[9] evaluated 34 MS cases at 7 T and found ~70% of cases had thalamic lesions, including focal lesions and diffuse confluent signal at the thalamus-ventricle border. Interestingly, focal thalamic lesion burden was associated with progressive clinical disease and correlated with cortical lesion burden, suggesting that GM lesions, regardless of location, may share a common pathophysiology.

Cortical lesions have been described in pathologic studies for decades. Early work by Brownell and Hughes[10] noted widespread cortical abnormality in MS, and later characterization of

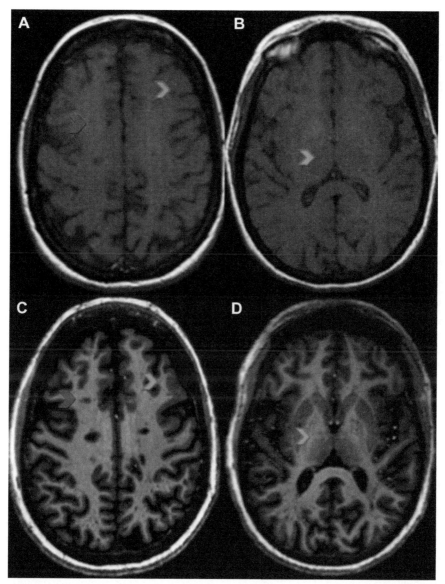

Fig. 1. Representative slices of a T1-weighted scan of a 62-year-old woman with relapsing-remitting MS. (*A, B*) Obtained using the spin-echo sequence on a 1.5-T magnet (TR [repetition time] 600, TE [Echo Time] 16 ms, 1 × 1 × 3-mm resolution). (*C, D*) Obtained using the MP2RAGE at 7 T (0.7-mm isotropic resolution). Improved contrast between WM and GM (*blue chevrons*) is evident. Lesion detection is also improved at 7 T (*red chevrons*).

lesion subtypes[11] focused on characterizing patterns of lesion distribution, but imaging correlates of these pathologic findings have proven difficult to come by. This difficulty was attributed to many factors, including lower amounts of inflammation in cortical lesions and small size of the lesions, both of which contribute to low contrast of lesions relative to normal cortical GM.

UHF imaging has enabled both ex vivo and in vivo observation of cortical lesions. Initial studies show improved detection of cortical lesions at 7 T compared with 3 T as well as the ability to differentiate their pathologically defined subtypes.[4,5,12–20] **Fig. 2** shows cortical lesions seen on T1-weighted MP2RAGE and T2*-weighted gradient echo. A leukocortical lesion can be seen in the primary motor cortex of the left hemisphere.

Most 7-T cortical lesion studies use a single imaging modality for cortical lesion detection, or simply make comparisons across sequences in order to identify the optimal approach, but each sequence has its own limitations and advantages. Sequences are constantly and iteratively being optimized. In one study, which used 3 different

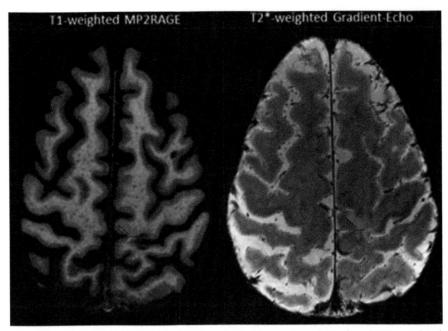

Fig. 2. Representative T1-weighted MP2RAGE (500-mm isotropic voxel resolution) and T2*-weighted GRE image (210 mm × 210-mm in-plane resolution) from a person with relapsing-remitting MS. A leukocortical lesion involving both cortex and subjacent juxtacortical WM is located in the central sulcus (*red arrows*).

pulse sequences, only 25% of lesions were detectable on all sequences, with particularly low concordance for intracortical lesions.[21] In addition, histopathological-radiological correlation studies still show that UHF MR imaging, even using the most sensitive imaging techniques, still misses cortical lesions seen on abnormality.[16,19,22,23]

The subpial type of cortical lesions remains the most challenging to image by MR imaging, but with improvements in acquisition and postprocessing quantitative analysis, even these lesions are starting to be visualized. Mainero's group[24] recently showed that quantitative mapping of the T2* relaxation time within the cortical layers can provide evidence of pathologic changes that are most prominent in the outer layers of the cortex. The extent, depth, and distribution of the laminar changes in T2* relaxation were different depending on the clinical stage of MS, suggesting a radiological correlate to what had been described previously only by pathology studies. However, it is important to appreciate that signal changes seen on T2*-weighted images, and indeed on all MR imaging sequences at all field strengths, represent an average of multiple, sometimes competing, processes. Iron deposition and loss of myelin, both of which occur pathologically in MS, cause opposite effects on T2*-weighted sequences, highlighting the disconnection between imaging physics and biology and making in vivo interpretation

sometimes difficult. Moreover, many advanced techniques require complicated postprocessing and hence are difficult to translate to the clinic.

The addition of summary measures of cortical lesion burden to WM lesion burden has also improved the modest correlation of MR imaging lesion number and volume with disability measures.[24,25] However, volumetric and numeric measures of MS lesions still do not capture the heterogeneity of disability seen in clinical practice. Even with perfect resolution of all MS lesions, it is evident that the full extent and range of clinical disability will not be completely captured by lesion number and/or volume. As pulse sequences and spatial resolution continue to improve, the limitations of UHF imaging on MS lesion detection remain unknown. However, detecting more MS lesions may be a futile measure, because improvements in sensitivity ignore the import in differences between MS lesions, which may ultimately be more important than lesion number or volume. In addition, MR imaging scans are snapshots in time, limiting the ability to fully appreciate the dynamic and complex biological processes that occur in MS.

CENTRAL VEINS

Beyond improvements in detection of MS lesions, UHF imaging has been instrumental in improving the detection of pathologic features of MS lesions, such as the presence of a central vein. The perivenular configuration of MS lesions was described in autopsy specimens by JD Dawson in 1916. These veins are very small in caliber and are thus rarely detectable on conventional MR imaging. Magnetic susceptibility effects increase with field strength, allowing improved visualization of small anatomic structures based on susceptibility differences between blood, iron, and myelin. In particular, T2*-weighted gradient-echo (GRE) imaging is exquisitely sensitive to deoxyhemoglobin within veins. UHF studies have shown that detecting a central vein within MS lesions is greatly improved at 7 T compared with 3 T,[4,26–29] and visualization of small veins is difficult at 1.5 T. **Fig. 3** shows images from a T2*-weighted GRE and demonstrates multiple MS lesions that surround a central vein. The vein is easily visualized due to the prominent loss of signal from deoxyhemoglobin found in greater amounts in veins.

The usefulness of central vein identification goes well beyond recapitulating a pathologic phenomenon, as the presence (or absence) of a central vein is a particularly important feature that can help differentiate MS from other diseases with overlapping imaging features. Studies have shown that greater than 90% of lesions in people with MS have a central vein, whereas other disorders with prominent neuroinflammation but different therapeutic approaches, including Susac syndrome[30] and neuromyelitis optica,[31] do not. In addition, common radiologic mimics, such as migraine[32] and small vessel ischemic disease,[29] are less commonly characterized by WM lesions with a central vein. Differentiating non-perivenular small vessel ischemic lesions or other nonspecific WM lesions from new MS lesions is important to limit unnecessarily changing disease-modifying therapy and exposing patients to more potent, and riskier, drugs. The "central vessel sign" has been proposed to be part of the diagnostic criteria for MS,[33,34] but recent evidence-based guidelines by the MAGNIMS and NAIMS groups recommend further inquiry into its use.[35,36]

ACUTE LESION EVOLUTION

Opening of the blood-brain barrier (BBB), as seen on MR imaging by contrast leakage on

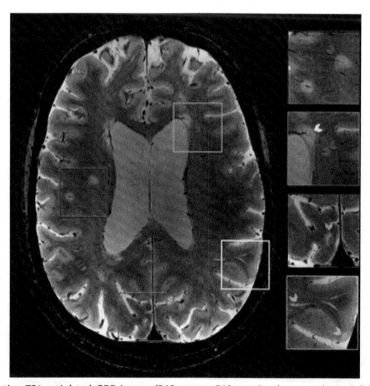

Fig. 3. Representative T2*-weighted GRE image (210 mm × 210-mm in-plane resolution) from a person with relapsing-remitting MS. Magnified boxes highlight different types of MS plaques: deep WM lesions with a central vein (*red chevrons in red and green boxes*), a periventricular lesion with branching veins (*yellow chevron in green box*), a subcortical lesion near a cortical vein (*green chevron in blue box*), and an intracortical lesion with a possible central vein (*orange chevron in yellow box*). Note also the elongated perivascular spaces around some vessels (*light blue chevron in yellow box*).

T1-weighted sequences, is accepted as an early event in lesion formation and radiologically defines active inflammatory demyelination.[37,38] These early studies found nodular and ring-enhancing morphologies in MS lesions, and for years the 2 types were thought to be entirely distinct. Imaging techniques, including dynamic contrast-enhanced (DCE) imaging, in which images are collected before, during, and after intravenous injection of a contrast agent, have disclosed the spatial-temporal dynamics of lesion enhancement. As first observed at 3-T MR imaging, contrast-enhancing MS lesions can display a centrifugal pattern of enhancement that starts at the central vein and fills outward, or a centripetal pattern that starts at the lesion periphery and fills inward.[39] The enhancement pattern can change from centrifugal to centripetal, indicating that enhancement is a dynamic process that may represent different pathophysiologic processes depending on the age of the lesion.

DCE imaging at UHF confirmed the findings seen at 3 T and demonstrated that small lesions typically show a centrifugal enhancement pattern originating from around the central vein, whereas larger lesions and leukocortical lesions display the centripetal enhancement pattern.[40] A study in a larger cohort of patients, followed up to 1 year (or more) after the detection of a new enhancing lesion, showed that the enhancement pattern on

DCE corresponds to concurrent and subsequent changes seen in images made from the phase of the T2*-weighted GRE signal.[41] Indeed, phase imaging is sensitive to changes both during lesion formation, corresponding to the location of the centripetal enhancement, and following resolution of enhancement, such that in some lesions, phase contrast remains abnormal at the periphery of chronic lesions (see later discussion). This finding may have important ramifications in characterizing lesion outcomes.

LESION OUTCOMES
Qualitative Imaging

Many techniques have been applied to image MS lesions and brain regions at UHF, particularly pulse sequences tuned to changes in iron content (including susceptibility weighted imaging and its parent sequence, T2*-weighted GRE). Iron-sensitive techniques have proved extremely useful for visualization of the central vein, as described above. Also, as myelin has a large component of iron, demyelination within MS lesions can be visualized and quantified as changes in signal intensity on iron-sensitive sequences.

An early observation was the heterogeneity of MS lesions on GRE images. The GRE technique obtains magnitude and phase images (**Fig. 4**). Susceptibility shifts, whether paramagnetic or

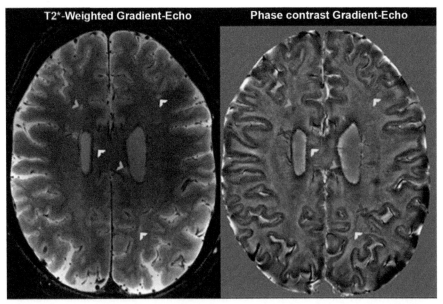

Fig. 4. Representative T2*-weighted magnitude and phase contrast GRE images (210 mm × 210-mm in-plane resolution) from a person with MS. On the magnitude image (*left*), lesions are hyperintense, and susceptibility shifts lead to signal loss. Lesions can display heterogeneous patterns on phase contrast (*right*), such as hypointense rims with isointense core (*red chevrons*) and uniform hypointensity (*green chevrons*). Some lesions are poorly detected on phase contrast (*yellow chevrons*).

diamagnetic, cause signal loss on magnitude images, and the direction of the shift can be determined from the phase image. Interestingly, MS lesions showed heterogeneous characteristics on phase and magnitude images.[42] In this first published analysis of changes in GRE at 7 T in 18 MS patients, 403 lesions were detected on GRE, with 52% seen both on phase and magnitude images, 22% on phase images only, and 26% on magnitude images only. In this study, 8% of lesions had a rim on the phase images, suggesting a population of MS lesions that is potentially pathologically distinct from other lesions. In a longitudinal study, both nodular and rim lesions were stable in appearance over the 2.5 years of follow-up imaging.[43]

Radiological-histopathological correlation studies have verified the presence of iron in phase-rim lesions, suggesting that iron within phagocytic macrophages and/or microglia is the histologic basis for this radiological finding.[16,44–46] Importantly, chronic phase-rim lesions also display characteristics suggesting greater tissue destruction (longer T1 relaxation values and larger size) compared with non–phase-rim lesions, supporting the notion that these lesions are important in the clinical pathophysiology of MS.[46]

The factors that influence if, when, and in whom these lesions develop are not yet fully understood, but these lesion characteristics could well provide an important radiological biomarker to identify a unique subset of MS lesions, that is, those with chronic inflammatory activity. Pathologically, chronic active lesions show active, often mild demyelination, with myelin breakdown products evident within microglia and/or macrophages. Autopsy studies have described this finding in a small percentage of MS lesions, and from these studies, chronic immunologic activity within lesions is hypothesized to engender lesion expansion. The extent to which this process is associated with clinical progression is a subject of current research. Importantly, inflammation in chronic active lesions is probably distinct in character from inflammation within new or newly contrast-enhancing lesions, and as such, is likely to require different treatment approaches. In principle, identifying chronic active lesions could identify patients at risk for more aggressive disease or progression and usher in new treatments focused on stopping this type of inflammation.

It is important to reiterate that iron-sensitive sequences are also sensitive to changes in tissue density, water, fiber orientation, and other types of abnormality. In addition, recent studies using quantitative susceptibility mapping (QSM) may assist in detecting changes at the periphery of MS lesions, because QSM removes some of the nonlocal contributions (such as the dipolar patterns) that can complicate interpretation of phase images,[47] sometimes at the expense of image quality. Such technical issues highlight the inherent problems associated with reliance on a single sequence or quantitative postprocessing technique. Combining information gained from the different iron-sensitive imaging techniques may improve upon the interpretation of a given lesion or region of interest.[48]

Quantitative Imaging

As described above, substantial advances in the understanding of MS lesion formation and evolution have resulted from UHF MR imaging followed by careful observation, as well as through the use of histopathological findings to drive radiologic techniques that recapitulate those findings. Radiologic techniques have also driven the field of MS research, particularly at UHF. A specific technique in MR imaging that has garnered much attention is quantitative iron imaging. UHF imaging with sequences sensitive to iron, particularly T2*-weighted sequences, goes beyond characterizing lesion subtypes, but have been used to study changes in iron within lesions, within the normal-appearing white matter, and within the deep gray nuclei. This technique can also be used to derive quantitative values related to iron concentration, including the R2* relaxation rate and QSM.

As iron is a major component of myelin, there have been attempts to provide a quantitative value of the extent of tissue injury in MS using UHF pulse sequences that can quantify iron content in MS lesions. In addition, some studies have reported abnormally high levels of iron within structures, such as the deep gray nuclei, in both MS and CIS.[49] In one study of people with MS compared with age-matched healthy controls, increased iron concentration in the deep GM correlated with a functional measure associated with the affected nuclei.[50] These findings were tempered by the fact that the specific nuclei affected were not consistent across sequences, complicating the interpretation.

Other studies have used quantitative iron imaging as a way of probing changes in the extralesional WM. Using a multiecho GRE sequence and fitting the T2* decay curve to a 3-component model, subtle changes in extralesional WM were reported in MS, potentially indicating widespread loss of myelin.[51] Extending this model to MS lesions, Li and colleagues[52] reported reduced myelin water fraction in both enhancing and non-enhancing MS lesions, indicating that this technique can be sensitive to detecting demyelination.

Although intriguing, these studies, and others like them, also highlight the limitations of quantitative techniques, as the derived iron concentrations are often affected by extraneous features such as concentration of deoxyhemoglobin in blood vessels, orientation of the brain during the imaging session, and the presence or absence of lesions. Interpreting radiological findings in the context of MS is often extremely difficult and has led to disparate ideas about whether iron drives, plays a minor role, or is simply a bystander in MS pathophysiology.

SPINAL CORD

UHF imaging is also being optimized for spinal cord imaging, albeit slowly. In principle, the increased SNR and higher spatial resolution of UHF imaging could be marshaled to improve identification of spinal cord inflammatory demyelination. Imaging the spinal cord at any field strength is difficult given its small size and propensity to artifacts related to respiratory- and cardiac-induced motion, which together severely limit lesion identification. However, recent studies have used UHF sequences to produce high-resolution images of MS spinal cord lesions. In a small pilot study, both resolution of the normal spinal cord anatomy and lesion detection were improved at 7 T compared with 3 T.[53] In addition, myelin water imaging was applied to an MS spinal cord postmortem, albeit on a preclinical scanner,[54] showing reductions of the myelin water fraction in regions with histologically proven MS lesions. Of course, application in vivo presents difficulties beyond image sequence, but at least in proof of principle, this sequence, and others, may be feasible at UHF.

LIMITATIONS AND CHALLENGES

Even with important advances in the understanding of MS pathophysiology, 7-T MR imaging has proven difficult to apply in all contexts. Limitations from artifacts, patient motion, additional safety concerns, and patient comfort have all made application of 7-T imaging less universal. New techniques, such as integrated navigator for motion correction, are needed before large-scale 7-T clinical application.[3] Nonetheless, many of these problems existed at 1.5 T and 3 T and were subsequently overcome, leading to widespread clinical adoption of higher magnetic field strength systems. Although 7-T magnets are regarded as investigational tools at this time, one manufacturer (Siemens) recently stated its intent to produce 7-T magnets for clinical use. Clinical UHF scanners mark the next advance in clinical MR imaging and will lead to much larger cohort studies of neuroinflammatory disorders, and with luck they will lead to new insights into MS pathophysiology.

FUTURE DIRECTIONS

UHF is a relative term, because advances in technology continue to press the boundaries of MR imaging field strength, shrinking the voxel size toward microscopic resolution. Advances in pulse sequences and new technology to overcome motion artifacts will allow MS researchers ever more detailed glimpses at the biology of MS lesion formation and evolution. Technological advances will also allow better in vivo spinal cord imaging.

What new information will the next generation of UHF scanners be able to resolve that we are missing today? In the newly forming MS lesion, BBB leakage is detected by gadolinium leakage, which is a nonspecific marker of BBB disruption. Biochemical and cellular changes presumably precede this event, but these changes are not yet detectable. Microglial nodules are described in pathology specimens as clumps of inflammatory cells surrounding a vessel, and one hypothesis is that this is an early sign of impending lesion formation. These nodules are too small to image currently, but once detectable, they may become an important biomarker of lesion development or treatment effectiveness. In addition, in place of gadolinium contrast, new, more specific, contrast agents capable of attaching to specific receptors or cells are on the horizon. High-field-strength scanners can be useful for detecting the changes caused by these agents, particularly if the changes are spatially restricted. In addition to acute MS lesions, there is much not known about what underlies the profound heterogeneity in disability and pathologic expression of MS. Imaging degrees of tissue destruction and repair, and in particular where and when those features are liable to be detected, will provide insights into how MS is different across patients and will potentially revolutionize clinical decision making.

ACKNOWLEDGMENTS

The authors thank Dr Martina Absinta for her help in editing figures included in the article.

REFERENCES

1. Young IR, Hall AS, Pallis CA, et al. Nuclear magnetic resonance imaging of the brain in multiple sclerosis. Lancet 1981;2(8255):1063–6.

2. Duyn JH. The future of ultra-high field MRI and fMRI for study of the human brain. Neuroimage 2012; 62(2):1241–8.

3. Federau C, Gallichan D. Motion-correction enabled ultra-high resolution in-vivo 7T-MRI of the brain. PLoS One 2016;11(5):e0154974.

4. Kollia K, Maderwald S, Putzki N, et al. First clinical study on ultra-high-field MR imaging in patients with multiple sclerosis: comparison of 1.5T and 7T. AJNR Am J Neuroradiol 2009;30(4):699–702.

5. Sinnecker T, Mittelstaedt P, Dörr J, et al. Multiple sclerosis lesions and irreversible brain tissue damage: a comparative ultrahigh-field strength magnetic resonance imaging study. Arch Neurol 2012;69(6): 739–45.

6. Mistry N, Tallantyre EC, Dixon JE, et al. Focal multiple sclerosis lesions abound in 'normal appearing white matter'. Mult Scler 2011;17(11):1313–23.

7. Marques JP, Kober T, Krueger G, et al. MP2RAGE, a self bias-field corrected sequence for improved segmentation and T1-mapping at high field. Neuroimage 2010;49(2):1271–81.

8. Vercellino M, Masera S, Lorenzatti M, et al. Demyelination, inflammation, and neurodegeneration in multiple sclerosis deep gray matter. J Neuropathol Exp Neurol 2009;68(5):489–502.

9. Harrison DM, Oh J, Roy S, et al. Thalamic lesions in multiple sclerosis by 7T MRI: clinical implications and relationship to cortical pathology. Mult Scler 2015;21(9):1139–50.

10. Brownell B, Hughes JT. The distribution of plaques in the cerebrum in multiple sclerosis. J Neurol Neurosurg Psychiatry 1962;25:315–20.

11. Peterson JW, Bö L, Mörk S, et al. Transected neurites, apoptotic neurons, and reduced inflammation in cortical multiple sclerosis lesions. Ann Neurol 2001;50(3):389–400.

12. Metcalf M, Xu D, Okuda DT, et al. High-resolution phased-array MRI of the human brain at 7 Tesla: initial experience in multiple sclerosis patients. J Neuroimaging 2010;20(2):141–7.

13. Cohen-Adad J, Benner T, Greve D, et al. In vivo evidence of disseminated subpial T2* signal changes in multiple sclerosis at 7 T: a surface-based analysis. Neuroimage 2011;57(1):55–62.

14. Nielsen AS, Kinkel RP, Madigan N, et al. Contribution of cortical lesion subtypes at 7T MRI to physical and cognitive performance in MS. Neurology 2013;81(7): 641–9.

15. Abdel-Fahim R, Mistry N, Mougin O, et al. Improved detection of focal cortical lesions using 7T magnetisation transfer imaging in patients with multiple sclerosis. Mult Scler Relat Disord 2014;3(2):258–65.

16. Pitt D, Boster A, Pei W, et al. Imaging cortical lesions in multiple sclerosis with ultra-high-field magnetic resonance imaging. Arch Neurol 2010;67(7): 812–8.

17. Mainero C, Benner T, Radding A, et al. In vivo imaging of cortical pathology in multiple sclerosis using ultra-high field MRI. Neurology 2009;73(12):941–8.

18. Schmierer K, Parkes HG, So PW, et al. High field (9.4 Tesla) magnetic resonance imaging of cortical grey matter lesions in multiple sclerosis. Brain 2010; 133(Pt 3):858–67.

19. Kilsdonk ID, Jonkman LE, Klaver R, et al. Increased cortical grey matter lesion detection in multiple sclerosis with 7 T MRI: a post-mortem verification study. Brain 2016;139(Pt 5):1472–81.

20. Sethi V, Yousry T, Muhlert N, et al. A longitudinal study of cortical grey matter lesion subtypes in relapse-onset multiple sclerosis. J Neurol Neurosurg Psychiatry 2016;87(7):750–3.

21. Tallantyre EC, Morgan PS, Dixon JE, et al. 3 Tesla and 7 Tesla MRI of multiple sclerosis cortical lesions. J Magn Reson Imaging 2010;32(4):971–7.

22. Yao B, Hametner S, van Gelderen P, et al. 7 Tesla magnetic resonance imaging to detect cortical pathology in multiple sclerosis. PLoS One 2014;9(10): e108863.

23. Bagnato F, Hametner S, Pennell D, et al. 7T MRI-histologic correlation study of low specific absorption rate T2-weighted GRASE sequences in the detection of white matter involvement in multiple sclerosis. J Neuroimaging 2015;25(3):370–8.

24. Mainero C, Louapre C, Govindarajan ST, et al. A gradient in cortical pathology in multiple sclerosis by in vivo quantitative 7 T imaging. Brain 2015; 138(Pt 4):932–45.

25. Harrison DM, Roy S, Oh J, et al. Association of cortical lesion burden on 7-T magnetic resonance imaging with cognition and disability in multiple sclerosis. JAMA Neurol 2015;72(9):1004–12.

26. Tallantyre EC, Brookes MJ, Dixon JE, et al. Demonstrating the perivascular distribution of MS lesions in vivo with 7-Tesla MRI. Neurology 2008;70(22): 2076–8.

27. Tallantyre EC, Morgan PS, Dixon JE, et al. A comparison of 3T and 7T in the detection of small parenchymal veins within MS lesions. Invest Radiol 2009;44(9):491–4.

28. Tallantyre EC, Dixon JE, Donaldson I, et al. Ultra-high-field imaging distinguishes MS lesions from asymptomatic white matter lesions. Neurology 2011;76(6):534–9.

29. Kilsdonk ID, Wattjes MP, Lopez-Soriano A, et al. Improved differentiation between MS and vascular brain lesions using FLAIR* at 7 Tesla. Eur Radiol 2014;24(4):841–9.

30. Wuerfel J, Sinnecker T, Ringelstein EB, et al. Lesion morphology at 7 Tesla MRI differentiates Susac syndrome from multiple sclerosis. Mult Scler 2012; 18(11):1592–9.

31. Sinnecker T, Dörr J, Pfueller CF, et al. Distinct lesion morphology at 7-T MRI differentiates neuromyelitis

optica from multiple sclerosis. Neurology 2012; 79(7):708–14.

32. Solomon AJ, Schindler MK, Howard DB, et al. "Central vessel sign" on 3T FLAIR* MRI for the differentiation of multiple sclerosis from migraine. Ann Clin Transl Neurol 2016;3(2):82–7.

33. Kau T, Taschwer M, Deutschmann H, et al. The "central vein sign": is there a place for susceptibility weighted imaging in possible multiple sclerosis? Eur Radiol 2013;23(7):1956–62.

34. Mistry N, Dixon J, Tallantyre E, et al. Central veins in brain lesions visualized with high-field magnetic resonance imaging: a pathologically specific diagnostic biomarker for inflammatory demyelination in the brain. JAMA Neurol 2013;70(5):623–8.

35. Rovira A, Wattjes MP, Tintoré M, et al. Evidence-based guidelines: MAGNIMS consensus guidelines on the use of MRI in multiple sclerosis-clinical implementation in the diagnostic process. Nat Rev Neurol 2015;11(8):471–82.

36. Sati P, Oh J, Constable RT, et al. The central vein sign and its clinical evaluation for the diagnosis of multiple sclerosis: a consensus statement from the North American Imaging in Multiple Sclerosis Cooperative. Nat Rev Neurol 2016;12(12):714–22.

37. McFarland HF, Frank JA, Albert PS, et al. Using gadolinium-enhanced magnetic resonance imaging lesions to monitor disease activity in multiple sclerosis. Ann Neurol 1992;32(6):758–66.

38. Frank JA, Stone LA, Smith ME, et al. Serial contrast-enhanced magnetic resonance imaging in patients with early relapsing-remitting multiple sclerosis: implications for treatment trials. Ann Neurol 1994;(36 Suppl):S86–90.

39. Gaitan MI, Shea CD, Evangelou IE, et al. Evolution of the blood-brain barrier in newly forming multiple sclerosis lesions. Ann Neurol 2011;70(1):22–9.

40. Gaitan MI, Sati P, Inati SJ, et al. Initial investigation of the blood-brain barrier in MS lesions at 7 tesla. Mult Scler 2013;19(8):1068–73.

41. Absinta M, Sati P, Gaitán MI, et al. Seven-Tesla phase imaging of acute multiple sclerosis lesions: a new window into the inflammatory process. Ann Neurol 2013;74(5):669–78.

42. Hammond KE, Metcalf M, Carvajal L, et al. Quantitative in vivo magnetic resonance imaging of multiple sclerosis at 7 Tesla with sensitivity to iron. Ann Neurol 2008;64(6):707–13.

43. Bian W, Harter K, Hammond-Rosenbluth KE, et al. A serial in vivo 7T magnetic resonance phase imaging study of white matter lesions in multiple sclerosis. Mult Scler 2013;19(1):69–75.

44. Bagnato F, Hametner S, Yao B, et al. Tracking iron in multiple sclerosis: a combined imaging and histopathological study at 7 Tesla. Brain 2011;134(Pt 12):3602–15.

45. Yao B, Bagnato F, Matsuura E, et al. Chronic multiple sclerosis lesions: characterization with high-field-strength MR imaging. Radiology 2012; 262(1):206–15.

46. Absinta M, Sati P, Schindler M, et al. Persistent 7-Tesla phase rim predicts poor outcome in new multiple sclerosis patient lesions. J Clin Invest 2016; 126(7):2597–609.

47. Cronin MJ, Wharton S, Al-Radaideh A, et al. A comparison of phase imaging and quantitative susceptibility mapping in the imaging of multiple sclerosis lesions at ultrahigh field. MAGMA 2016; 29(3):543–57.

48. Li X, Harrison DM, Liu H, et al. Magnetic susceptibility contrast variations in multiple sclerosis lesions. J Magn Reson Imaging 2016;43(2):463–73.

49. Al-Radaideh AM, Wharton SJ, Lim SY, et al. Increased iron accumulation occurs in the earliest stages of demyelinating disease: an ultra-high field susceptibility mapping study in Clinically Isolated Syndrome. Mult Scler 2013;19(7):896–903.

50. Schmalbrock P, Prakash RS, Schirda B, et al. Basal ganglia iron in patients with multiple sclerosis measured with 7T quantitative susceptibility mapping correlates with inhibitory control. AJNR Am J Neuroradiol 2016;37(3):439–46.

51. Sati P, van Gelderen P, Silva AC, et al. Micro-compartment specific T2* relaxation in the brain. Neuroimage 2013;77:268–78.

52. Li X, van Gelderen P, Sati P, et al. Detection of demyelination in multiple sclerosis by analysis of [Formula: see text] relaxation at 7 T. Neuroimage Clin 2015;7:709–14.

53. Dula AN, Pawate S, Dortch RD, et al. Magnetic resonance imaging of the cervical spinal cord in multiple sclerosis at 7T. Mult Scler 2016;22(3):320–8.

54. Laule C, Yung A, Pavolva V, et al. High-resolution myelin water imaging in post-mortem multiple sclerosis spinal cord: a case report. Mult Scler 2016; 22(11):1485–9.

Index

Neuroimag Clin N Am 27 (2017) 367–370
http://dx.doi.org/10.1016/S1052-5149(17)30013-8
1052-5149/17

Moving?

Make sure your subscription moves with you!

To notify us of your new address, find your **Clinics Account Number** (located on your mailing label above your name), and contact customer service at:

Email: journalscustomerservice-usa@elsevier.com

800-654-2452 (subscribers in the U.S. & Canada)
314-447-8871 (subscribers outside of the U.S. & Canada)

Fax number: 314-447-8029

Elsevier Health Sciences Division
Subscription Customer Service
3251 Riverport Lane
Maryland Heights, MO 63043

*To ensure uninterrupted delivery of your subscription, please notify us at least 4 weeks in advance of move.

Printed and bound by CPI Group (UK) Ltd, Croydon, CR0 4YY

08/06/2025

01896875-0011